To the dancers—
our patients, colleagues, friends—
who embody the dream of dancing with
their commitment, passion and vision

Dance Medicine
A Comprehensive Guide

Allan J. Ryan, M.D.
Robert E. Stephens, Ph.D.

Co-published by Pluribus Press, Chicago, *and*
The Physician and Sportsmedicine, Minneapolis

Library of Congress Catalog Card Number:
87-60404

International Standard Book Number:
0-931028-92-2

Pluribus Press, Inc.
160 East Illinois Street
Chicago, Illinois 60611

Chapter 13 Illustrations: Susan Strawn

91 90 89 88 87 5 4 3 2 1

Printed in the United States of America

CONTENTS

ABOUT THE EDITORS

ALLAN J. RYAN, M.D., received his medical degree from Columbia University. He completed his internship at Kings County Hospital, Brooklyn, New York, and his medical residency at New Haven Hospital, Connecticut, and Long Island College, New York, New York. Dr. Ryan practiced general surgery at The Meriden Hospital, Connecticut, and served as chairman of the Department of Rehabilitation and athletic teams physician at the University of Wisconsin-Madison. Former editor-in-chief of *The Physician and Sportsmedicine,* Dr. Ryan is now director of Sports Medicine Enterprises in Minneapolis, Minnesota.

ROBERT E. STEPHENS, Ph.D., graduated from the University of Kansas Medical Center with doctoral honors in anatomy. Former principal dancer in Ballet Midwest, Dr. Stephens has been a dance medicine consultant to the San Francisco Ballet, Ballet West, Houston Ballet, New York City Ballet, American Ballet Theatre, Royal Ballet, Paris Opera Ballet and others. He has taught at the University of Kansas Medical Center, and is now associate professor of anatomy and director of sports medicine at the University of Health Sciences Medical School in Kansas City, Missouri.

CONTRIBUTORS

RICHARD M. BACHRACH, D.O., Director, The Center for Dance Medicine, New York, New York

JOAN BENSON, R.D., Consultant Dietitian, Center for Sports Medicine and Dance Medicine, St. Francis Memorial Hospital, San Francisco, California

JERALD L. COHEN, M.D., F.A.C.P., F.A.C.S.M., Chief, Echocardiographic Laboratory, Cardiology Section, Veterans Administration Medical Center, East Orange, New Jersey

JAMES G. GARRICK, M.D., Director, Center for Sports Medicine and Dance Medicine, Orthopedic Surgeon to the San Francisco Ballet Company, St. Francis Memorial Hospital, San Francisco, California

DONNA M. GILLIEN, M.S., Director, Wellness, Merritt Perralta Institute, Oakland, California

A.J.G. HOWSE, F.R.C.S., Physician to the Royal Ballet and the Royal Academy of Dancing, The Remedial Dance Clinic, London, England

BARNARD KLEIGER, M.D., Visiting Professor Emeritus, Albert Einstein College of Medicine, Attending Orthopedic Surgeon, Montefiore Hospital and Medical Center, Einstein-Weiler College Hospital, Bronx, New York; Consultant, Orthopedic Surgeon, Hospital for Joint Diseases, Orthopedic Institute, New York, New York. Dr. Kleiger died April 1987 while this book was in progress.

ALVIN R. LOOSLI, M.D., Center for Sports Medicine and Dance Medicine, St. Francis Memorial Hospital, San Francisco, California

LYLE J. MICHELI, M.D., Director, Sports Medicine Division, Children's Hospital, Physician to the Boston Ballet, Boston, Massachusetts

ANTHONY P. MILLAR, M.B., B.S., F.R.A.C.P., F.A.C.R.M., Institute of Sports Medicine, Lewisham Hospital, Petersham, Australia

MARIKA E. MOLNAR, M.A., R.P.T., Eastside Sports Physical Therapy, Eastside Dance Medicine Center, New York, New York

THOMAS M. NOVELLA, D.P.M., Diplomate, American Board of Podiatric Orthopedics; Fellow, American College of Foot Orthopedists, New York, New York

RONALD QUIRK, F.R.C.S., F.R.A.C.S., Royal Australian Ballet, Melbourne, Australia

G. JAMES SAMMARCO, M.D., F.A.C.S., Consultant to the Cincinnati Ballet Company; Associate Clinical Professor, Department of Orthopedic Surgery, University of Cincinnati Medical Center; Director, Performing Arts Center, Cincinnati, Ohio

DIANA SCHNITT, M.F.A., C.M.A., Chairman, Dance Department, Connecticut College, New London, Connecticut

JEROME M. SCHNITT, M.D., Assistant Clinical Professor, Psychiatry, Yale University School of Medicine, New Haven, Connecticut

JAY SEALS, Vice President, Sales, Robbins, Inc., Cincinnati, Ohio

RUTH SOLOMON, Director, Dance Theater Program, University of California-Santa Cruz, Santa Cruz, California

LEON SPEROFF, M.D., MacDonald Hospital for Women, Cleveland, Ohio

EIVIND THOMASEN, M.D., Professor-Dr. Med. Physician to the Royal Danish Ballet, Arhus C, Denmark

ERNEST L. WASHINGTON, M.D., Company Physician, Los Angeles Breakers Dance Company; Editor, Dance Medicine-Health Newsletter, Los Angeles, California

STEVEN WILLIAMS, M.D., University Hospitals of Cleveland, Cleveland, Ohio

INTRODUCTION

Allan J. Ryan, M.D.

O body swayed to music, O brightening glance,
How can we know the dancer from the dance?
—William Butler Yeats
"Among School Children"

DANCERS TEND TO BE wary of physicians for several reasons. They believe that physicians know very little about dance, other than social dancing, and cannot understand very well how and why the types of injury they encounter occur. Some have had the experience of consulting a physician regarding a dance injury only to be told to stop dancing. Others, seeking medical advice regarding weight control, may have been advised that they needed to gain rather than to lose weight. Some have consulted one or more of the nonmedical therapists who cluster around dance companies and who discourage them from seeking medical advice. This reluctance to consult physicians affects professional more than amateur dancers, but the latter are influenced by what they observe to be the practices of the former.

The most important thing the physician can do at the first encounter is to gain the dancer's confidence. This doesn't come easily, especially if the physician is not knowledgeable about the type or style of dance in which the dancer is involved, but manifesting a desire to learn about it makes a good beginning. When this approach is combined with caution in making a diagnosis and even more caution in making recommendations for specific treatment, there is good ground for establishing a comfortable working relationship between dancer and physician. Although the dancer probably expects some immediate feedback as far as treatment is concerned, it is better to offer too little than too much.

Injuries occur among dancers for many of the same reasons that they occur among athletes. Many dance movements are explosive in character, others require long sustained effort, some take the body through extreme ranges of motion, and all are characterized by patterns of motion that are repeated time after time on the same day and repeatedly day after day. Many top athletes have hours and days of demanding practice and other supporting workouts. Few, however, spend as many hours in practice (class for the classic dancer) and rehearsal for as many days a week or so continuously throughout a year as the professional dancer.

Because the majority of dancers' injuries are the result of overuse rather than of one particular accident or occurrence, the onset of symptoms and the appearance of disability tend to be insidious. Because of the lack of proper treatment or in spite of it, some of these injuries become chronic, with periodic exacerbations. These factors make it difficult to establish the occurrence of specific injuries over a given period of time or a particular set of circumstances, such as in class, in rehearsal, or in performance. Because the actions of professional dancers are so continuous, times and situations blend together, making it difficult to develop strategies for injury prevention based on exact data. After working with a group of dancers and having the opportunity to examine them physically and discuss their complaints over a considerable period of time, one may be able to say that certain injuries have occurred commonly and others infrequently in the group. This may not be of much help in determining why this was the case, however. A survey of all dancers in one company on a particular day would show that a certain number had signs, symptoms, or both of an acute or chronic injury and that others were partially or completely disabled from dancing on that day as a result.

Except with the large and well-established companies, records of injuries may be scanty or absent. Many smaller companies do not have a physician who sees their dancers regularly, and the only records might be of insurance payments for the medical care of dancers. The dancers are on their own as far as medical advice and care are concerned, and the records of this care are not brought together and analyzed. For the most part, the researcher is left only with personal reminiscences of dancers, physicians, teachers, other supervisors, and other persons who have performed some types of services for injured dancers.

Despite all of the above qualifications and limitations, some reports of the incidence and results of injuries among dancers of both sexes from different styles and schools and of varying ages can shed some light on the epidemiology of these injuries. These experiences, including those reported by the authors of some of the other chapters in this book, can provide some ideas about how these injuries can be reduced or prevented. The publication of these findings may additionally provide incentives to others to expand this research across other populations of dancers to provide an even better basis for preventive actions.

1

THE EPIDEMIOLOGY OF DANCE INJURIES

Allan J. Ryan, M.D., and Robert E. Stephens, Ph.D.

ALTHOUGH THE PUBLIC IS generally aware and appreciative of the art of dancing, it is not usually cognizant of the considerable physical, intellectual, and emotional demands of being a dancer. This lack of awareness is due in part to the private nature of learning, practicing, and creating dance movement—the turmoil of these endeavors is a deeply personal matter. In class and rehearsals, dancers scrutinize other dancers with only slightly less venom than they do themselves. Technique and body clash and mesh in unpredictable, impossible, imperceptible, and incredible battles. The merciless mirror provides an easy target for their constant admonitions. No one in dance escapes this harsh reality. These battles are not for the public to see. They view only the parade of victors and know not of their scars.

In another respect, the dancer prefers to bear this pain in silence. There is nothing glamorous or aesthetic about an injured dancer performing in pain. What is deemed admirable and courageous in sports would seem foolish and inappropriate in an art form. Nevertheless, dancers do practice and perform in pain for a variety of foolish and noble reasons. Their pain and disability is a private battle rarely discussed with the public, the uninformed physician, or other dancers. As a result, tales of injuries are usually anecdotal rather than epidemiological. This insular nature of the world of dance is one of the reasons that information regarding the incidence, type, and distribution of injuries in dance has not and is not readily forthcoming from this small, elite society that is largely closed to outsiders. Investigators are still amazed that there is a population of *artists* who suffer a number of injuries quite similar to those found among *athletes*. It is this odd analogy that seems to verify the worthiness of dance for study, not the sociocultural impact of the injured dancer as talent untapped and art lost.

Under properly controlled scientific circumstances, epidemiological studies can provide valuable information about the distribution and/or causes of injuries in the dance population.[1-3] This information can then help health professionals develop and implement effective injury prevention programs as well as deliver better medical services. Most studies of dance injuries simply report the number and type of injuries and omit critical information about the total number of dancers in that population (e.g., company or school) or their physical characteristics and working history and conditions. Without specific information about the size of the population and the conditions under which it was surveyed, one cannot accurately determine the incidence or etiology of injuries in that group. Many case history reports have described particular types of dance-related injuries with little or no indication as to their prevalence in a dance school, company, or population. All of the published surveys of dance injuries have difficulty defining the incidence of specific injuries in relation to the size and stratification of the dance population.

Dance is a hierarchical profession, and studying a local civic ballet company is quite different from studying the American Ballet Theatre. The type or style of dance as well as the caliber of dancer must also be considered in any assessment of the incidence of injuries in a given population of dancers. Whether Balanchine or Cecchetti techniques in classical ballet, Graham or Horton in modern, Tremaine or Fosse in jazz, Georgian or Spanish in character dancing, each style places a particular demand on the human body and may therefore contribute in some manner to the overall incidence of injury in a specific dance population.

The hierarchy of dance starts with the thousands of local dance studios at the base of the pyramid, followed by university dance departments, the preprofessional dance schools that are usually affiliated with a dance company, and finally, at the very apex, the dance companies. Dance companies may be nonprofessional, semiprofessional, or professional, depending upon payment for the dancer's services and, to a lesser degree, the dancer's membership in a labor union. Dancers in smaller civic dance companies are usually unpaid or paid by performance, whereas the dancers in regional and national companies are usually paid for rehearsals and performances or receive a salary. In most ballet companies, dancers are ranked as principals, soloists, corps de ballet, or apprentices, depending on their artistry, expertise, and seniority. Because the work loads and responsibilities may vary from one rank to another, there may be differences in the incidence of injury.

In the major ballet companies, the dancer's obligations to the company and, in some instances, the company's responsibility to the dancer are under the careful surveillance of dance unions such as the American Guild of Musical Artists (AGMA). In many respects, companies such as the New York City Ballet, American Ballet Theatre, San Francisco Ballet, Ballet West, and Houston Ballet not only represent the pinnacle of ballet but are the financial centers of dance in America. The conditions under which injuries occur in the various studios, schools, and companies within the hierarchy of dance are quite often qualitatively and quantitatively different. Under these diverse conditions and influences, broad surveys of dance injuries without specifying the particular dance style and technical proficiencies have little epidemiological value.

Epidemiological studies not only describe the incidence, type, and distribution of injuries but should also indicate the duration of study and the physical characteristics and conditions of that population of dancers. This chapter will concentrate on the reports and surveys dealing with the physical characteristics and work loads of ballet dancers and the incidence, severity, distribution, and type of injuries common in dance. Causal factors such as occupation, anatomy, biomechanics, training, technique, diet, nutrition, environment, and psychology are discussed in the next chapter.

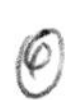

The Dancer

Physical Characteristics

Many different dance styles, from ballet to folk dance, are practiced by persons with an even wider variety of body types. Dance is for anyone who has the feeling and desire and capacity for movement. Graceful movement is not necessarily a function of a particular body type. On the other hand, whether ballet enthusiasts will pay to see chubby ballerinas punish their toes is a practical sociocultural issue of some concern to the aspiring performer. Over the centuries, dancers have always changed their forms in order to conform to the aesthetic ideals of a particular individual or society. The transformation of the dancer into its present-day ultralean androgenous form can be traced to the romantic ballets of the early nineteenth century. Although these early ballerinas would be unliftable by today's standards, they nevertheless sought the illusion of a fragile, ethereal sylph. This trend persists to this day in the dreams of most dancers and the gaunt reality of a few.

Health professionals should understand that the image of the tall, lean, narrow-hipped, long-limbed ballet dancer is not universally accepted in the dance world. There are thousands of wonderful dancers in many disciplines who hardly fit into this restrictive mold. Some dancers ignore and scorn such arbitrary barriers to the learning, creation, performance, and enjoyment of dance movement. However, physicians should be acutely aware of the dancer's preoccupation with thinness and body image when evaluating or discussing the amount of body fat in a dancer. Leanness is not only an artistic standard in many professional dance companies—it is an occupational absolute. Dancers constantly strive to perfect the form of the human body while they struggle with the trials of dance technique.

A number of scientific studies have been done on professional dancers from international, national, and regional ballet companies.[4-18] These reports demonstrate the amazing degree of homogeneity in the overall physical characteristics of top ballet dancers. The average female dancer in these companies was 23 years old, 5 ft. 5½ in. tall, and weighed 107 lb., with 13-16% body fat. The male dancers were 27 years old, 5 ft. 10 in., 153 lb., with 8-13% body fat (table 1-1). Obviously, the leanness of professional ballet dancers is comparable to that of top nonendurance athletes. Advanced students in the major ballet schools and studios also tend to approach these figures.[15]

Almost any dance company has examples of dancers who excel in spite of

Table 1-1: Physical Characteristics and Training, Work, and Injury Histories of Professional and Advanced Student Ballet Dancers*

	Professional Dancers		Student Dancers	
	Men	Women	Men	Women
Number of dancers	15	24	11	71
Age	27.3 ± 5.6	26.6 ± 3.7	21.0 ± 2.9	16.0 ± 1.8
Height (cm)	178.1 ± 3.3	166.1 ± 4.3	178.3 ± 6.9	163.6 ± 4.3
Weight (kg)	69.4 ± 5.5	48.7 ± 3.6	65.5 ± 8.5	47.4 ± 5.6
% Body fat	13.0 ± 2.3	15.7 ± 1.2	11.7 ± 2.9	16.6 ± 1.5
Starting age in dance	12.3 ± 4.2	8.6 ± 2.1	16.3 ± 2.1	7.3 ± 3.4
Total years of dancing	13.0 ± 4.8	12.7 ± 3.6	4.0 ± 2.7	8.2 ± 2.8
Years at this level	7.2 ± 3.4	5.1 ± 2.2	0.7 ± 1.1	2.7 ± 1.2
Classroom work load (hr.)	9.3 ± 0.9	10.2 ± 2.3	17.3 ± 7.7	13.6 ± 6.1
Rehearsal work load (hr.)	26.1 ± 6.2	26.6 ± 6.1	—	—
Performance work load (hr.)	9.5 ± 5.3	7.9 ± 3.6	—	—
Total work load (hr.)	44.9 ± 4.1	44.7 ± 4.0	—	—
Prevalence of injury	93.3%	87.5%	81.8%	60.6%
Prevalence of disability	63.6%	60.9%	45.4%	26.8%
Workmen's Compensation	40.0%	42.1%	—	—
Loss of salary	45.5%	15.0%	—	—

*Numbers are listed as means ± standard deviation.

the fact that they do not fit within the physical norm. Perhaps they are a bit bosomy, a little shorter, or thicker in the thighs, but they succeeded nevertheless despite some pretty fierce odds. By today's standards, these individuals represent the exception rather than the rule, and they know their career limitations and vulnerabilities very well. The major task of the "nonstandard" ballet dancer is slipping through the cattle-sorting at the beginning of a school or company audition and getting a chance to dance. The chances of this happening are roughly inversely proportional to the status of the school, studio, or company.

Training and Work Load

In terms of duration, frequency, and intensity, the rigor of a dancer's training has few rivals in the art or sport world. Training to become a dancer is comparable to a young boy's taking year-round batting and fielding practice 6 days a week from the age of 8 to 17. Serious ballet training typically begins at the age of 8 for females, but somewhat later for males (table 1-1). The tendency for American boys to start ballet training 4-9 years later than girls may reflect the sociocultural bias against dance as an acceptable occupation for men. However, the emergence of powerful, positive male role models in dance such as Mikhail Baryshnikov and Peter Martins has answered many of the public's serious doubts about the validity and masculinity of studying dance.

Over the course of about 10 years, the young dancer takes more and more 90-minute classes per week at progressively higher levels of intensity and proficiency. During this time, dancers may train in one particular style of ballet, such as Cecchetti, Russian, or Bournonville; however, most ballet dancers study more than one style. In addition, most dancers also train in modern, jazz, and character dance. Similarly, dancers in each of these other dance disciplines also commonly cross-train in other techniques and styles.

Selection for the ballet schools affiliated with the top companies occurs rather early in this training process, forcing the budding adolescent to make a commitment to the dance. While their peers by age are worrying about pimples and dates, young talented dancers are faced with a crucial career choice. Because many companies take most of their new dancers from their affiliated dance schools, it can be difficult—although not impossible—for a novice to enter the ranks of a large ballet company without having progressed through the school. More latitude exists in this regard in small companies and in other forms of dance, such as modern and jazz. Although a dancer may believe it was difficult getting into a company, it may be far more difficult to survive its grueling schedules and constant pressures.

When working with dancers, the physician needs to determine the amount of exposure to injury a dancer may have during the course of a week, month, season, or year. The number of hours per day devoted to class, rehearsal, and performance; the number of performances a week or in a season; and the number and length of seasons per year are all important epidemiological considerations, especially as they relate to overuse injuries. In addition, certain dance styles may influence the occurrence of injuries, and it is helpful to know which ones influence the training and choreography.

A typical work schedule during a season for a professional ballet dancer includes 9 hr. in class, about 26 hr. in rehearsal, and 8-12 hr. in performance, for a total of 43-48 hr. during a 6-day period (table 1-1).[4,9,15,19,20-22] The standard union contract is 36 weeks per year, but varies according to the tour schedules and bookings. The contract year is subdivided into 3-4 seasons, each having a varying number of rehearsals and performances. In many professional companies, the rehearsal and performance work load and working conditions are specified in the dancer's contract and monitored by the union.

In dance studios and schools there is, of course, no union to protect the student from his own youthful ambition to dance more and more. Studies of advanced female students indicate that they spend about 14 hr. a week in class, which was generally reported as 2 classes per day on a 5-day schedule.[15] Some male students spent as many as 30 hr. per week in class. This disproportionate classroom work load of some of the male students reflects their desire to accomplish specific goals in a shorter time, and it probably contributes to their rapid accumulation of injuries so early in their careers.

Prevalence of Dance Injuries

How injurious is dancing? If viewed from the broad perspective of the millions of individuals who participate in a wide variety of dance forms, it probably doesn't differ much from many other noncombative sporting activities. However, as one ascends the hierarchy of dance into the highly competitive nationally and internationally ranked dance schools and companies, dance-related injuries almost certainly become more prevalent and have more serious implications and repercussions. At this level, the disability of an injury not only disturbs the dancer's technique but it may also seriously affect present or future financial or job security.

Only a few publications provide information about the incidence or prevalence of injuries in dance, and these deal primarily with ballet dancers. A report on the New York City Ballet indicated that on any given day during the contract season, 17% (15/90) of the dancers were not dancing because of injuries.[18] In this company as well as others, the incidence of injury may vary with the work load and working conditions, but detailed studies need to be done.

The prevalence rate of dance-related injuries in ballet is much higher than the incidence rate and is much better documented. In 1982-83, a study of professional dancers from Ballet West and advanced student dancers from the Ballet West Summer Program indicated that almost 90% of the professional dancers (35/39) and 63% (52/83) of the students had had a dance-related injury at some time in their careers[15] (table 1-1). The professional dancers had almost twice as many injuries per dancer as the students, probably due to their greater work load and more years of training. About 62% of the professional dancers and about half of the students incurred some degree of temporary or permanent disability from their injuries. The professional dancers claimed that 41% of their injuries were severe enough to file for Workmen's Compensation and 26% resulted in a loss of salary.

Among the four groups of male and female student and professional dancers, the female students had the lowest injury rate (61%) and their injuries tended to be less severe (27%); they were also the youngest, i.e., 16 years of age. The injury frequency (82%) of the male students was almost the same as that of the professionals—quite high considering the fact that they had been dancing for an average of only 4 years and were the least experienced (table 1-1). These young male dancers also tended to have more disabling injuries at an earlier stage of their careers. This may be attributable to overtraining in their effort to compensate for a late start in dance.

More professional male dancers claimed a loss of salary from their injuries than did female dancers (table 1-1). This discrepancy may suggest that the women's injuries were not severe enough to prevent their dancing for more than 2 weeks, which is usually the maximum paid leave time for an injury. However, a more likely possibility is that they continued to dance despite their injuries because of the extreme competition for employment and dancing roles for women in the few major ballet companies in the United States.

The seriousness of ballet injuries has been confirmed in another major American ballet company, where there was an 80% chance of a dancer's filing for Workmen's Compensation for physical disability during a single season.[18] In addition to the physical and psychological implications of an injury, disabled dancers are often forced, consciously or subconsciously, to return to dancing too soon. In some cases, if rehabilitation requires more than 2 weeks, the dancer may become unemployed and may not receive Workmen's Compensation, since not all injuries are covered by the program. Such a case is discussed in detail in chapter 2. Clearly, in such instances the tendency is to return to dancing before rehabilitation is complete rather than add more financial insecurity to a profession that has very little in the first place.

Distribution of Dance Injuries

In the past 20 years, almost 7,000 dance injuries have been reported in 9 major surveys on the distribution and type of injuries in ballet,[15,23-26] modern,[27] theatrical,[28,29] and university-based[30,31] dancers. These data are summarized in table 1-2. It is not surprising that the vast majority of dance-related injuries occurred in the lower extremities. Regardless of the type of dance, most studies reported that 60-80% of these injuries involved the ankle, foot, or knee. The specific order of distribution varied somewhat according to the type of dance (ballet, modern, or theatrical), style (such as Cecchetti, Russian, or Bournonville in ballet; or Graham, Horton, or Limon in modern), experience, and sex of the population.

In all of the studies, ankle and foot injuries were collectively more frequent than knee injuries. In two of the studies of theatrical and modern dance, knee injuries were more common than either ankle or foot injuries.[27,28] Also, more back injuries were reported in these dance forms than in ballet. In the Ballet West study, ankle, foot, and back injuries, in that order, resulted in the greatest number of Workmen's Compensation claims.[15] The frequency of leg injuries also ranked in the top five in most of these studies. Other sites of injury have also been reported, although with much less frequency and a bit more curious origins.

Although the injuries to the lower extremities in dance are not pathologically different from those in sports, they may, of course, differ in their etiology and significance. For example, an errant landing in either ballet or basketball may result in a lateral inversion ankle sprain and subsequent chronic ligamentous laxity. In a basketball player, the ankle may be stabilized by strapping; however, this is not feasible for a ballet dancer. Even the most basic ballet technique requires extreme dorsiflexion and plantarflexion of the foot. In the next section, some of the more common injuries of the lower extremity are mentioned, along with a few of the conditions under which they occur.

Ankle and Foot Injuries

Feet are to a dancer what hands are to the pianist—absolutely critical to the performance of the art. A ballet dancer with poorly pointed, turned-in, or clumsy feet receives no mercy from just about any other dancer. These useless distal appendages are the "locker room" jokes of the dance scene. Dancers constantly strive to make them supple enough to absorb the shock of numerous jumps and strong enough to propel the dancer smoothly into space. All the while, they must maintain the 180° external rotation of the lower extremities ("turn-out") as well as display the extended line of fully pointed feet the instant they leave the floor. Technically, the dancer's ankles and feet perform the functions of dorsiflexion/plantarflexion and pronation/supination *in extremis.* All too often, they bear the bad results with the good.

Excessive pronation frequently results in tenosynovitis of the tibialis posterior, flexor digitorum longus, and/or flexor hallucis longus tendon sheaths. Chronic inflammation may also lead to calcific tendinitis. Plantar fasciitis, calcaneal spurs, and sesamoiditis are also triggered by dancing on hard floors.

Table 1-2. Summary of Surveys on Distribution of Injuries in Dance

	Foot		Ankle	Leg	Knee	Thigh	Hip	Lumbar	Neck	Other	No./ Injuries	Injury Rate
Ballet dancers												
Stephens (15)**												
Professionals	27.5		38.9	8.0	6.7	0.7	6.0	9.4	—	2.7	149	90
Students	22.0		24.4	14.9	15.5	8.9	5.4	7.1	—	1.8	168	70
Quirk (23,24)	20.1		22.3	7.5	17.3	4.3	8.6	8.5	—	11.4	2113	—
Thomasen (25)												
Male		36.4 +		—	34.0	—	—	—	—	39.2	760	—
Female		46.2		—	26.7	—	—	—	—	27.2		—
Volkov (25)												
Male		23.0		—	38.5	—	—	—	—	20.1	240	—
Female		71.0		—	12.2	—	—	—	—	16.5		—
Micheli (26)		24.1		20.5 + +	38.6	—	—	13.3	—	3.6	83	—
Modern dancers												
Solomon (27)	7.0		19.6	7.0	20.1	4.8	11.3	15.3	4.4	2.6	229	—
Theatrical dancers												
Rovere (29)	14.8		22.2	5.4	14.5	—	14.2	17.6	3	11.4	352	84.9
Washington (28)												
Individual	10		13	14	14	—	7	12	5	18	414	—
Group reports	21		21	—	34	—	7	6	1	7	1248	—
University students												
Clanin (31)	13		13	8	6	9	2	6	1	—	335	59.3
Shaw (30)		64.6		10.7	17.7	—	—	—	—	—	798	—
										Total:	6889	

* All numbers in percent.
** Numbers in parentheses refer to references.
+ Includes injuries of foot and ankle.
+ + Includes injuries of leg and thigh.

Functional gastroc-soleus equinus and failure to allow the heels to load during landing keeps the foot in a nonshock-absorbing supinated position. This may result in Achilles tendinitis, partial or complete rupture of the Achilles tendon, subluxation and tenosynovitis of the peroneus longus tendon at the level of the lateral malleolus, medial ankle tenosynovitis, metatarsal stress fractures, and/or osteochondritis dissecans of the superior dome of the talus.

Inversion or lateral ankle sprains constitute the most common injury in the ankle region; in one study, they also ranked first in the number of Workmen's Compensation claims.[15] Jones fractures or avulsion fractures of the peroneus brevis from the base of the fifth metatarsal are also inversion injuries. Eversion or medial ankle sprains are rather unusual among dancers.

Forced dorsiflexion or plantarflexion of the foot may result in anterior or posterior talar impingement syndromes, respectively. The presence of an os trigonum may further exacerbate the latter syndrome. Hallux rigidus is stimulated by hyperdorsiflexion of the first metatarsophalangeal joint in *demi-pointe.* Forcing the turn-out causes pronation of the foot and abduction of the big toe, which may subsequently lead to the development of hallux valgus or bunion deformities. Improperly fitting shoes may cause hammer toe deformity, calcanceal bursitis, Morton's neurinoma, soft corns, of subungual hematomas.

Leg Injuries

In ballet, 8-12% of all injuries occurred in the leg region (table 1-2). The dorsiflexors and evertors of the foot and extensors of the toes are located anteriorly and laterally, and the plantarflexors and invertors of the foot and flexors of toes are attached to the posterior side of the tibia and fibula. It is the posterior group—and to a lesser extent the lateral group—of muscles that are usually involved in leg injuries.

Certainly the most common injury is posterior compartment "shin splints," which is probably a periostitis or fasciitis near the origin of the flexor digitorum longus muscles about 6 in. above the medial malleolus along the posteromedial edge of the tibia. It is often due to excessive pronation while jumping on a hard floor. Tibia stress fractures may also evolve from these conditions. Anterior compartment syndrome is quite rare in dancers, probably because the tibialis anterior muscle plays a very active role in maintaining the heels on the floor during the *plié* and is, therefore, in excellent condition.

Occasionally, dancers complain of pain on the lateral aspect of the distal third of the fibula. Most of these injuries are peroneal tendinitis, but cases of fibular stress fractures have been reported. Both of these injuries may be secondary to a functional equinus condition (see chapter 2).

Knee Injuries

Dancers often complain of knee pain, most of which is associated with "forcing the turn-out." Under normal circumstances, turn-out, or external rotation of the lower extremities, occurs principally at the hip joint. If the external rotation at the hip is less than 55°, a dancer may dangerously compensate by bending the knees slightly, placing the freshly rosined feet in 90° external rotation, then slowly straightening the knees. This sequence is a common sight in almost any ballet class. During the final lockout phase of this extension, the knee joint normally rotates the leg internally. The shear forces between the knee joint's need to internally rotate and the sticky foot's stubborn demand for external rotation place extraordinary stresses upon and may strain or damage the medial collateral ligaments and the medial menisci. In modern and theatrical dance, where knee injuries are slightly more frequent than in ballet, knee injuries do not arise so much from problems of turn-out as from the patellofemoral compression of severe extension and floor work, and sudden twisting or turning movements of the extremity.[27]

Patellofemoral syndromes such as chondromalacia patellae are usually due to trauma to the patella. Genu valgum and a poor alignment of the quadriceps extensor mechanism (Q angle $> 10°$) may also contribute to chondromalacia patellae or subluxation and dislocation of the patella. Other knee disorders include patellar tendinitis (jumper's knee), Osgood-Schlatter disease, and infrapatellar bursitis.

Thigh Injuries

Generally, strained or pulled thigh muscles are not very frequent in trained dancers. Their flexibility and excellent quadriceps/hamstring balance usually prevent such injuries. When they do occur, the most frequent are hamstring and adductor strains. The sartorius muscle, which is used extensively in ballet as an external rotator of the thigh, may be involved in injuries. Strains of the proximal end of the sartorius muscle often occur during repetitive movements involving flexion, abduction, and external rotation of the thigh as in the *passé* position. During its acute phase of inflammation, the swelling within the damaged sartorius may compress and later entrap the lateral femoral cutaneous nerve, which may course through the proximal head of this muscle. The result is meralgia paresthetica of the anterolateral aspect of the thigh. In rare cases, the femoral nerve may be stretched or compressed behind the femoral sheath due to a damaged iliopsoas muscle.

Hip Injuries

Dancers require an extreme amount of range of motion at the hip joint: a minimum of 90° of flexion, extension, abduction, and circumduction. It is, therefore, a wonder that there are not more serious injuries in this region. Dancers often complain of a temporary restriction of hip range of motion (hip binding) or unusual clicking sounds associated with certain dance movements, such as abducting the entire extremity at hip level, *à la seconde à la hauteur.* The precise origin of these noises and bindings is not known. In some cases, it may be the greater trochanter catching on the edge of the gluteus maximus muscle. Deeper clicks may occur as the rim of the femoral head slips across the iliofemoral ligament. Most of these noises are asymptomatic and harmless.

Deep pain in the hip region may also be attributable to inflammation of the bursa between the hip joint and the psoas muscle. The iliopsoas muscle is active in many dance movements as a flexor of the hip, lateral flexor of the lumbar spine, or a minor external rotator of the thigh. In some cases, repeated trauma from dancing on hard floors and years of forcing the range of motion of the hip has led to the development of osteoarthritis of the acetabulum.

Back Injuries

Because posture is the framework for all movement, one might suspect that the stress of dancing may place a significant amount of stress upon the spine. Modern and jazz dancing require a much more extensive use and range of motion of the spine than ballet, and therefore have a somewhat greater rate of injury. The spine plays primarily a supporting role in the ballet dancer, and therein lies the problem. If supporting means balancing an 110-lb. ballerina on one's right shoulder or lifting her gently off the floor a few dozen times per dance, all sorts of havoc to the lumbar spine can result. Indeed, lower back syndrome is a common complaint among dancers, especially male ballet dancers who partner frequently. Some cases may become quite severe and actually involve varying degrees of nerve impingement, spondylolysis, and/or spondylolithesis.

Although irritation of the cervical spine is frequently due to the whip-like rotation ("spotting") of the head during pirouettes, cervical injuries in ballet are not common. In one instance, a male dancer had to be taken to the hospital in a neck brace and backboard when he dropped his partner on his head during an overhead lift. In this case, his embarrassment fortunately was more severe than the strain to his cervical muscles.

Miscellaneous Injuries

A whole collection of other injuries involve other bodily regions. For example, a dancer may fall out of a turn or from a lift and sustain a wrist fracture or shoulder dislocation. Female dancers often complain about bruised ribs from rough handling by their partners. On the other hand, the men occasionally sprain a finger while controlling their partner's rapid spins and swirling costume. Finally, in addition to the physical injuries, dancers also suffer from psychological injuries such as "burnout," depression, and eating disorders. These maladies affect dancers at all levels, shaking an untold number from their dream to dance.

Summary

Just how injurious is dancing? Does it present unnecessary or unreasonable hazards or liabilities for children and adults? In the vast majority of instances, dance is a very safe and healthy physical activity with no long-lasting results other than proud, humorous or slightly embarrassing memories of achievement or ineptness. Certainly, there are hazards and injuries as a result of participation in dance. Some dance teachers demand too much of fragile bodies, some companies have punitive rehearsal schedules, some theaters have rock-hard stage floors. These *unreasonable* risks frequently yield *unacceptable* results.

Nevertheless, there are risks involved in art and sport. Risks that create new styles and generate impressive records and achievements may also be the same risks that cause injuries, whether physical or psychological. It is the conflict between *reasonable* risks and *exceptional* results that is not always easily resolvable in medical, scientific, or legal terms. The conflict extends much deeper than that, centering on the uniquely human desire to sacrifice something of oneself for an abstract, indescribable feeling of accomplishment. Whether it is the purest expression of emotion in movement or running the world's fastest mile, these are human accomplishments that are at once intensely personal, yet publicly shared. Indeed, some people do falter in that final turn, perhaps never to finish. But never taking that first step for fear of failure is to deny the human need to move, and by that movement leave a legacy for a moment or more. Long after the final performance, a dancer still dances, an athlete still competes. Beautiful dances and great races are memories of movement.

References

1. Powell KE, Kohl HW, Caspersen CJ, Blair SN. An epidemiological perspective on the causes of running injuries. Phys Sportsmed 1986; 14(6):100-14.
2. Walter SD, Sutton JR, McItosh JM et al. The aetiology of sports injuries: a review of methodologies. Sports Med 1985; 2(Jan-Feb):47-58.
3. Michael M, Boyce WT, Wilcox AJ. Biomedical bestiary: an epidemiologic guide to flaws and fallacies in the medical literature. Boston: Little, Brown and Co., 1984.
4. Calabrese LH, Kirkendall DT, Floyd M et al. Menstrual abnormalities, nutritional patterns, and body composition in female classical ballet dancers. Phys Sportsmed 1983; 11(2):86-98.
5. Calabrese LH. The dancer disabled: other miseries of the dance. Emerg Med 1982; May 30:52-64.
6. Cohen JL, Chung SK, May PB et al. Exercise, body weight and amenorrhea in professional ballet dancers. Phys Sportsmed 1982; 10(4):92-101.
7. Cohen JL, Gupta PK, Lichstein E, Chadda KD. The heart of a dancer: noninvasive cardiac evaluation of professional ballet dancers. Am J Cardiol 1980; 45(5):959-65.
8. Cohen JL, Kim CS, May PB et al. Exercise, body weight, and amenorrhea in professional ballet dancers. Phys Sportsmed 1982; 10(4):92-101.
9. Cohen JL, Potosnak L, Oscar F, Baker H. A nutritional and hematologic assessment of elite ballet dancers. Phys Sportsmed 1985; 13(5):43-54.
10. Cohen JL, Segal KR, McArdle WD. Heart rate response to ballet stage performance. Phys Sportsmed 1982; 10(11):120-33.
11. Cohen JL, Segal KR, Witriol I, McArdle WD. Cardiorespiratory responses to ballet exercise and the $\dot{V}O_2$ max of elite ballet dancers. Med Sci Sports Exerc 1982; 14(3):212-17.
12. Mostardi RA, Porterfield JA, Greenberg B, Goldberg D, Lea M. Musculoskeletal and cardiopulmonary characteristics of the professional ballet dancer. Phys Sportsmed 1983; 11(12):53-61.
13. Schantz PG, Astrand PO. Physiological characteristics of classical ballet. Med Sci Sports Exerc 1984; 16(5):472-76.
14. Dolgener FA, Spasoff TC, St. John WE. Body build and body composition of high ability female dancers. Res Q Exerc Sport 1980; 51:599-607.
15. Stephens RE. The biomechanical aspects of injuries in elite ballet dancers. La recherche en danse. Universite de Paris-Sorbonne, 1986 (in press).
16. Stephens RE. Biomechanical aspects of ballet and ballet injuries (slide cassette). Minneapolis: MacGraw-Hill, 1982.
17. Stephens, RE. The etiology of injuries in professional ballet dancers. La recherche en danse. Universite de Paris-Sorbonne, 1986 (in press).

18. Vincent LM. Competing with the sylph: dancers and the pursuit of the ideal body form. Kansas City, KS: Andrews and McMeel, 1979.

19. Stephens RE. Biomechanical and nutritional aspects of ballet. 3rd Int Symp on Orthop and Med Aspects of Dance (speech). University of Paris-Sorbonne, Oct 1983.

20. Miller EH, Schneider HJ, Bronson JL, McLain D. A new consideration in athletic injuries: the classical ballet dancer. Clin Orthop 1975; 111:181-91.

21. Micheli LJ, Gillespie WH, Walaszek AA. Physiologic profiles of female professional ballerinas. Clin Sports Med 1984; 3(Jan):199-209.

22. Kirkendall DT, Bergfeld JA, Calabrese L et al. Isokinetic characteristics of ballet dancers and the response to a season of ballet training. J Orthop Sports Phys Ther 1984; 5(4):207-11.

23. Quirk R. Ballet injuries: the Australian experience. Clin Sports Med 1983; 2(Nov):504-514.

24. Quirk R. Injuries in classical ballet. Aust Fam Phys 1984; 11(Nov):802-04.

25. Thomasen E. Diseases and injuries of ballet dancers. Denmark: Universitetsforlaget I Arhus, 1982:88-96.

26. Micheli LJ. Back injuries in dance. Clin Sports Med 1983; 2(Nov):473-84.

27. Solomon RL, Micheli LJ. Technique as a consideration in modern dance injuries. Phys Sportsmed 1986; 14(Aug):83-92.

28. Washington EL. Musculoskeletal injuries in theatrical dancers: size, frequency and severity. Am J Sports Med 1978;6:75-98.

29. Rovere GD, Webb LX, Gristina AG, Vogel JM. Musculoskeletal injuries in theatrical dance. Am J Sports Med 1983; 11(4):195-8.

30. Shaw JH. Survey of dance injuries (masters thesis). Salt Lake City: Univ of Utah, 1977.

31. Clanin DR, Davidson DM, Plastino JG, Ascher MS. Injury patterns of university dance students. Dance Med Health Newsletter 1984; 3(2):6-7.

32. Garrick J. Back injuries in dance (speech). Annu Dance Med Symp Cincinnati, 1983.

2

THE ETIOLOGY OF INJURIES IN BALLET

Robert E. Stephens, Ph.D.

DANCERS PAY A HEAVY price for their art. Despite the obvious aesthetic rewards of being a professional dancer, the enormous physical and psychological stresses without financial security make the art of dancing one of the most demanding of occupations. Dancers constantly face the possibility of serious injury and disability, and very few dancers escape the tragedy of careers cut short by injury. Indeed, there is every indication that the length of a professional dancer's career is steadily declining. Previously, a dancer could expect a career to last into the 30s or 40s, perhaps even longer.[1] Now there are many careers that end in the mid-20s.

The dancer's "Achilles heel" is a reluctance to face the need for effective injury prevention programs before the onset of the first injury. To do so would admit to one's own vulnerabilities—a disturbing thought when one is preoccupied with the ferocious demands of acquiring and maintaining ballet technique. Yet, injured dancers return to performing like lemmings to the sea, without any accounting for the cause of injury, but with the ultimate result of clearing the way for a new generation of dancers. Very often, it is not just one cause, but a cluster of complex interrelated factors that lead to a preventable injury.

During the past few years, research has begun to elucidate the various factors affecting the levels of technical performance of dancers and their predisposition to injury.[2,3,4] This chapter is based extensively on the author's work with dancers from Ballet West, the San Francisco Ballet and School, Ballet Midwest, Indiana University, the Ballet West Summer Program, American Ballet Theatre, Joffrey Ballet, Houston Ballet, Royal Ballet, and the New York City Ballet. Their evaluations and comments in examinations, questionnaires and interviews, along with the author's experiences as a leading dancer, dance teacher, consultant, and scientist, constitute the basis of this analysis of the occupational, training and technique, anatomical, biomechanical, environmental, nutritional, and psychological factors that contribute to dance-related injuries.

Occupational Factors

Professional dancers work in a highly pressurized, closely scrutinized, competitive occupation. There is a constant, unrelenting impetus by teachers, staff, other dancers, and the audience to exceed previous aesthetic standards. Any treatment program that runs counter to the occupational demands and needs of the artist poses a major dilemma for the dancer. Pain and injury management of tragically short careers is the all-too-frequent result. Inevitably, after many years of training and a few years of performing, all dancers must eventually start new careers.

> A 24-year-old male dancer* in the corps of one of the top ballet companies in the United States approached the author in the wings of the opera house during a Sunday matinee performance of *Western Symphony.* Between his brief appearances on stage, he complained of severe pain in the midtibial region, which prevented him from jumping. Indeed, during one entrance, his double *tours en l'air* were barely off the floor. Upon palpation, a large bony callous was felt at the point of pain. He reluctantly admitted to the diagnosis of a tibial stress fracture 6 months prior to this time. I recommended that he see his physician on Monday and consider a hiatus from dance to allow for healing. He explained to me that he was cast in the soloist's role of Benvolio in Tuesday's opening night performance of *Romeo and Juliet*. It was the "big break" in his career. He didn't know how much of an ironic twist of the truth that was. Needless to say, he never saw a physician, and went on to dance the part.
>
> Two years later, I heard from one of his colleagues that the progressive pain and disability had become too much for him and the company. He retired from dance and now manages a retail clothing shop.

In addition to having to cope with a disabling injury, dancers are often forced, consciously or subconsciously, to return to dancing too quickly. Many union contracts permit only 2 weeks of rehabilitation with pay. Subsequently, the dancer must file for Workmen's Compensation or unemployment insurance. The interval between filing the claim and receiving the money frequently leaves the dancer without financial support. According to a year-long Performing Arts Center for Health survey, 75% of the dancers in New York City were unemployed at some time during the year, had a median income of $8,714, and did not have adequate medical care services available to them.[1] One state threatened to eliminate unemployment insurance for dancers by classifying

*The case histories presented in this chapter are derived from the author's 12 years of experience as a dancer, dance teacher, consultant, and scientist. In some cases, minor details have been changed in order to protect the identity of the dancer.

them as seasonal workers. All of these circumstances—the poor pay and scant medical and occupational support services—often cause the dancer to return to dancing without adequate rehabilitation, which invariably contributes to the development of chronic injuries.

Even the process of getting started in ballet may be injurious. Most female ballet dancers start serious ballet training at about age 8, as compared to 12-16 for men (table 2-1).[4] Initially, this preparation would include the development and proper execution of a complete set of barre exercises and center work during a 1½-hr. class. As a dancer progresses, the number of classes and the level of technical difficulty gradually increase. Eventually, the professional dancer will take 6 classes per week at an extremely advanced level. More than ever before, there is an intensely competitive push among dancers, teachers, and directors to develop formidable, astonishing technique at a very early age. America loves its "baby ballerinas."

Most major ballet companies take almost 80% of their dancers from their company schools. After a few auditions and summer workshops, a 17-year-old dancer has or has been given a very clear idea about the chances of entering a major ballet company. The tremendous pressure to "make it" in a major company by the late teens often results in increased work loads in an effort to accelerate the development of technique. The current wave of interest in national and international ballet competitions further exacerbates the situation—dancers and their schools measuring themselves by their medals.

Training and Technique

Professional dancers attribute many of their injuries to improper ballet technique and/or training.[4] The weekly work load of the dancers in Ballet West and the Ballet West Summer Program is summarized in table 2-2. In interviews, the dancers listed 7 major factors related to training and technique that contributed to their injuries. These factors included: (1) inadequate warm-up, (2) lack of training specificity, (3) poor preseason condition, (4) rehearsal and

Table 2-1. Training History of Ballet Dancers*

Dancers	Starting Age	Total Years of Training	Years at This Level
Female professionals N = 24	8.6 ± 2.1	12.7 ± 3.6	5.1 ± 2.2
Male professionals N = 15	12.3 ± 4.2	13.0 ± 4.8	7.2 ± 3.4
Female students N = 77	7.3 ± 3.4	8.2 ± 2.8	2.7 ± 1.2
Male students N = 11	16.3 ± 2.1	4.0 ± 2.7	0.7 ± 1.1

*In years

performance schedules, (5) improper teaching of technique, (6) starting ballet training too late, and (7) development of muscle imbalances.

Inadequate Warm-Up

Many dancers claimed that a shortened or absent warm-up prior to class, rehearsal, or performance contributed to their injury. During interviews, they often failed to indicate a knowledge of effective methods of preparing their body for dancing. In addition, they complained of difficulty in keeping their muscles warm and ready during a long rehearsal when they are active only periodically, and then only in short bursts. Logistically, it may be difficult and at times unavoidable to efficiently schedule and accurately predict the temporal constraints of multiple simultaneous rehearsals. In these situations, dancers should not be required to dance full-out during lengthy rehearsals, or should be given adequate warning prior to participation.

Lack of Training Specificity

To benefit from practice, a dancer must specifically train in the technique to be used in the performance. For example, dancers from the highly respected San Francisco Ballet were practicing a very strict Russian technique by day in the classroom but performing a neoclassical Balanchine repertoire in the evening. There were numerous complaints about the physical strain and injuries this type of conflict causes.

Poor Preseason Conditioning of the Dancer

The standard union contract of dancers in the United States is about 32 weeks, usually divided into three 10- to 12-week seasons. During these intervals, a dancer must recover from the previous season and prepare for the next by taking classes. Occasionally, a dancer will begin a season in poor physical condition and sustain an overuse injury during the prolonged, strenuous rehearsal schedule. Although these are relatively minor acute injuries such as tendinitis, tenosynovitis, or muscle strains, they frequently plague the dancer throughout the remainder of the season. If these injuries are allowed to become chronic, they will probably reduce the length and productivity of the dancer's career.

Scheduling of Rehearsals and Performances

The tendency in certain ballet companies has been to reduce the amount of rehearsal time and increase the number of performances, or to have both occurring at the same time. For these companies, rehearsals represent the absence of income from performances and an obligation for paying dancers to practice. Because American dancers are paid by the company for only 30-36 weeks per year, companies have frequently attempted to schedule performances for as many weeks as possible. For the dancer who is returning from a long vacation to a strenuous rehearsal and performance schedule, this situation may cause overuse injuries very early in the season. Unfortunately, there is not much time to recover from these injuries during the season without increasing the dancer's chances of losing a position, dancing roles, or even a job.

Improper Performance and Teaching of Technique.

Dancers are always concerned with the development, maintenance, and improvement of their ballet technique. Nevertheless, mistakes do happen—consciously or unconsciously. The male dancer may lift his partner without sufficient upper body and abdominal strength, or the budding ballerina may do a *fouetté rond de jambe en tournant* before she is ready.

Ballet technique is a highly evolved art and science. Over the past 400 years, several major schools of technique have grown out of the stylized court dances of Catherine de Médicis and Louis XIV. Forming the historical, artistic, and pedagogical heritage of modern ballet are the Russian style radiating from the Vaganova school in Leningrad, the Cecchetti method based at the Royal Ballet School in London, the Bournonville style at the Royal Danish Ballet, the Balanchine style from the American School of Ballet, and the French school from the *École de Danse du Théâtre National de l'Opéra.*

Although there is little scientific evidence to demonstrate safety of any one technique over another, this doesn't stop the dance community from having intense and sometimes unqualified opinions about the hazards of the various styles. For example, the technique taught at the American Ballet School and performed in the New York City Ballet has received considerable criticism in the past few years, primarily because the heels are not allowed to load (bear weight) during the *plié.* However, for those dancers who have been trained in a particular technique from an early age with a reasonable physical facility and who continue to perform in that style, the risks are probably similar to other styles. Of course, most dancers don't have such a pure pedigree; they often represent an amalgamation of techniques, physiques, training, and choreographic styles. There are also those proponents who simply don't care about the hazards of their beloved technique, always pointing to examples of famous survivors.

Although most teachers of professional dancers have a good knowledge of basic technique, they do not always understand or compensate for the physical limitations of their students. Some teachers tend to interpret technique as an absolute that does not allow for an imperfect instrument (i.e., the body). They suggest that if dancers do not have a perfect body for ballet, then they should select another career. Naturally, dancers will try to compensate in order to achieve the appearance of good technique, often to the detriment of their bodies. The forcing of turn-out from the knees and feet rather than from the hips is the most flagrant example of violating physical restrictions for the sake of technique. Teachers should remember that many great artists had some physical limitations and technical faults, yet ballet has survived and continues to progress.

Starting Ballet Training Too Late

In America, men tend to start classical ballet training at a later age than they do in Europe or Russia, where dance is a more respected profession for men. This impression, as well as the late start, seems to be changing in America. However, it is not uncommon for men to have started as late as the age of

16 (table 2-1), 8 years later than female dancers. As a result of this late start, the men often take an extraordinary number of classes in an effort to compensate for their late start (table 2-2).

A 17-year-old male beginning ballet student was practicing some new leaps he had learned in intermediate jazz class. He had just finished a 2½ hr. class that morning. While coming down from a jump, he landed on the outside of his right forefoot, and a loud snapping noise was heard by the author, who was about 50 ft. away. There was immediate swelling at the base of the fifth metatarsal. After ice was applied, the student was taken to the emergency room. X-rays indicated a Jones fracture or avulsion fracture of the base of the fifth metatarsal near the insertion of the peroneal brevis tendon. However, this came as no surprise to the young man; he had known the diagnosis at the moment of the injury. He had had the same fracture a year before under similar circumstances, but on the other foot.

Excessive training, combined with fatigue, unsupervised rehearsals, and attempting steps beyond the individual's level of technical ability, significantly predispose the dancer to injuries in the early stages of his career.

Development of Muscle Imbalances

A well-balanced ballet class emphasizes movement in all directions—right, left, forward, backward, up, down, and turning. As a result, good training will develop the muscles of the lower extremities symmetrically. In some instances, however, excessive training and improper technique may cause imbalances of the hip rotator musculature and triceps surae. Limitation of the amount of external rotation affects a dancer's ability to turn out, a fundamental part of ballet technique. Attempts to compensate or perform ballet steps with this poor alignment may result in injuries of the hip, knee, ankle, and foot. Tightness of the triceps surae or functional equinus tends to decrease the shock-absorbing capacity of the foot during jumps. It also decreases the *plié,* the most frequent movement in ballet. The detailed biomechanics of these muscle imbalances are discussed in the section below on biomechanical factors.

Table 2-2. Training Work Load of Ballet Dancers*

Dancers	Class	Rehearsal	Performance	Total
Female professionals N = 24	10.2 ± 2.3	26.6 ± 6.1	7.9 ± 3.6	44.7 ± 4.0
Male professionals N = 15	9.3 ± 0.9	26.1 ± 6.2	9.5 ± 5.3	44.9 ± 4.1
Female students N = 77	13.6 ± 6.1	**	**	**
Male students N = 11	17.3 ± 7.7	**	**	**

*In average hours of participation per week
**Rehearsal and performance work loads for advanced students were not included.

Anatomical Factors

The dancer's dilemma is the imperfect body in the perfect art. Many dancers complain that ballet technique imposes "unnatural" positions, movements, and therefore stresses upon the body. Anyone who has ever attempted taking a ballet class knows of this frustrating and sometimes painful struggle. As the dancer ascends to the highest levels of technique, there is progressively less tolerance of anatomical or aesthetic variations.

In the general dance population, anatomical factors are more likely to contribute to an injury than in highly selected preprofessional and professional dancers. Among leading dancers, variations in measurements of limb segment lengths and circumferences are usually slight (< 8 mm), and major osseous variations in the alignment of the lower extremity are rarely seen.[3,4,5] By the time dancers reach this level, anatomical factors have long since sorted out the meek, the frail, and the physically unsuitable. Anatomical factors do play a role in the injuries of these dancers, but they are more likely to be more subtle and supplementary to other factors, such as technique. On rare occasions, a dancer may have a leg length difference, scoliosis, or excessive external tibial torsion, and this often has significant implications for the proper performance of technique. Key anatomical factors that influence the dancer's proper performance of ballet technique include: (1) somatotype, (2) femoral angle, (3) femoral torsion, (4) genu recurvatum, (5) tibial torsion, (6) ankle joint plantarflexion, and (6) foot development and type.

Somatotype

Currently, the aesthetically "ideal" body type in many major professional ballet companies in the United States comprises long, lean lines formed by a long neck and limbs, a short torso, and a relatively small head (figure 2-1).[6,7] Dancers with this somatotype were the favorite of the late George Balanchine, director of the New York City Ballet, and are often referred to as "Balanchine bodies." Other characteristics of the Balanchine dancer include an ability for excellent turn-out, a high-arched foot capable of overarching on *pointe,* and a lean, androgenous appearance.

Although this type of body may be aesthetically favored in certain companies, it is not necessarily the most durable anatomical framework for dancing. For example, in *arabesque* the long lower extremity can act as a powerful lever on the lower back, where the force may not be dissipated by the short torso and relatively weak abdominal muscles (figure 2-1). The emphasis in ballet on higher extension of the thigh at the hip may further exacerbate the forces on the lower spine and lead to lower back syndrome. About 12% of the Ballet West dancers complained of lower back syndrome.[4]

Femoral Angle

In the hip, the femoral angle of inclination is formed by the neck and shaft of the femur. It is normally 125°, but varies in inverse proportion to the development of the width and stature of the pelvis.[8] In a wider gynecoid pelvis, which is more common in women, the femoral angle approaches a right angle

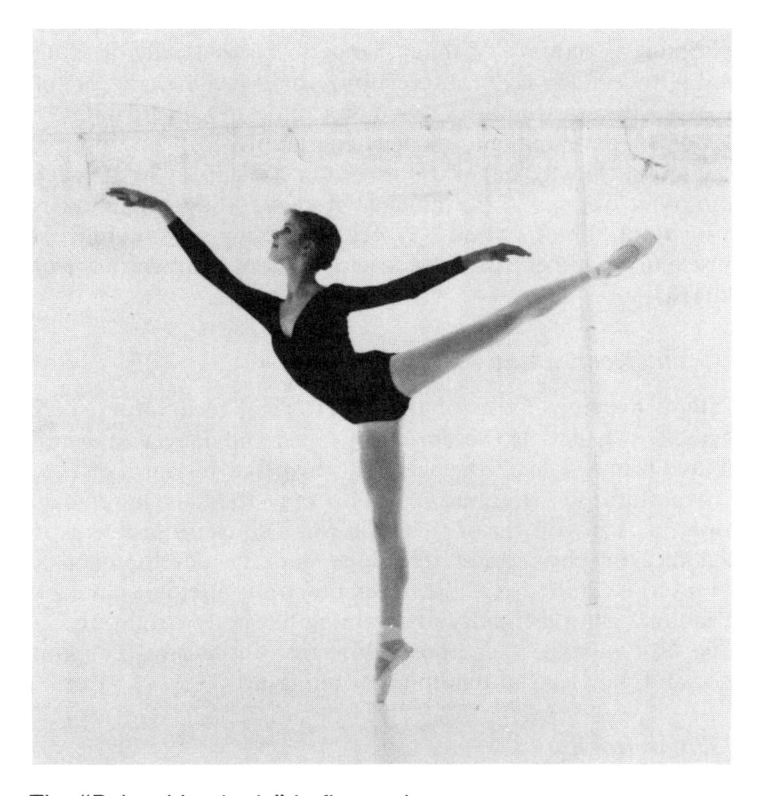

Figure 2-1. The "Balanchine body" in first arabesque.

and may be associated with a genu valgum.[5,9,10] This "knock-kneed" alignment may lead to patellofemoral tracking problems, medial knee strain, and excessive pronation of the foot.[10-12] The excessive pronation may, in turn, cause a variety of injuries such as plantar fasciitis, medial ankle tenosynovitis, Achilles tendinitis, and posteromedial tibial shin splints. Pronation also internally rotates the leg and may strain the medial aspect of the knee.[5,9] More obtuse femoral angles ($>125°$) are more characteristic of android pelvises and genu varum, or "bowlegs."[8,10] Of the two types of genu configurations, a slight genu varum may be favored, primarily because it creates a wider opening or separation of the legs during *petite batterie*. Excessive genu varum is, of course, aesthetically and technically undesirable.

Femoral Torsion

The angle of anatomical femoral torsion determines the amount of external rotation (femoral retroversion) and internal rotation (femoral anteversion) intrinsic to the femur. Normally, adults have about 12-14° of anteversion.[8] Excessive femoral anteversion and the associated squinting patellae and "pigeon-toed" gait is anathema in ballet because of the demand for extreme external rotation (i.e., turn-out). Individuals with femoral retroversion tend to walk "duck-footed," a characteristic that is either a fortuitous genetic windfall or an occupational affectation of many dancers. Theoretically, a relative degree of femoral retroversion (< 10° anteversion) would facilitate the 90° of external rotation of the lower extremities that a dancer desires for turn-out.[5,11,13] Although genes, normal development, and certain pathological conditions affect the angle of femoral torsion, ballet training does not appear to increase the amount of femoral retroversion.[13] Inasmuch as students who start younger tend to have better turn-out (tables 2-1 and 2-3),[13] early training may minimize some of these osseous changes and enhance the development of ligamentous laxity in the hips and knees.

Genu Recurvatum

Slight hyperextension of the knees (genu recurvatum) of about 10° is fashionable in ballet. However, it may cause the dancer to stand with weight distributed primarily over the heels, tilt the pelvis forward, and sway the lower back (hyperlordosis) (figure 2-2).[10] This may result in lower back syndrome. Improper body alignment of this type will also cause problems in the correct performance of basic ballet technique and the development of technique-related injuries.[5,7,10] For example, when on *pointe* a female dancer with genu recurvatum may have difficulty maintaining her body weight over her foot (i.e., "pulling off" *pointe*). This poor alignment overstresses the plantarflexors of the foot and may lead to tendinitis or tenosynovitis.

Tibial Torsion

Normally, the tibia is externally twisted about 12° along its length.[5,14,15] Excessive external tibial torsion (> 20°) may result in patellofemoral and knee disorders, because the dancer cannot align the knees over the toes during the *pilé*. The inward rotation of the thigh over the externally rotated leg creates tracking problems with the patella, shear forces in the knee, and pronatory forces on the foot. The "pigeon-toed" gait characteristic of excessive internal tibial torsion (< 10°) results in severe pronation of the foot. This inward alignment of the distal extremity is contrary to the need for extreme external rota-

Table 2-3. Total Rotational ROM of the Hip Joint

Dancers	Control Values	Hip Neutral		Hip Flexed
Female professionals N = 48	90-100°	75.4 ± 11.1	*	80.8 ± 10.2
		**		*
Female students N = 144	90-100°	80.6 ± 10.2	**	86.6 ± 10.6
Male professionals N = 30	90-100°	70.2 ± 11.1		72.8 ± 10.6
Male students N = 22	90-100°	65.2 ± 10.4		70.3 ± 7.9

*P<0.05
**P<0.01

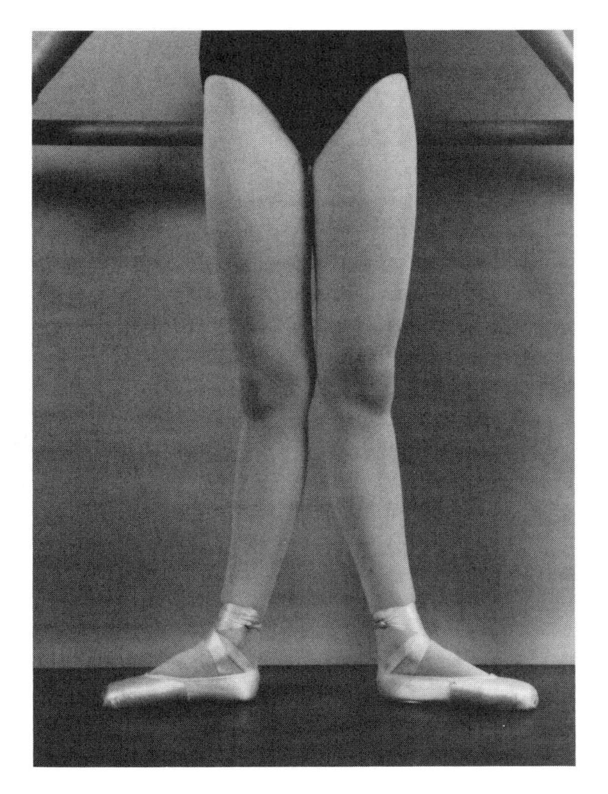

Figure 2-2. Genu recurvatum may not allow the heels to approximate in first position, thereby giving the appearance of a slight second position. The line of gravity is located between the heels rather than through the feet, tending to pull the dancer off *pointe* when *en relevé.*

tion in ballet movements, and individuals with the condition should consider other forms of dance.

Ankle Joint Plantarflexion

Osseous limitation of ankle joint plantarflexion, or a poor *pointe,* virtually bars employment in a professional ballet company. The strongly pointed, if not overarched, foot is an essential element in the aesthetic and technique of ballet (figure 2-3). With limited ankle plantarflexion, female dancers cannot reach the complete on *pointe* position, and men cannot obtain *demi-pointe,* both essential positions in the performance of most ballet movements. Frequently, limited plantarflexion may be due to impingement of the posterior joint margin or posterior tubercle of the talus and the posterior edge of the tibia at the tibiotalar joint during extreme plantarflexion. An os trigonum near the posteriolateral tubercle of the talus is present in about 7% of the cases of posterior talar impingement syndrome,[16-18] and may result in tarsal tunnel syndrome.[19-21]

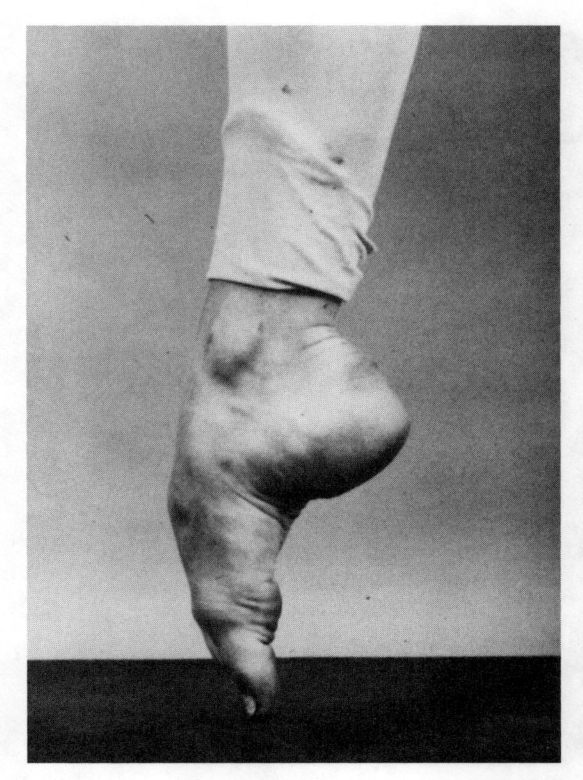

Figure 2-3. Plantarflexed cavus foot. At least 90° of plantarflexion is required when pointing the foot. This ideal example demonstrates a perfectly pointed, high-arched foot, an aesthetic standard in ballet.

Foot Development and Types

Osseous development of the foot is also a consideration in the causes of injuries in young female dancers.[10] Dance teachers should be aware of the anatomic, technical, and legal implications of starting a female dancer on *pointe* too early. *Pointe* work should not be permitted before the age of 10 years, and should be strictly limited to a gradually progressive series of exercises between the ages of 10 and 12. Because of the possibility of compression injuries to the epiphyseal plates, x-rays of the feet should be taken if there is any question as to the skeletal maturity, especially of the first and second metatarsals and digits. The level of technique and overall musculoskeletal maturity are additional factors when considering the proper age to start *pointe* work. As long as the dancer is learning and practicing good ballet technique, a one- or two-year delay in starting full-time *pointe* work should not be a detriment.

An 11-year-old girl of Indian descent was referred to the author by her dance teacher and physician to determine if she should begin *pointe* work. Prior physical examination revealed an intelligent, healthy prepubescent female of normal height and weight for her age. She had severely pronated feet and significant bunion deformities, bilaterally. X-rays confirmed these observations and indicated that the epiphyseal plates were still quite active. After review of the medical evidence, discussions with the teacher, the dancer, and her mother (who had the same foot type as her daughter's), and observing the girl in ballet class, it was unanimously decided to omit *pointe* work as a part of her ballet training. Although naturally disappointed, the young girl was satisfied that a concerted effort was made to determine the short- and long-term effects of *pointe* work on her feet. She is now a prelaw student at a state university and enjoys participation in ballet as recreation.

The Greek forefoot, in which the second digit is longest, may result in a hammer-toe deformity of that digit or depression of the head of the second metatarsal. Usually this does not affect dancing. The most dangerous foot type for the female dancer is the Egyptian forefoot, in which the first metatarsal and digit are the longest. When standing on *pointe,* this foot type exposes the first metatarsophalangeal joints to unnecessary valgus stresses. Bunion deformities, fractures of the hallux, onycholysis, or subungual hematomas may result.[22,23] *Pointe* work may exacerbate certain congenital forefoot conditions such as bilateral bunion deformities in the child and is, therefore, contraindicated.[24] Other forms and expectations of dance should be encouraged.

Although anatomical factors may limit the amount and caliber of participation and, perhaps, the career possibilities a young person may have in ballet, they should not hamper the individual's desire to dance within the limits of one's own abilities, discipline, talent, and pain-free enjoyment.

Biomechanical Factors

Neither ballet nor the dancer understands or has any use for "normal" range of motion; minimal function is often minimal dancing—something that doesn't sell many tickets. Ballet movements require full range of motion of the joints, especially of the lower extremity. The dancer's expectations are always at the extreme of any biomechanical or artistic consideration. In many instances, there is an almost inseparable interrelationship among anatomy, biomechanics and ballet technique, and the development of injuries. A study of 54 biomechanical measurements and assessments indicated that, in the final analysis, five critical biomechanical factors were associated with the development of dance-related injuries: (1) muscle imbalances of the rotator musculature of the hip, (2) gastroc-soleus equinus, (3) foot plantarflexion, (4) hallux rigidus, and (5) foot type.[3,4]

Muscle Imbalances of the Hip

Normally, there is 45-50° of internal and external rotation of the hip (technically referred to as femoral torsion), with a total range of motion of 90-100°.[14,15,25-27] Femoral torsion is evaluated by using a gravity goniometer to measure the degrees of internal rotation, external rotation, and total range of motion (ROM) of the femur in the acetabulum (figure 2-4).[14,25] These measurements may also indicate the amount of anatomical femoral torsion (i.e., anteversion or retroversion), the presence of soft tissue limitation such as muscle

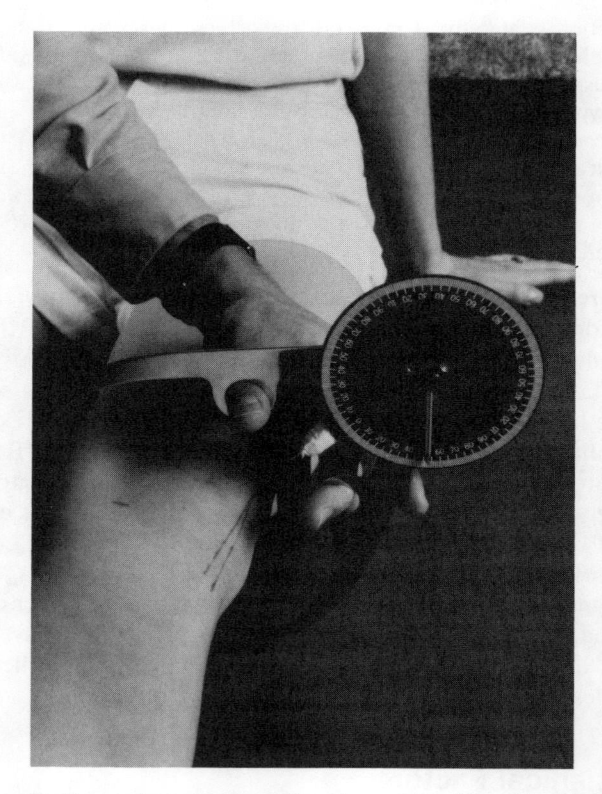

Figure 2-4. Testing external range of motion of the hip with a gravity goniometer. Most professional dancers have 55-70° of external rotation of the hip. Some dancers have a muscle imbalance of the deep hip rotators, probably due to their extensive amount of use in ballet without stretching.

imbalances, or the asymmetries of the ROM of each extremity. The internal and external ROM are measured with the dancer in the supine (or hip neutral) and sitting (or hip flexed 90°) positions. Internal and external rotation as well as the total ROM should be bilaterally symmetrical and equal in both testing positions.

Measurements of femoral torsion have demonstrated a significantly greater amount of total hip ROM in top female professional and student dancers than in the corresponding male groups ($p < .05$).[3] In addition, the total hip ROM in all of the groups was generally less than control values (table 2-3).[14,26,27] The female student dancers had the greatest total ROM, followed by the female professionals, the male professionals, and the male students. This was the same range order as their starting ages in studying dance (table 2-1).

A study of the Cincinnati Ballet suggested a correlation between the age that a person started dancing and the ability to turn out.[13] Since the x-rays of these dancers did not indicate a significant amount of femoral retroversion, the study attributed this relationship to changes in the restrictiveness of the ligaments of the hip and knee rather than actual osseous restructuring. The capacity to develop these changes apparently diminishes rapidly between the ages of 10 and 14.

The female dancers also had significant increases in the total hip ROM when the hip was in the flexed position versus the supine position (table 2-3; $p < .05$). In this situation, the degrees of femoral retroversion cannot be calculated accurately using goniometers when there is a difference between the total ROM in the two testing positions.[14,15] However, a difference between the total ROM in the two testing positions usually indicates a soft tissue limitation associated with a muscle imbalance of the rotator musculature of the hip.[14,15] This may be attributable to the constant use of the hip rotator muscles in ballet. Although dancers are concerned only with turn-out, they would also agree that ballet requires efficient movement in all directions—a direct product of fluid, complete, and balanced ROM of all the joints of the lower extremities. A series of hip exercises developed by the author has been very effective in correcting these muscle imbalances[28] as well as alleviating some dancers' complaints of clicking noises or binding in the hip.[29]

External rotation was normal (44-50°) in all of the groups, but was lowest in the male student group (39°). The dancers also demonstrated some degree of limitation of internal rotation (range: 24-37°). Limitation of internal rotation may be due to the tightness of the external rotator musculature, ligamentous restrictions, or the degree of femoral retroversion.

Limitation of hip rotation, especially external rotation, can have a profound effect upon a dancer's technique and vulnerability to injury. A dancer may attempt to compensate for limited turn-out by tilting the pelvis, increasing the lordotic curvature of the lumbar spine, twisting the knees, or abducting the forefoot (figure 2-5). This is known among dancers as "forcing the turn-out." Dancers with inadequate turn-out may also use rosin or slight moisture on the shoes to increase friction, place their feet in fifth position *demi-plié,* and slowly straighten the legs. Howse appropriately referred to this as "screwing the knee."[11] The inward torque of the hip rotators on the fixed, externally rotated foot is devastating to the medial aspect of the knee. A dancer with pain in this region should be suspected of forcing turn-out. The resultant compensatory mechanisms also increase the amount of stress placed upon the joints of the lower extremities, prevent proper alignment, and increase pronation of the foot. In the author's experience, therapeutic exercises can minimize or eliminate hip limitation due to muscle imbalances, thus allowing the dancer to use the complete range of motion at the hip.[29]

TURN-OUT

Although "perfect" turn-out theoretically involves 90° of external rotation at each hip, few dancers have as much as 70° (figure 2-6). Yet, many dancers can demonstrate adequate turn-out in the basic ballet positions. Turn-out involves a sufficient amount of external rotation at the hip (55-70°), about 10° of external rotation at the knee, tibial torsion (12°), and abduction of the forefoot at the midtarsal joint.

During a *grand plié,* the external rotation of the hip is superimposed

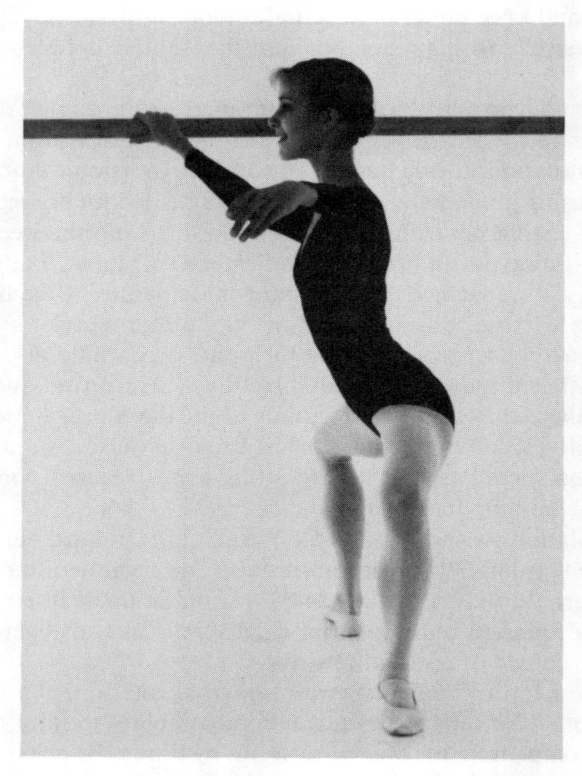

Figure 2-5. Poor turn-out in second position. In order to compensate for poor turn-out, dancers frequently tilt the pelvis to increase the external ROM of the hip. The resultant hyperlordosis and poor body alignment are not only amusing, but also quite dangerous.

upon the simultaneous actions of flexion and abduction of the thigh at the hip joint (figure 2-6). The abduction of the thigh may allow for an additional amount of external rotation at the hip joint. This movement is not accounted for during the conventional testing of femoral torsion. In addition, dancers with soft tissue limitation of the hip will often compensate for decreased external rotation by tilting the pelvis (i.e., flexing the hip), which increases the ROM (figure 2-5). The evidence indicates that the relative amount of anatomical femoral retroversion is less of a factor than the complex compensatory mechanisms of the entire lower extremity and spine.[10,13] The *plié* also illustrates the fact that basic ballet movements are complex biomechanical activities that extend beyond normal uniplanar joint motion.

Gastroc-Soleus Equinus

The range of motion at the ankle joint is assessed using a standard goniometer to measure the number of degrees of dorsiflexion of the neutral foot with the knee extended and flexed.[14,25] These two positions primarily test the

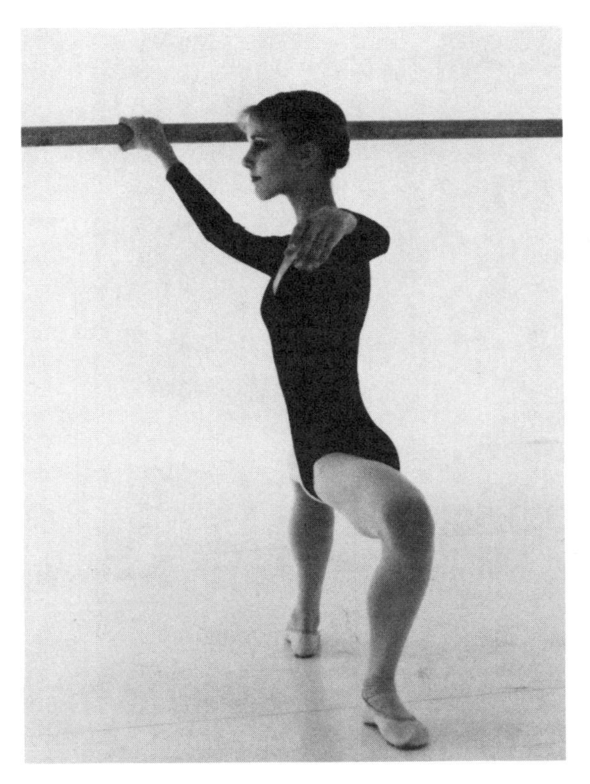

Figure 2-6. Perfect *plié* in second position. Dancers dream of having turn-out and a *plié* like this. Notice the perfect alignment of feet, knees, and body. A few years later, this 14-year-old became an international prize winner and a leading dancer with a major ballet company.

flexibility of the gastrocnemius and soleus muscles, respectively. Normal values for ankle dorsiflexion are between 10-13° when the knee is straight and about 20-23° when the knee is flexed.[14,15,26,27,32] A minimum of 10° of ankle joint dorisflexion is essential for the normal biomechanics of the foot (figure 2-7).[15,25,32] In some cases, dorsiflexion of the ankle may be blocked by anterior tibiotalar impingement syndrome[30,31] or tight calf muscles.

Both male and female professional dancers demonstrated about a 10° limitation of ankle dorsiflexion in both testing positions (table 2-4).[3,4] This indicated the presence of a gastroc-soleus equinus, a functional dynamic muscle imbalance of the posterior calves.[32,33] It is a common biomechanical problem among professional, advanced university, and aerobic dancers as well as many competitive endurance athletes, such as runners, and is related to the frequency, duration, intensity, and technique of training.[32,34]

Professional dancers may acquire a functional equinus condition from years of extensive daily use of the calf muscles without a proportional amount of calf stretching, or technical faults such as the failure to allow the heels to contact the floor during the landing and takeoff phases of the *plié*. Functional

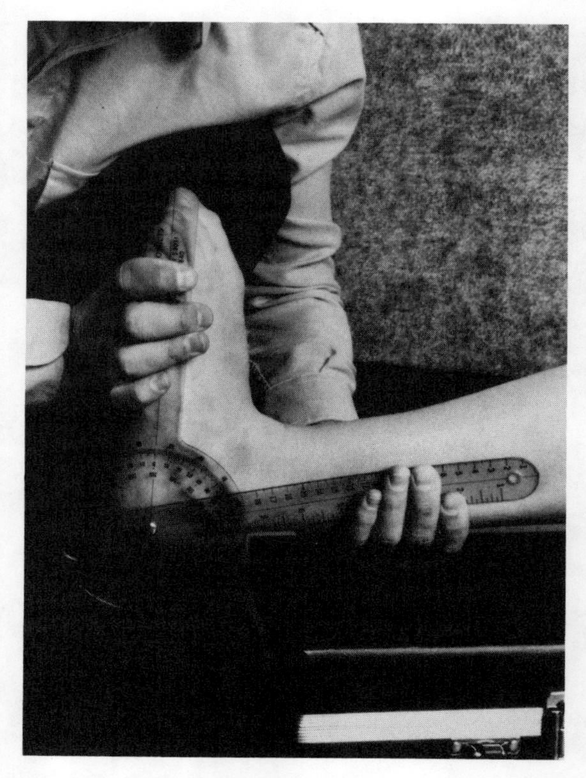

Figure 2-7. The ROM of ankle joint dorsiflexion is tested with a standard goniometer. This dancer has 15° of dorsiflexion; a minimum of 10° is necessary for normal function of the foot.

equinus alters the normal biomechanics of the foot during the fundamental movement of the *plié* and seriously predisposes the dancer to injury.

A 16-year-old advanced female student in a major ballet school was referred to the author by the director. At the time of the initial complaint, six weeks before, she had been taking class every day and rehearsing *Les Patineurs* as an understudy. Her injury had been diagnosed as severe acute peroneal tendinitis and was treated with anti-inflammatory medication and reduced activity. Three weeks after the diagnosis, she started taking *barre,* and two weeks later began center work. After one week, the pain was beginning to return. It was at this point that I first saw her.

Biomechanical evaluation revealed a slight bilateral gastroc-soleus equinus, which was more prominent on the left. I observed her in class and noted that she repeatedly failed to allow the heels to contact the floor during the *plié,* and that she usually performed more movements on her left foot ("her turning leg"). *Petit allegro* combinations were especially irritating. With her physician's approval, she was taught an extensive stretching and strengthening program for her calves and feet, which she performed approximately 6 times a day. She was told the importance of

Table 2-4. Ankle Joint Dorsiflexion

Dancers	Control Values		Knee Neutral	Control Values		Knee Flexed
Female professionals N = 48	10-13°	*	1.4 ± 5.2	20-23°	*	11.7 ± 6.2
Male professionals N = 30	10-13°	*	-0.7 ± 3.8	20-23°	*	8.0 ± 3.5
Female students N = 144	10-13°		4.1 ± 9.5	20-23°		14.2 ± 6.7
Male students N = 22	10-13°		6.3 ± 7.2	20-23°		14.5 ± 7.6

$^{*}P<0.05$

loading the heels in the *plié* and to concentrate on this principle during all phases of the class. Three weeks later, she was completely asymptomatic, although *petit allegro* was still frustrating.

BIOMECHANICS OF THE PLIÉ WITH FUNCTIONAL EQUINUS

During the initial phase of the *plié,* the tibia must be free to move forward the first 10° on a neutral foot (figure 2-8).[15,32,35,36] Functional equinus reduces this forward movement while inverting the calcaneus. Concurrently, the internal rotation of the tibia caused by flexion at the knee tends to pronate the subtalar joint. The peroneal muscles may be activated in an attempt to evert the rearfoot and balance the powerful effect of the triceps surae muscles.[37,38] The opposition of these muscle groups may be the mechanism for the development of lateral leg pain, peroneal tendinitis, and fibular stress fractures due to the extensive attachment of the peroneal muscles to the fibula.[13]

From the available evidence, it is possible to postulate two theories, not necessarily mutually exclusive, on how the foot responds to the functional equinus condition in dancers.[9,32,36-41] One theory suggests that during the initial phase of the *plié,* the foot pronates because of the internal rotation of the tibia, the eversion of the rearfoot by the peroneal muscles, and abduction of the forefoot. These factors release the midtarsal joint and permit dorsiflexion of the forefoot upon the rearfoot, thereby deepening the *plié.* When a dancer with functional equinus does not allow the heels to load properly during the *plié,* the foot will remain flexible and ineffective as a lever arm instead of resupinating during the propulsive phase of the *plié.* Therefore, the lower extremity must absorb abnormal amounts of pronatory and propulsive forces.

The second theory maintains that functional equinus creates an abnormal opposition of everting (peroneal muscles) and inverting (triceps surae muscles) forces in the rearfoot as suggested in the first theory. However, in this battle over the control of the rearfoot, the powerful triceps surae predominate, thus keeping the foot supinated and the midtarsal joint locked. This makes the foot an effective rigid lever arm during the *plié* but a poor shock absorber. Observations of classroom technique indicate that as the

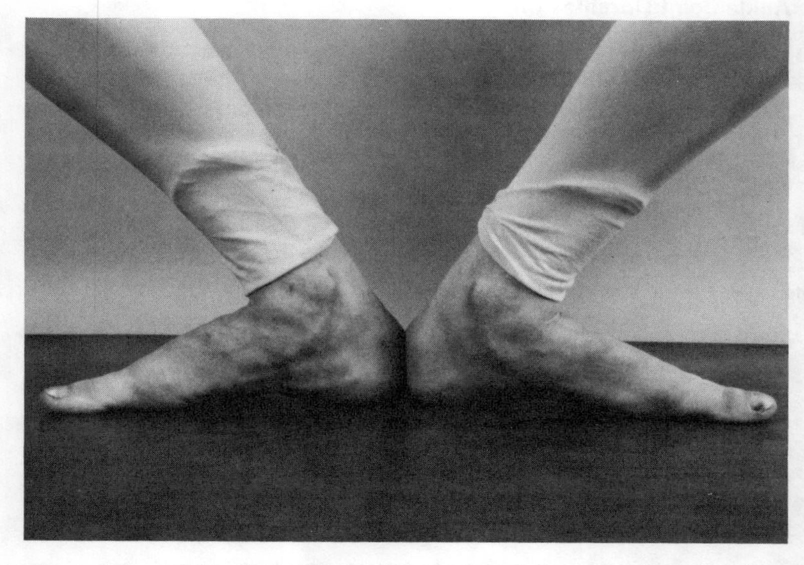

Figure 2-8. *Plié* in first position. During the *plié*, the first 10° of dorsiflexion must occur on a neutral foot. Gastroc-soleus equinus or tightness of the triceps surae muscles limits dorsiflexion and adversely affects the shock-absorbing capacity of the foot.

tempo of *petit allegro* increases, dancers are more likely to prevent the heels from loading during the *plié*. This decreases the latency time between the pronation phase of landing and the resupination phase of the propulsive takeoff by keeping the foot supinated.

There may also be a relationship between the varus rearfoot condition produced by functional equinus in dancers and the incidence of metatarsal stress fractures, medial ankle tenosynovitis, peroneal tenosynovitis, and Achilles tendinitis.[35,40] A correlation between stress fractures in female athletes and various degrees of rearfoot varus alignment has been reported in the literature.[42]

In an individual dancer, the presence of functional equinus, a technique that does not permit the heels to contact the ground, and a cavus foot type, which is relatively nonshock-absorbing but very fashionable these days, represents a serious predisposition to injuries of the foot, ankle, and leg.[9,40]

> While the author was performing injury prevention evaluations for a company-affiliated ballet school, a young woman in her early 20s appeared at the door with a burly male escort and sweetly but firmly requested an immediate evaluation. Not knowing whether she was a dancer (she "looked" like a dancer), I explained the nature of the exam, and proceeded with the evaluation. The biomechanical evaluation showed significant bilateral gastroc-soleus equinus, high-arched cavus feet, and an unusual pattern of calluses on her feet that indicated either a very tight *pointe* shoe box or the practice of Chinese foot binding. The results indicated that she was inordinately predisposed to Achilles tendinitis,

medial ankle tenosynovitis, and, most seriously, metatarsal fractures. With each word, she and her friend became more upset, until she finally burst into tears. Her friend then informed me that she was the star principal dancer with a major ballet company and that she indeed had all of these problems, including three metatarsal stress fractures.

Later, we discussed at length effective methods of minimizing the chances of the recurrence of her injuries: wider boxes in her *pointe* shoes, calf stretching exercises, loading the heels during the *plié,* and better nutrition (she exhibited anorexic behavior, and almost certainly had caloric, protein, vitamin, and mineral deficiencies). Nevertheless, the conversation often returned to the premise that the company would take care of everything. She was their star; they wouldn't let anything happen to her. Her world was about fantasy—Odette/Odile and sylphs at midnight—not physical and financial reality. In the final analysis, she believed in denial and the company as a surrogate parent. By the age of 24 she was retired from dance because of chronic injuries—disenchanted with the betrayal of ballet.

The increasing demands in ballet for faster allegro combinations, along with the lack of calf-stretching exercises proportional to the amount of their use, will continue to make functional equinus an important consideration in the etiology of ballet injuries. Ankle joint plantarflexion, first metatarsophalangeal joint dorsiflexion, and the foot type also play significant morphological, biomechanical, and clinical roles in the functional and aesthetic aspects of the foot.

Ankle Joint Plantarflexion

In professional ballet companies, a dancer must be able to plantarflex (i.e., point or extend) the foot in such a way that the dorsum of the forefoot falls in a direct line from the anterior edge of the tibia (figure 2-9). In the *demi-pointe* or on *pointe* positions, this aligns the foot in a manner that allows the *bones* to bear the weight properly—not the ligamentous and musculotendinous structures of the foot and ankle.

Although overarching of the foot is currently popular in many ballet companies, it can create biomechanical problems. On *pointe,* the extension of the line of gravity in front of the foot, increases the amount of stress on the ligamentous and tendinous structures on the dorsum of the foot (figure 2-10). In one study, about 40% of top female dancers had the ROM necessary to overarch the foot.[3] An appreciable number of these dancers complained about various strains on the dorsal aspect of the foot.

As mentioned previously, in some cases plantarflexion may be limited by posterior talar impingement or other factors.[16,17] This causes the line of gravity to fall directly beneath the heel rather than over the metatarsal heads or through the phalanges (figure 2-11). This alignment increases the amount of stress placed upon the muscles, tendons, and ligaments of the posterior, medial, and lateral aspects of the ankle, thus increasing the vulnerability of these areas to injuries such as tendinitis, tenosynovitis, and shin splints. Evidence also indicates that the forefoot is able to abduct while supinated in the on *pointe* position.[24] This may allow a degree of pronation and shock absorption in the foot, but it may hasten the development of bunion deformities.

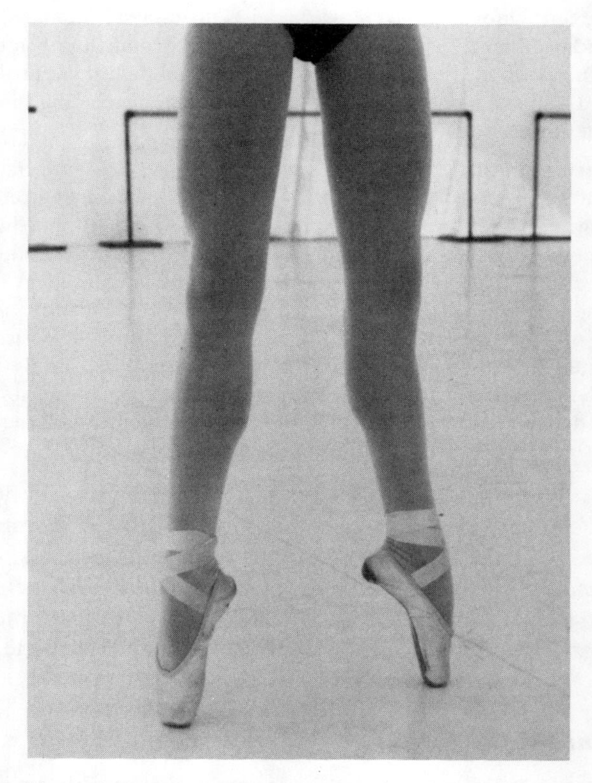

Figure 2-9. Normal feet *sur les pointes.* The line of gravity for each foot should extend through the tibia and bones of the foot to the tips of the toes.

Limited plantarflexion is an unsatisfactory condition in professional dancers mainly due to fairly uncompromising aesthetic standards for beautifully pointed feet. A slightly dorsiflexed foot destroys the elongating illusion of the fully extended extremity. Female dancers must have linear plantarflexion in order to perform on *pointe,* and men need it for *demi-pointe.* Functionally, limited plantarflexion may also appear in dancers who are overweight and having difficulty rising to full *pointe* position. These conditions are not acceptable in most professional ballet companies in the United States.

Hallux Rigidus

In ballet, 90° of dorsiflexion at the first metatarsophalangeal joint (MPJ) is important in the normal function of the foot on *demi-pointe* (figure 2-12). It is a more significant factor in male dancers, who use the *demi-pointe* position more frequently, than it is in women, who work primarily on *pointe.* Studies have indicated that 30-40% of professional dancers had varying degrees of unilateral or bilateral hallux rigidus.[3] In the *demi-pointe* position, plantarflexion of the ankle joint is limited by the amount of dorsiflexion of the first metatarsophalangeal joint. In cases of hallux rigidus, the line of gravity passes behind

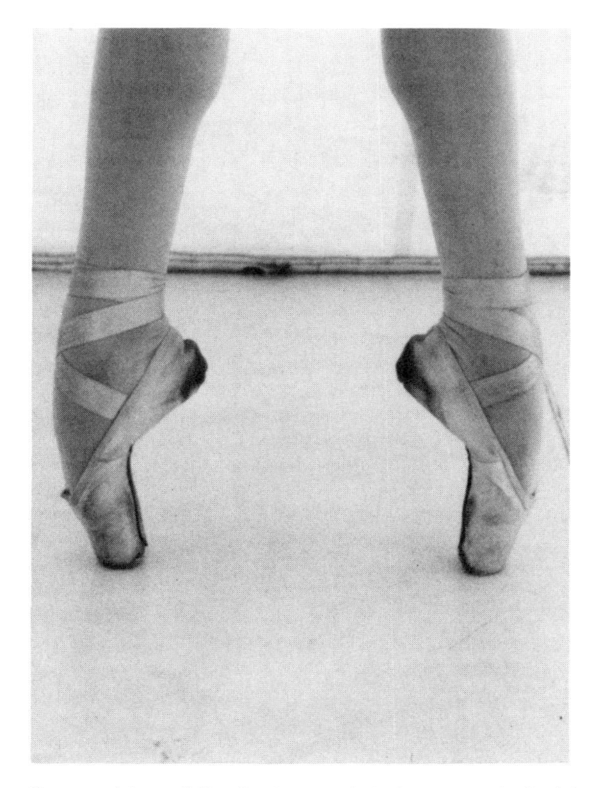

Figure 2-10. Overarching of the foot on *pointe* is currently fashionable in ballet. However, overarching may stress the ligaments on the dorsum of the foot as well as damage the toenails, because the line of gravity falls on a point anterior to the dorsum of the foot rather than through the foot.

the metatarsal heads, thus creating the same biomechanical problems as mentioned with limitation of ankle joint plantarflexion (figure 2-11). When a dancer is unable to reach the full *demi-pointe* position, the foot must be evaluated separately for hallux rigidus and/or limitation of ankle joint plantarflexion.

A 26-year-old male principal dancer in a regional ballet company experienced needle-sharp pain in the back of the right ankle when he pointed his foot. During a dress rehearsal of *Giselle,* the abrupt pain from a *relevé* to pirouette caused his leg to reflexively relax, and he collapsed on stage. Examination of the right leg demonstrated limited plantarflexion (figure 2-11), which was painful when passively pointed to its limit. In addition, he had hallux rigidus and severe crepitus and chronic tenosynovitis of the medial ankle tendons, especially the flexor hallicus longus. One year later, the right ankle required surgery to remove an impacted posterior tubercle/os trigonum of the talus and the calcified sheaths of the flexor hallicus longus tendons. Although rehabilitation was successful, the dancer never returned to a full rehearsal/performance schedule. He is now pursuing a career in medicine.

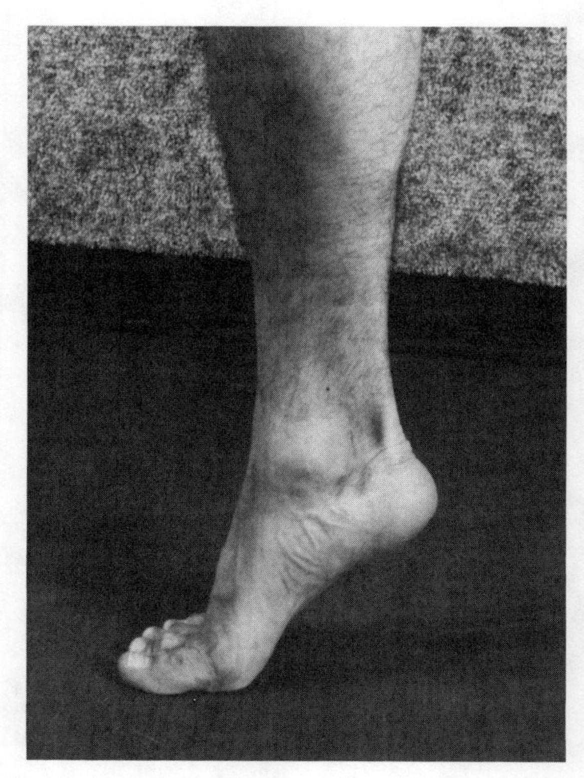

Figure 2-11. Abnormal *demi-pointe.* This dancer demonstrates limited plantarflexion due to posterior impingement and hallux rigidus. In dancers, ankle joint plantarflexion and first metatarsophalangeal dorsiflexion must be analyzed separately.

The impingement of the dorsal margins of the joint associated with hallux rigidus frequently results in inflammation of the joint capsule and the development of dorsal exostoses.[23] Often, a dancer with hallux rigidus will roll toward the lateral side of the foot ("sickle the foot") during the *relevé* to *demi-pointe* or while performing movements on *demi-pointe.* Female dancers who have this condition may have difficulty rolling down through the foot from the on *pointe* position, or rising (*relevé*) to the on *pointe* position.

Pes Planus and Cavus

Another important factor about the ballet dancer's foot is the foot type: pes planus or pes cavus.[9,40] Currently, the cavus foot is the aesthetic favorite in ballet, although it is by no means a requirement (figure 2-3). Biomechanically, this foot type is relatively rigid and nonshock-absorbing.[43] In addition, the cavus foot may be associated with a short Achilles tendon and concomitant equinus condition. The combination of the cavus foot, functional equinus, and

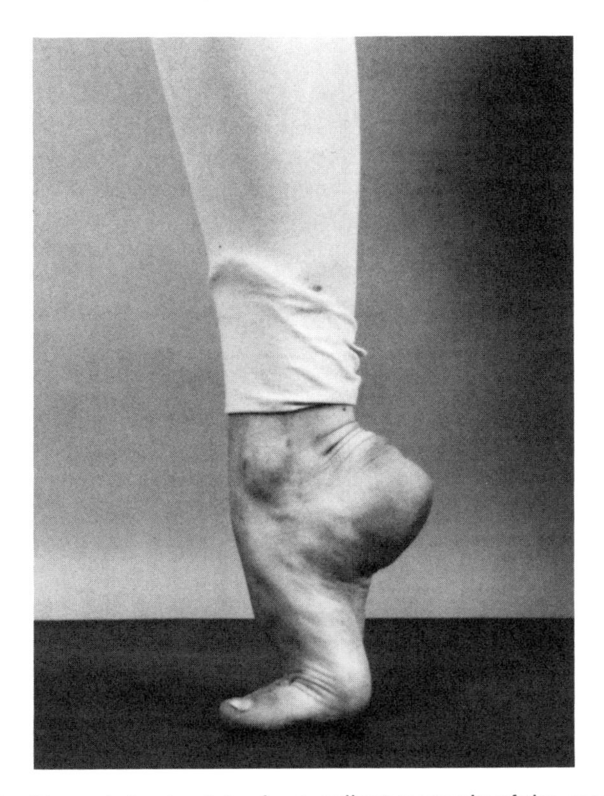

Figure 2-12. Normal *demi-pointe.* An excellent example of the amount of ROM in the ankle joint and first metatarsophalangeal joint in the *demi-pointe* position. The weight is distributed directly to the heads of the metatarsals. Male dancers use the *demi-pointe* position extensively, especially during pirouettes.

a ballet technique that does not permit the heels to load in the *demi-plié* represents a serious potential injury situation for the dancer.

Pes planus is commonly caused by forefoot varus.[44,45] Pronation allows the medial aspect of the forefoot to contact the ground and compensate for the forefoot varus. In addition, the general ligamentous laxity characteristic of the pronated foot overworks the flexors of the toes and the plantarflexors of the foot in a futile effort to stabilize the arches of the foot.[43,46,47] This predisposes these tendons and their associated synovial sheaths and attachments to injuries such as posteromedial shin splints, flexor hallucis longus tenosynovitis, or plantar fasciitis. Excessive pronation may also be due to hypermobile, dorsiflexed first rays that often splay when loaded.[48] This increases the load on the remaining metatarsals, predisposing them to stress fractures.[49,50] Pronation also internally rotates the leg against the external rotation of the hip, possibly resulting in knee and patellofemoral problems.[5,12] In ballet, however, excessive pronation is usually a functional result of forcing the turn-out in compensation for limited external ROM of the hip.[51]

Environmental Factors

Environmental factors that contribute to dance injuries may range from the ridiculous to the subtle: the famous case of the prima ballerina in *On Your Toes* being knocked off her toes and seriously injured by a wayward stage batten, or the case of the dancer with a crippling sesamoiditis due to the placement of the seam on the sole of his ballet slipper. Sometimes it is a long, cramped bus ride followed by a quick warm-up and performance in an unfavorable studio and theater. In fact, climate control and dance floors in the studio and on stage are common contributors to dance-related injuries.[4]

Climate Control

Dancers frequently report that studios and theaters are either cold or drafty. In some cases, classes or performances may be outdoors in pavilion tents or amphitheaters; both cold and hot weather are obvious hazards. Cool temperatures make it difficult to warm up properly or stay warmed up. Dehydration, heat cramps, exhaustion, or stroke are possible both outdoors and indoors.

> Prior to a performance of *Les Patineurs,* a graceful and amusing parody of the pleasures and perils of ice skating, the theater management waited until a half-hour before the audience arrived to turn on the air conditioner. Within 10 minutes of the opening curtain, 200,000 watts of stage lighting and 2,000 warm bodies had overcome the air conditioner and created a 100° plus sauna on stage. Many of the sweating dancers, dressed in heavy waistcoats and long dresses, suffered from dehydration, heat cramps, or exhaustion. On the lighter side, the finale was a sight to see. Amidst the gently falling snowflakes, the spinning dancers looked like lawn sprinklers in a blizzard.

Floors

The resiliency and surface of the studio and stage floors can be critically important. The long- and short-term effects of performing on hard, nonresilient floors can be disastrously disabling even in the absence of any other contributing factors. A number of injuries of the lower extremities, such as posteromedial shin splints, medial ankle tendinitis and tenosynovitis, Achilles tendinitis, plantar fasciitis, and tibial and fibular stress fractures are attributable to dancing on hard floors.[52] Dancers learn to adapt to hard floors by minimizing their exposure by "marking" (using gestures for certain movements) and increasing their *plié.*

> I learned the best lessons about the resiliency of dance floors when I first started dancing solos. The male variation in the "Bluebird Pas de Deux" requires 32 grueling *brisé volés* crossing diagonally from upstage left to downstage right. Initially, the concert hall floor was soft and compliant—almost buoyant—and I was flying. Midstage was the dancer's equivalent to "hitting the wall": The heavy steel stage traps sucked every ounce of energy from my thighs. Every step shook my bones. The final stretch of stage was soft—a marathon run in the sand. Only sheer willpower and fear made me finish. It was not until after the performance that I realized that I was injured. The next day the problem was diagnosed as os-

teochondritis dissecans of the superomedial surface of the talus. After that, I learned to watch out for those traps.

Hard, noncompliant floors or stages can be especially dangerous if they are located in important studios or theaters. The dancer may be compelled to dance on these hard surfaces because of the prestige of the studio or theater. A notorious example was the stage at Kennedy Center in Washington, D.C. Dancers complained for years about the hard stage and the resultant injuries. Finally, after the dancers' union threatened to boycott performances, a new floor was installed. Some union contracts now require a wood floor suspended over a five-tiered lattice (cross-stringer system).[53,54] (The proper characteristics and construction of dance floors are discussed in chapter 19.)

Dancers have their preferences as to natural wood, linoleum, or synthetic floor surfaces, depending upon the individual style of dance and previous experience. Most dance studios have wooden floors and permit the dancers to use rosin for friction. Many companies use a vinyl surface for performances, yet frequently will not use vinyl in the studio. Uniform traction, the absence of rosin or splinters, and in some cases, a slight degree of additional resiliency make synthetic dance floor surfaces highly desirable in the ballet studio and on the stage. Any surface must be kept clean, smooth, and free from irregularities or imperfections that may cause the dancer to slip or trip.

A few years ago, a famous ballerina told me a nightmarish story about her dance injury. After many years of self-imposed exile, George Balanchine had returned to his native country with his superb company, the New York City Ballet. On opening night at the Bolshoi Theatre, many eyes in the audience were looking for this extraordinarily talented young woman. Unfortunately, during her entrance, she slipped and fell on the slick floor and was knocked unconscious. The curtain had to be lowered in order to revive her. After a brief intermission, she was able to perform.

In retrospect, she told me that nothing could match the fear and horror she felt during that fall—the hopes and dreams of so many people dashed in an instant. Yet she recovered and so did everyone else. Both the company and she went on to astonishing success. Today she is widely considered to be one of the greatest ballerinas of all time.

Dietary and Nutritional Factors

The female ballet dancer is probably more of a reflection of a particular society's perspective of women than we would casually like to admit. Dancers epitomize in our own minds the self-awareness, frustrations, and distortions of our fat-conscious culture. Practical medical guidelines and aesthetic criticisms of the ultralean "Balanchine" dancer have not changed the critical expectations of the staff and public. As one principal dancer stated, "Ballet is a visual art, and therefore we have a certain responsibility to look presentable to the paying public. Currently, there is absurd and dangerously unhealthy pressure from the public, staff and peers to be too thin, despite the intelligence of knowing how bad it is."

Several nutrition-related situations may contribute to an injury: (1) overweight, (2) underweight, (3) fatigue and anemia, and (4) muscle spasms due to electrolyte imbalances.

Overweight

Generally, overweight is a more significant factor among university and private studio dancers than among professional dancers. "To be a dancer is to be thin," and an overweight dancer is virtually unemployable in a professional ballet company in the United States. In addition, a dancer who is overweight may have problems in controlling his or her technique, such as rising on *pointe*. Nevertheless, about 40% of female Ballet West dancers believed that it was more healthful to be slightly overweight or of average weight than to be underweight.[4]

> A 19-year-old, slightly overweight semiprofessional female dancer in a civic ballet company came to me during a rehearsal of *The Nutcracker*. During the brisk hopping movements of the marzipan dance, she developed a sharp pain in the right big toe. Examination of her toe indicated chronic damage to the medial edge of the toenail, thickening of the nail, and fresh blood under the nail. There was point tenderness of the proximal phalanx of the right hallux. The digit was packed in ice and the dancer was taken to the emergency room. Radiographs indicated a fracture of the proximal phalanx of the right hallux.
>
> Later examination of her nearly new *pointe* shoes showed the collapse (more accurately, crushing) of the medial portion of the shoe box. Older pairs were even worse. Clearly, she had not been standing squarely on *pointe*. The director commented that her *pointe* problems had progressively worsened as she gained weight. During her recovery and rehabilitation, the dancer was started on a balanced dietary program, lost 8 lb. (to 17% body fat) and worked on proper body alignment in class. Her stance on *pointe* greatly improved, and *relevé en pointe* was also easier with less weight—much to the relief of her big toe.

Underweight

America's obsession with leanness is epidemic in dance and is further compounded by the enormous occupational bias in favor of thin dancers. In fact, 60% of the Ballet West dancers and advanced students thought it was more healthful to be underweight—not always a safe or reasonable assumption. Over the past 12 years, the author's experience with dancers at all levels of participation, from small studios, universities, and company-affiliated schools to civic, regional, national, and international ballet companies, clearly places the problem of excessively lean dancers at the top of each hierarchy. In general, the impetus for and occurrence of excessively underweight dancers are directly proportional to the competitiveness and professional status of the school or company. The top dancers in highly competitive national or international ballet schools or companies are much more likely to be excessively lean than are members of local studios or nonprofessional troupes. In fact, the latter more typically reflect the trends in the general population for that age group, and quite often overweight is a more significant problem.

Studies have shown that many dancers who are excessively lean are often protein and carbohydrate deficient.[6,55,56] This, of course, makes it difficult for the body to build, maintain, and repair tissue—essential events for optimal physical performance and rehabilitation. Despite the fact that none of the Ballet West dancers were overweight, half thought that they had a weight problem, and 70% of the dancers were dieting. However, skinfold measurements of body fat using electronic calipers indicated that the female professional and advanced student dancers had 15.7 and 16.6% body fat, respectively (Sloan formula),[57] and the male professionals and students had 13.0 and 11.7%, respectively (Durnin formula)[58] (table 2-5). These measurements correlate very well with studies from other ballet companies.[6,59-65] Despite these optimal values of body fat for men and women, the dancers were still inordinately concerned with dieting and considered themselves overweight from the perspective of the dance company or school.[4]

There is a possibility that ultraleanness, along with the associated nutritional deficiencies and physical demands of ballet, may contribute to delayed menarche and the development of menstrual irregularities. Delayed menarche and menstrual abnormalities have been reported in dancers from Ballet West (38%),[66] American Ballet Theatre (47%),[67] and the Cleveland Ballet (50%).[55,68] There is evidence that highly athletic women with absent or irregular menses have an almost 3-fold increased risk of stress fractures,[69] perhaps due to the negative effects of a reduction of circulating E_2 on bone density.[70] Dietary calcium deficiency may further compound this situation.[55,56]

Fatigue and Anemia

In dance, fatigue is most commonly due to the long hours of practice and performance, but it may also be attributable to calorie- and iron-deficient diets.[71] The dancers from Ballet West and the Ballet West Summer Program reported an average daily intake of only 1,420 and 1,760 calories, respectively. This caloric deficiency corresponds with studies of the Cleveland Ballet (1,358 cal./day) and American Ballet Theatre (1,673 cal./day).[55,56] All corroborate the fact that female professional dancers consume an inadequate amount of calo-

Table 2-5. Physical Characteristics of Ballet Dancers

Dancers	Age	Height*	Weight**	Percent Body Fat
Female professionals N = 24	22.6 ± 3.7	166.1 ± 4.3	48.7 ± 3.6	15.7 ± 1.2
Male professionals N = 15	27.3 ± 5.6	178.1 ± 3.3	69.4 ± 5.5	13.0 ± 2.3
Female students N = 77	16.0 ± 1.8	163.6 ± 4.3	47.4 ± 5.6	16.6 ± 1.5
Male students N = 11	21.0 ± 2.9	178.3 ± 6.9	65.5 ± 8.5	11.7 ± 2.9

*In centimeters
**In kilograms

ries and are also protein and carbohydrate deficient. Although sports-related anemia due to hemolysis, hematuria, or other factors does not seem to be a factor,[72,73] low ferritin levels have been reported in 33-75% of 22 American Ballet Theatre dancers.[56]

Muscle Spasms

Muscle spasms may be due to localized microtrauma, lactic acid accumulation, or electrolyte imbalances. Although many dancers take multivitamin and mineral supplements, electrolyte imbalances of calcium or potassium have been documented in some groups of dancers.[6,55,56] Transient exercise-induced hypokalemia may be a factor in triggering muscle spasms, along with inadequate dietary intake, self-abusive eating behavior such as vomiting, or the use of laxatives or diuretics.[6,55]

Psychological Factors

Participation in dance can be the harshest look in the mirror an individual will ever take. Youth, health, beauty, and physical performance seem to ferment the type of creative narcissism and personal discipline necessary to excel in the highly competitive dance world. In order to survive and ascend, a dancer must be self-analytical and self-critical virtually to a fault. For dancers, dance is more than an art; it is an all-consuming life-style. The aesthetic, the technique, the teachers, and perhaps most important, the dancer himself, constantly push to exceed, to overcome, to persist and to persevere. The love of dance and desire to dance are intrinsic to dancers of all levels and talent. Many have sacrificed a great deal just to have those few moments of pure movement where the physical price was no measure of the artistic reward—a price so often paid in pain.

Competition

Out of hundreds of thousands of young dancers, only a very select few will become professional dancers. There are probably only about 500 positions for dancers in the major ballet companies in the United States and perhaps a few hundred additional jobs in regional and civic companies. Not all of these jobs pay enough for the dancer to live on year-round. The competition for the few top positions in most prestigious companies is extremely severe. It is not unusual for a dancer to continue to dance in spite of injuries because of the extreme competition for employment and dancing roles with the few major ballet companies.

Pressure from Staff and Dancers

Ballet companies may induce dancers to perform under hazardous conditions or with injuries through implied and real threats to their jobs. In these circumstances, dancers' unions such as the American Guild of Musical Artists (AGMA) may offer some support. However, there are other ways to motivate dancers. In the major ballet companies, the dancers are well aware that there is a reservoir of younger—and generally healthier—dancers in the company-affiliated school. Senior student dancers usually learn much of the basic corps and soloist repertoire either on their own or in class (i.e., at no expense to the company) and may even serve as apprentices to the company. The company's leverage is this prerehearsed, dance-like-there-is-no-tomorrow senior class. These other dancers are always in the wings ready and eager to step in at a moment's notice.

There are other, more insidious ways of motivating an injured dancer to perform. For example, while the company is on tour, other dancers may consciously or subconsciously encourage the disabled dancer to perform. They are well aware that the injured dancer's absence from the stage increases their work load and their chance of injury. If the other dancers are successful at convincing the injured dancer to perform, they remain healthy while the injured dancer develops chronic disability and must stop dancing. Eventually, the other dancers will get the disabled dancer's roles when they return home from the tour.

Anorectic Behavior

Currently, anorexia nervosa is a very sensitive and oversensationalized subject in America. Clinical anorexia nervosa is probably as rare in professional dancers as it is in the general population.[74] Nevertheless, some dancers exhibit certain anorectic characteristics, such as the distortion of body image, preoccupation with excessive leanness, and self-abusive behavior such as semi-starvation, self-induced vomiting, and laxative abuse.[6,11,75,76] Anorectic behavior, found mostly in the highly competitive professional ballet schools and companies, may have disastrous physical, psychological, and financial consequences for the affected dancer.

A real need exists, however, to define the elements of the spectrum from healthy leanness to anorectic behavior to clincial anorexia.[11] Although many dancers are extremely lean, it is the author's experience that they are not necessarily unhealthy or anorectic. The incidence of anorectic behavior in most dance companies and studios is probably not significantly different from that in the general population or among other female athletes when adjusted for age, level of activity, and social status.[77]

Psychological Burnout

Many professional dancers grew up under the dominant influence of a ballet studio, school, or academy. For those dancers who lived at a professional ballet school, the school becomes their surrogate parent, nurturing their growth into professional dancers. Most of their waking lives is concerned with becoming dancers. Eventually, some individuals become psychologically fatigued and can take no more; they are "burned out." The associated physical fatigue, along with mental malaise and inattentiveness, can expose the dancer to unnecessary errors of technique, training, or judgment.[78]

Other Psychological Factors

Dancers don't always stop dancing because of physical injuries. With age, the technique may slowly slip away, and with it the allegiance of an adoring, appreciative public. When the disparity between the "imperfect instrument" and the "perfect art" becomes too great, it is time to flee to other careers that are more respected, stable, or secure.

Performing is full of contrasts and contradictions—the elation of entertaining and the strain of training every day: at one moment, attention and adulation; at another, anonymity and depersonalized criticism. Postperformance depression is part of the dancer's reality. In one survey, more than 70% of the professional dancers experienced depression, 12% used tranquilizers, and 30% were seeking psychological counseling.[1] The well-publicized suicide of a principal dancer with the New York City Ballet was a tragic reminder of these pressures.

Although the world of ballet is very glamorous, steeped in centuries of tradition and smug elitism, the life of a professional dancer can be an insular, almost asocial, life-style. There is precious little time for social activities or relationships. These things are often set aside for after the career. Academic and emotional growth may also be delayed. For some young, discerning dancers, the austere life of the artist is not very attractive, and their talents are best expressed elsewhere.

Some dancers may stop dancing because of a sense of betrayal by the company (see earlier case history). The benevolence of the professional ballet school is replaced by the harsh realism of the company. Talented young dancers who are trained as artists become a commodity in a very difficult business.

Summary

Although dance is a graceful and expressive art form, its enormous physical and psychological demands make it comparable to the most strenuous sports. After many years of training and a few years of performing, all dancers must eventually start new careers. If a physician was told that after all of his years in school he would be able to practice for only a few years, would he still want to become a physician?

Ballet is also big business. Ballet companies in the United States are multimillion-dollar corporations in which the dancer is frequently viewed as an expendable commodity. A large ballet company may spend $200,000 or more per year caring for and replacing disabled dancers. Many of these tragic injuries could have been prevented if a fraction of that money had been spent on effective etiological and injury prevention programs.[28]

A 28-year-old male soloist dancer in a major professional ballet company came to the author for consultation. His chief complaint was severe pain in the lateral aspect of his left leg during jumps. Point tenderness was present on the fibula approximately 4 in. above the lateral malleolus. Biomechanical evaluations demonstrated a muscle imbalance of the hips that limited his turn-out. This was more prominent on the left. He admitted forcing his turn-out at the foot in order to compensate. Training history indicated that the pain began 6 months previously while he was performing on a hard stage in Denver and that he had been dancing steadily ever since. It was concluded that the pain was caused by the dynamic muscle imbalance in the hips, forcing the turn-out, the hard dance floor, and the heavy work load. He was referred to a physician, and a diagnosis of a fibular stress fracture was made after bone scans.

Four months later, I was contacted by the dancer, who was suing the state's Workmen's Compensation Board for wages lost during his recovery. Because the injury did not occur at a finite place and time relative to work, the board claimed it owed no compensation. I prepared a statement documenting the work load and physical demands of dancing. It read in conclusion:

"Without any doubt, Mr. W. sustained his injury while dancing, not jogging or playing tennis. The issue of the time of onset is irrelevant, since there are many infamous precedents for awarding compensation for long-term exposure to occupational hazards. When did the coal miner get black lung disease? On the first or 10,000th inhalation? Or the asbestos worker asbestosis? The board seems to be saying to dancers, 'When you get a real job in the real world and become a real person, we'll talk about real compensation.' What we are witnessing is selective discrimination against dance as a serious occupation for adults."

Because of his unwillingness to accept the inequities of the system, this bold dancer settled his dispute and established a precedent for fair and equitable job treatment for all dancers in the state. After his recovery, he worked hard to incorporate effective injury prevention techniques and exercises into his training, and he was promoted to principal dancer. He is still performing today.

Dance research has provided a new perspective and respect for dancers as artists and workers. Now, it's time to apply this knowledge in developing effective injury prevention and rehabilitation programs. Every effort must be made to address the medical and occupational needs of this precious human resource.

The author acknowledges the participation or contributions of the following organizations and individuals: Ballet West, Ballet Midwest, Ballet Aspen, San Francisco Ballet, Skyndex Corp., the University of Health Sciences, David Barnes, and Pat Schudy.

References

1. PACH survey. Dance Med Health Newsletter 1983;2(1):3.
2. Stephens RE. Biomechanical aspects of ballet and ballet injuries (slide cassette). Minneapolis: McGraw-Hill, 1982.
3. Stephens RE. The biomechanical aspects of injuries in elite ballet dancers. La recherche en danse. Universite de Paris-Sorbonne, 1986 (in press).
4. Stephens RE. The etiology of injuries in professional ballet dancers. La recherche en danse. Universite de Paris-Sorbonne, 1986 (in press).
5. Hardaker WT, Erickson L, Myers M. The pathogenesis of dance injury. In: Shell CG, ed. The dancer as athlete. Olympic Sci Conf Proc. Champaign, IL: Human Kinetic Press, 1984; 8:11-29.
6. Vincent LM. Competing with the sylph: dancers and the pursuit of the ideal body form. Kansas City, KS: Andrews and McMeel, 1979.
7. Gelabert R. Preventing dancer's injuries. Phys Sportsmed 1980; 8(4):69-76.

8. Gray H. Gray's anatomy of the human body, 29th ed. (Am). Goss CM, ed. Philadelphia: Lea & Febiger, 1973; 239.
9. Subotnick SI. Structural and functional lower extremity abnormalities which produce abnormal foot function. In: Podiatric sports medicine. Mount Kisco, NY: Futura, 1975;83-85.
10. Sparger C. Anatomy and ballet, 5th ed. London: A and C Black, Ltd., 1970.
11. Bergfeld JA, Hamilton WG, Micheli LJ et al. Medical problems in ballet: a round table. Phys Sportsmed 1982;10(3):98-114.
12. Clippinger-Robertson KS, Hutton RS, Miller DI, Nichols TR. Mechanical and anatomical factors relating to the incidence and etiology of patellofemoral pain in dancers. In: Shell CG, ed. The dancer as athlete. Olympic Sci Conf Proc. Champaign, IL: Human Kinetic Press, 1984;8:53-72.
13. Miller EH, Schneider HJ, Bronson JL, McLain D. A new consideration in athletic injuries: the classical ballet dancer. Clin Orthop 1975;111:181-91.
14. Root ML, Orien WP, Weed JH, Hughes RJ. Clinical biomechanics, Vol 1: Biomechanical examination of the foot. Los Angeles: Clinical Biomechanics Corp, 1971.
15. Root ML, Orien WP, Weed JH. Clinical biomechanics, Vol 2: Normal and abnormal function of the foot. Los Angeles: Clinical Biomechanics Corp, 1977.
16. Howse AJG. Posterior block of the ankle joint in dancers. Foot Ankle 1982;3(2):81-84.
17. Quirk R. Talar compression syndrome in dancers. Foot Ankle 1982;3(2):65-68.
18. Brodelius A. Osteoarthritis of the talar joints in footballers and ballet dancers. Acta Orthop Scand 1961;30:309-14.
19. Hamilton WG. Stenosing tenosynovitis of the flexor hallucis longus tendon and posterior impingement upon the os trigonum in ballet dancers. Foot Ankle 1982;3(2):74-80.
20. Sammarco GJ. Forefoot conditions in the dancer: part 2. Foot Ankle 1982;3(2):93-98.
21. Havens RT, Kaloogian H, Thul JR, Hoffman S. A correlation between os trigonum syndrome and tarsal tunnel syndrome. J Am Podiatr Med Assoc 1986;76(8):450-54.
22. Snijders CJ, Snijders JGN, Philippens MMGM. Biomechanics of hallucis valgus and spread foot. Foot Ankle 1986;7(1):26-39.
23. Sammarco GJ. Forefoot conditions in the dancer: part 1. Foot Ankle 1982;3(2):85-92.
24. Kravitz SR, Huber S, Murgia CJ, Fink KL, Shaffer M, Varela L. Biomechanical study of bunion deformity and stress produced in classical ballet. J Am Podiatr Med Assoc 1985;75(7):338-45.
25. Burns LT, Burns MJ, Burns GA. A clinical application of biomechanics: part 1. J Am Podiat Assoc 1973; 63(8):394-400.
26. Boone DC, Azen SP. Normal range of motion of joints in male subjects. J Bone Joint Surg (AM) 1979;61A(July):756-59.
27. American Academy of Orthopedic Surgeons. Joint motion: method of measuring and recording. Chicago: American Academy of Orthopedic Surgeons, 1965.
28. Stephens RE. The development of effective injury prevention programs for ballet dancers (speech). 2nd Int Cong on Dance Res. University of Paris—Sorbonne, Oct 2, 1986.
29. Allan WC, Harper MC. The snapping hip syndrome. Am J Sports Med 1984;12(5):361-65.
30. Kleiger B. Anterior tibiotalar impingement syndrome in dancers. Foot Ankle 1982;3(2):69-73.
31. Subotnick SI. Anterior impingement exostosis of the ankle. J Am Podiatr Med Assoc 1976;66(12):958-63.
32. Subotnick SI. Dynamic muscle imbalance (runner's equinus). In: Podiatric sports medicine. Mount Kisco, NY: Futura, 1975;83-5.

33. Whitney AK, Green DR. Pseudoequinus. J Am Podiatr Med Assoc 1982; 72(7):365-371.
34. Stephens RE. Unpublished data on dancers at Indiana University and aerobic dancers in Kansas City.
35. Gans A. The relationship of heel contact in ascent and descent from jumps to the incidence of shin splints in ballet dancers. Phys Ther 1985; 65(Aug):1192-96.
36. Kotwick JE. Biomechanics of the foot and ankle. Clin Sports Med 1982;1(Mar):19-34.
37. Jahss MH. The subtalar complex. In: Jahss MH, ed. Disorders of the foot. Philadelphia: WB Saunders, 1982;728.
38. Mann RA. Biomechanics. In: Jahss MH, ed. Disorders of the foot. Philadelphia: WB Saunders, 1982:44.
39. Subotnick SI. The biomechanics of running. In: Podiatric sports medicine. Mount Kisco, NY: Futura, 1975;83-85.
40. Subotnick SI. Foot types and injury predilections. In: Podiatric sports medicine. Mount Kisco, NY: Futura, 1975;83-85.
41. Mann RA, Inman VT. Phasic activity of intrinsic muscles of the foot. J Bone Joint Surg 1964;46A:335.
42. Taunton JE, Clement DB, Webber D. Lower extremity stress fractures in athletes. Phys Sportsmed 1981;9(1):77-86.
43. Hsu JD, Imbus DE. Pes cavus. In: Jahss MH, ed. Disorders of the foot. Philadelphia: WB Saunders, 1982;463-85.
44. Rose GK. Pes planus. In: Jahss MH, ed. Disorders of the foot. Philadelphia: WB Saunders, 1982; 486-520.
45. Subotnick SI. The flat foot. Phys Sportsmed 1981; 9(8):85-89.
46. Vincent LM. The dancer's book of health. Kansas City, KS: Sheed Andrews and McMeel, 1978.
47. Subotnick SI. Shin splint syndrome of the lower extremity. In: Podiatric sports medicine. Mount Kisco, NY: Futura, 1975;79-81.
48. D'Amico JC, Schuster RO. Motion of the first ray. J Am Podiatr Med Assoc 1979;69(1):17-23.
49. Irvin R, Steven R. Sports medicine prevention, evaluation, management and rehabilitation. Englewood Cliffs, NJ: Prentice Hall, 1983;404.
50. Kravitz SR, Murgia CJ, Huber S, Saltrick KR. Biomechanical implications of dance injuries. In: Shell CG, ed. The dancer as athlete. Olympic Sci Conf Proc. Champaign, IL: Human Kinetic Press, 1984;8:43-51.
51. Ende LS, Wickstrom J. Ballet injuries. Phys Sportsmed 1982; 10(7):101-108.
52. Weiker G. Dancers for the American Ballet Theatre may have more stress fractures (abstract). Phys Sportsmed 1981;9(5):36.
53. Seals JG. A study of dance surfaces. In: Sammarco GJ, ed. Symposium on injuries to dancers. Clin Sports Med 1983;2(3):557-61.
54. Werter R. Dance floors: a causative factor in dance injuries. J Am Podiatr Med Assoc 1985;75(7):355-58.
55. Calabrese LH, Kirkendall DT, Floyd M et al. Menstrual abnormalities, nutritional patterns, and body composition in female classical ballet dancers. Phys Sportsmed 1983;11(2):86-98.
56. Cohen JL, Potosnak L, Oscar F, Baker H. A nutritional and hematologic assessment of elite ballet dancers. Phys Sportsmed 1985;13(5):43-54.
57. Sloan AW, Burt JJ, Blyth CS. Estimation of body fat in young women. J Appl Physiol 1962;17:967-70.

58. Durnin JV, Womersley J. Body fat assessed from total body density and its estimation from skinfold thickness. Br J Nutr 1974;32(Jul):77-97.

59. Cohen JL, Gupta PK, Lichstein E, Chadda KD. The heart of a dancer: nonivasive cardiac evaluation of professional ballet dancers. Am J Cardiol 1980;45(5):959-65.

60. Cohen JL, Kim CS, May PB, et al. Exercise, body weight, and amenorrhea in professional ballet dancers. Phys Sportsmed 1982;10(4):92-101.

61. Cohen JL, Segal KR, McArdle WD. Heart rate response to ballet stage performance. Phys Sportsmed 1982;10(11):120-33.

62. Cohen JL, Segal KR, Witriol I, McArdle WD. Cardiorespiratory responses to ballet exercise and the VO_2 max of elite ballet dancers. Med Sci Sports Exerc 1982 ;14(3):212-17.

63. Mostardi RA, Porterfield JA, Greenberg B, Goldberg D, Lea M. Musculoskeletal and cardiopulmonary characteristics of the professional ballet dancer. Phys Sportsmed 1983;11(12):53-61.

64. Schantz PG, Astrand PO. Physiological characteristics of classical ballet. Med Sci Sports Exerc 1984;16(5):472-76.

65. Dolgener FA, Spasoff TC, St. John WE. Body build and body composition of high ability female dancers. Res Q Exerc Sport 1980;51:599-607.

66. Stephens RE. Biomechanical and nutritional aspects of ballet. 3rd Int Symp on Orthop and Med Aspects of Dance (speech). University of Paris—Sorbonne. Oct 1983.

67. Cohen JL, Chung SK, May PB et al. Exercise, body weight and amenorrhea in professional ballet dancers. Phys Sportsmed 1982;10(4):92-101.

68. Calabrese LH. The dancer diabled: other miseries of the dance. Emerg Med 1982: May 30:52-64.

69. Lloyd T, Triantafyllou SJ, Baker ER, Houts PS et al. Women athletes with menstrual irregularity have increased musculoskeletal injuries. Am J Sports Med 1986;18(4):374-79.

70. Cann CE, Martin MC, Gerrant HK, Jaffe RB. Decreased spinal mineral content in amenorrheic women. JAMA 1984;251:626-29.

71. Peterson MS. Nutritional concerns for the dancer. Phys Sportsmed 1982;10(3):137-43.

72. Carlson DL, Mawdsley RH. Sports anemia: a review of the literature. Am J Sports Med 1986;14(29):109-12.

73. Eichner ER. The anemias of athletes. Phys Sportsmed 1986; 14(9):122-30.

74. Malhoney MJ. Anorexia nervosa and bulimia in dancers: accurate diagnosis and treatment planning. In: Symp on Injuries to Dancers. Clin Sports Med 1983; 2(3):549-55.

75. Braisted JR, Mellin L, Gong EJ, Irwin CE. The adolscent ballet dancer: nutritional practices and characteristics associated with anorexia nervosa. J Adolesc Health Care 1985; 6(Sep):365-71.

76. Szmukler GI et al. The implications of anorexia nervosa in a ballet school. J Psychiatr Res 1985;19(2-3):177-81.

77. Rosen LW, McKeag DB, Hough DO, Curley V. Pathogenic weight control behavior in female athletes. Phys Sportsmed 1986; 14(1):79-86.

78. Rowland TW. Exercise fatigue in adolescents: diagnosis of athlete burnout. Phys Sportsmed 1986; 14(9):69-77.

3

TRAINING THE YOUNG DANCER

Lyle J. Micheli, M.D., and Ruth Solomon

THE EARLY TRAINING OF the young dancer lays the groundwork for the progressive development of strength and technique from which may come a glamorous professional career or many years of enjoyable and healthful recreational dance. Unfortunately, this early training may also lay the groundwork for injuries that can plague the professional or recreational dancer for the rest of a dance career.

Recent research and the experience of training young dancers for many years suggest to the authors that the development of aesthetically effective dance style and the prevention of injury through proper technique can, and indeed must, coexist in the training of the young dancer.

The tragedy of all too many injuries to young dancers is that they are potentially preventable, often by merely paying attention to early warning signs and instituting relatively simple preventive measures. Those in charge of the training must understand not only how injuries occur in dancers—the mechanism of injury—but also must appreciate the unique characteristics of young dancers that may make them particularly susceptible to injury. The significance of this observation can be illustrated by an analogy: At first meeting, the doctor and the new patient and the dance teacher and the new student are likely to share certain concerns in common. Most essentially, the doctor will take note of those anatomical characteristics—e.g., swayed back (lumbar lordosis), bowed legs (genu varum), rolling in or out on the foot (pronation or supination)—that may have contributed to the patient's current condition or are likely to cause problems in the future. The teacher will regard these same characteristics as factors to be considered in assessing the student's ability to dance. Unhappily, this comparison tends to break down quickly: The doctor will continue to treat the dancer's body in compliance with what he understands of its individual structure and, all too often, the teacher will subordinate individual needs to external demands. For the dance teacher serves an art form. The technique class the teacher conducts is intended to strengthen and train the body for performance. Also, especially if the genre in question is classical dance, the class provides a yardstick against which both student and teacher can measure progress. Those students who demonstrate the abilities required by the form may continue with the training. Those who do not are likely to drop out.

Mechanism of Injury

Along the way, those who are talented and those who are not, those with bodies equipped by nature to withstand the rigors of training and those less perfectly endowed—all are subjected to the same regimen day after day. Virtually all dance training is based on repetition, and in a discipline such as ballet, tradition allows for little variance in the type and order of material presented. All injuries to the structural components of the body—the bones, joints, muscle tendon units, and ligaments—are the result of either single-impact macrotrauma (the so-called acute injuries, such as a sprained ankle from an improper landing) or of repetitive microtrauma (the so-called overuse injuries, which include tendinitis, bursitis, "dancer's knee," and stress fractures). These overuse injuries are usually the result of repetitive activity of any kind, such as running, jumping or performing a *plié.* In children, there were very few overuse injuries until repetitive training activities in organized dance or organized sports became popular. It is now these overuse injuries that occur most frequently in the young dancer and are most amenable to prevention if the preconditions for injury are recognized early enough.

Population at Risk

The process of growth itself, and the presence of special growth tissue, is unique to the child and is, in fact, what makes the child a child. As long as one is growing, one is a child. Once longitudinal growth has ceased and the specialized tissue responsible for it—the growth cartilage—has disappeared, childhood has ended.

The child, we now know, has a special risk of injury because of the presence of this growth cartilage and because of the growth process itself. This growth cartilage is more susceptible to mechanical injury than adult tissue, particularly during periods of rapid growth. The growth cartilage is actually present at three sites: the growth plate, near both ends of the long bones; the joint cartilage, the smooth lining covering the insides of the joints; and at the point of insertion of the major muscle tendon units into bone, the growth apophyses.

An injury to the growth plate, such as a fracture through it, may be catastrophic, with growth stopping at the site of fracture. There may be a loss of length of the affected extremity of as much as 4 in. At the joint surface, injury to the lining cartilage as it grows may cause chips to form in the joint, resulting in early arthritis as an adult. We have seen this process—called osteochondritis —occur in both the knees and ankles of young dancers, eliminating them from dancing. Finally, injury to the growth cartilage tendon insertion sites, with repetitive microtrauma causing a tiny pulling away or avulsion of the tendons at this weak spot, can result in painful prominences at these sites, such as at the tibial tubercle just below the knee (Osgood Schlatter disease), or at the back of the heel (Haglund disease).

As noted above, the growth process itself—particularly during periods of accelerated growth, as in early adolescence—also may increase the chance of injury. Because growth occurs in the bones alone, and the soft tissues spanning the bones (the muscles, tendons, and ligaments) do not grow directly, they become relatively tighter during a growth spurt. At the time of the adolescent growth spurt in particular, when the child may grow as much as 3/4 in. in a month, there may be a dramatic loss of flexibility, thus temporarily increasing the chance of injury.

In dealing with children's dance injuries, we have learned to look for certain "risk factors" that may have been involved in the occurrence of the injury and that must be corrected to prevent further injury or reinjury. In the child dancer, these factors are: (1) faults of training, especially changes in its duration or intensity; (2) technique; (3) anatomic malalignment; (4) muscle-tendon imbalance; (5) shoe wear; (6) dance surface; and (7) changes in growth rate. Careful assessment of every injury is necessary in order to prevent the chance of further or ongoing problems. Frequently, two or more different risk factors may be involved in the onset of a given injury.

Training errors, particularly too rapid changes in the duration or intensity of training, appear to be involved in at least half of all dance injuries we see. The serious young dance student taking 4 or 5 classes a week who suddenly is taking 4 or 5 hr. of intense training per day at a summer dance program may be prime for a new injury or the recurrence of an old one. It might be wise, indeed, if there were a graded, slow, and progressive increase in the intensity of training over the first week, at least, in such programs.

Dance technique, of course, is frequently indicated as the cause of injury.[1] Perhaps of greatest importance for the teacher is adapting technique to the particular makeup of each individual dancer; for example, not allowing or encouraging increased turn-out below the knee or excessive swaying of the lower back. Additionally, in the early years it is important that balanced training be maintained, using the muscles on both the inner and outer, front and back, of all major bones and encouraging stable and balanced alignment of the lower back and pelvis.

The third factor, anatomic malalignment, can be an important contributor to the occurrence of a dance injury, but sometimes it may be overemphasized. Certainly, a child who has much more internal rotation than external rotation at the hip (increased femoral anteversion) may have difficulty with ballet technique, in attaining turn-out or in jumping, and may have an increased risk of injury because of this. At the knee, a child with excessive knock-knee (genu valgum) may also be at risk of injury unless certain compensatory train-

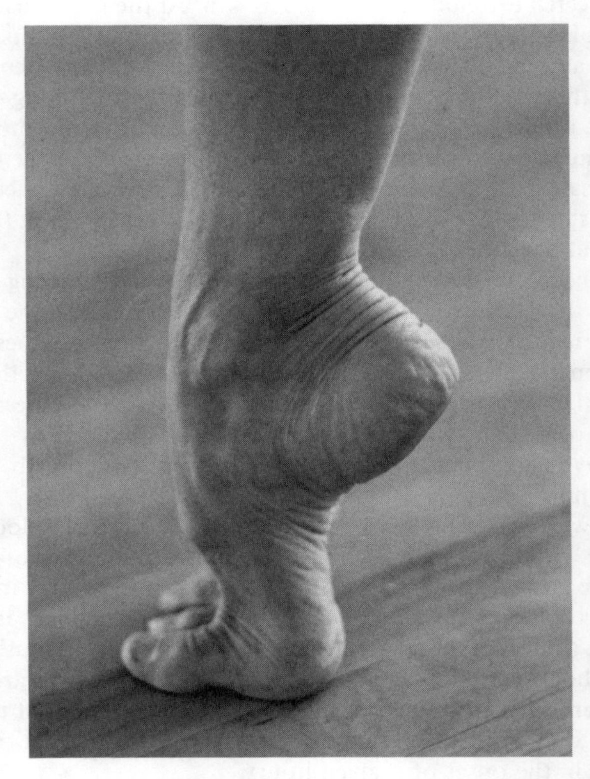

Figure 3-1. Cavus foot, with weight born too much on the first metatarsal.

ing is done. At the foot, the child with a high-arch, stiff foot (cavus foot) may also have increased risk of injury (figure 3-1), whereas a child with a flexible flat foot, with proper strengthening of the muscles about the foot, can safely and effectively dance. In summary, even in classical ballet training, individuals with a wide range of body structures can, with careful supervision, pursue dance safely and effectively.

Muscle-tendon imbalances may be a more frequent contributor to injury than we realize, particularly in ballet. We have learned from our studies of many sports injuries that imbalances of muscle strength and flexibility can be frequent contributors to injury. Our own studies of the muscle strength and flexibility of a group of first-rank ballet dancers have suggested that ballet training itself contributes to muscle imbalances unless additional compensatory exercises are used.[2] For example, in ballet dancers the muscles in the back of the calf that extend the foot may be 4-5 times stronger than the muscles in the front and sides of the foot that raise and rotate it. This degree of imbalance may well contribute to the occurrence of tendinitis in both the young and the professional dancer. Similarly, ballet dancing tends to make the outer side of the thigh muscles (vastus lateralis) stronger than the inside portion (vastus medialis), and this also can contribute to the occurrence of injury by causing the patella to ride to the outside of its groove. Compensatory exercises that specifically aid in strengthening the inner portion of the thigh muscle are often needed in a young dancer who complains of kneecap or "dancer's knee" pain.

As noted, shoe wear and the dance surface are additional risk factors that must be considered in the occurrence of injury. A dancer who has recently changed to a different type of toe shoe, in particular, may complain of pain that is found to result from the different positioning of the foot in the new shoe. Dancing on a hard surface is well known as a precipitator of injury in the dancer. This is a particular risk for the young dancer, who frequently performs in church basements or on gym floors that are improperly sprung and padded.

Finally, as noted above, growth itself can be a risk factor. The young dancer who is involved in a very significant growth spurt, particularly at adolescence, will develop tightness of major muscle groups and imbalances that must be corrected by directed physical therapy. Otherwise, the risk of injury while dancing may be dramatically increased. At such times, the intensity of dance technique—the amount of jumping, in particular—should be decreased.

The Teacher's Responsibility

Once the factors involved in injury are understood, it becomes clear that injuries can be minimized by heightening one's awareness of the demands being made on the dancer's body and adjusting the training accordingly. On the one hand, the dance teacher needs to cultivate an eye for the anatomical peculiarities of the students—a way of seeing that we have already suggested is similar to the doctor's when examining a patient. As in the case of the doctor, this requires knowledge of anatomy. On the other hand, the teacher must understand the technique being taught implicitly, not only with regard to the movements themselves, but in terms of an intimate knowledge of what is happening inside the body performing those movements. This, too, points to an anatomical approach to teaching.

A simple example may serve to illustrate the teacher's responsibility as we conceive it. Virtually all ballet classes (and many modern dance classes as well) begin with a series of standing *pliés* (figures 3-2, 3-3). This simple movement is one of the cornerstones of the art form, as it is an integral part of practically every other movement the dancer performs. Properly executed, it enhances the dancer's ability to do everything else properly: to pirouette, to *jeté,* to land properly (and safely) from jumps, etc. It is not surprising, then, that tradition has assigned the *plié* a preeminent position in the studio routine.

The *plié* is very demanding in anatomical terms, however. Specifically, proper alignment of the quadriceps mechanism and of the tracking of the patella in its groove are essential for a strong and injury-free *plié.* Each time the student starts down into *plié,* the legs must be aligned in such a way that a straight line could be drawn from the hip socket through the knee and ankle and to the second toe. This in turn relates to the alignment of the lower leg relative to the femur and the hip joint. Furthermore, the dancer's weight must be distributed mainly through the first, second, and third metatarsals rather than dropping onto the fourth and fifth. All of this can be determined by observing the use of the foot as well as the alignment and use of the pelvis.

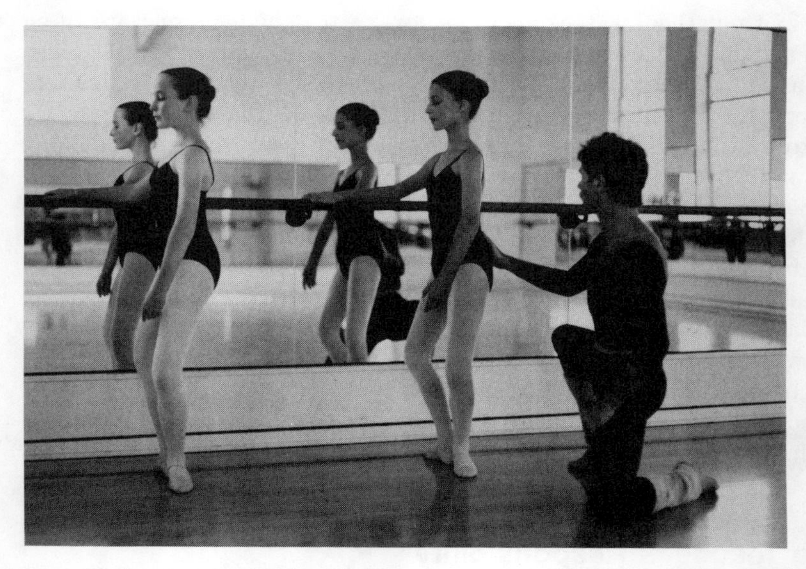

Figure 3-2. *Demi-plié* in first position; the beginning of class at the barre.

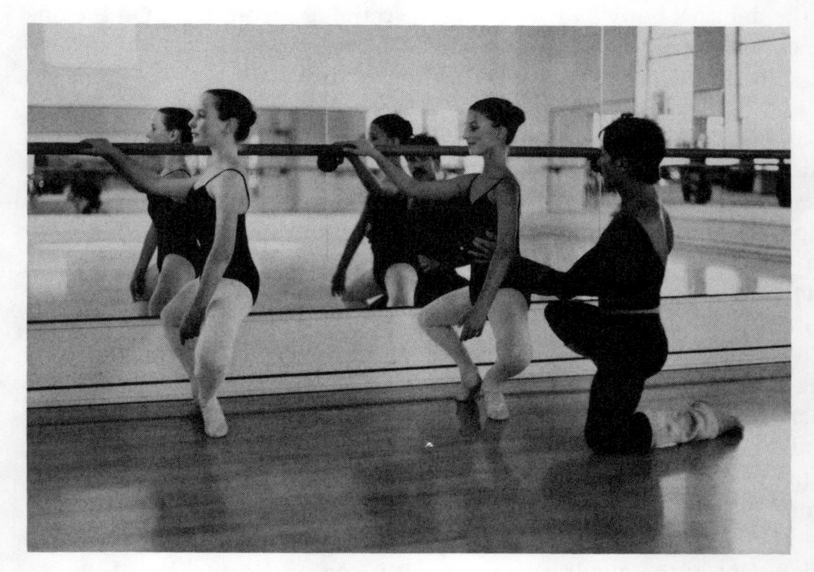

Figure 3-3. *Grand plié,* working on alignment of the pelvis, knee, ankle, and second toe.

When we say that the *plié* "must" be performed in the way described, we have in mind primarily the vulnerability to injury that comes from performing it improperly (that is, we are only secondarily concerned with the fact that performing the movement economically and accurately from a physiological point

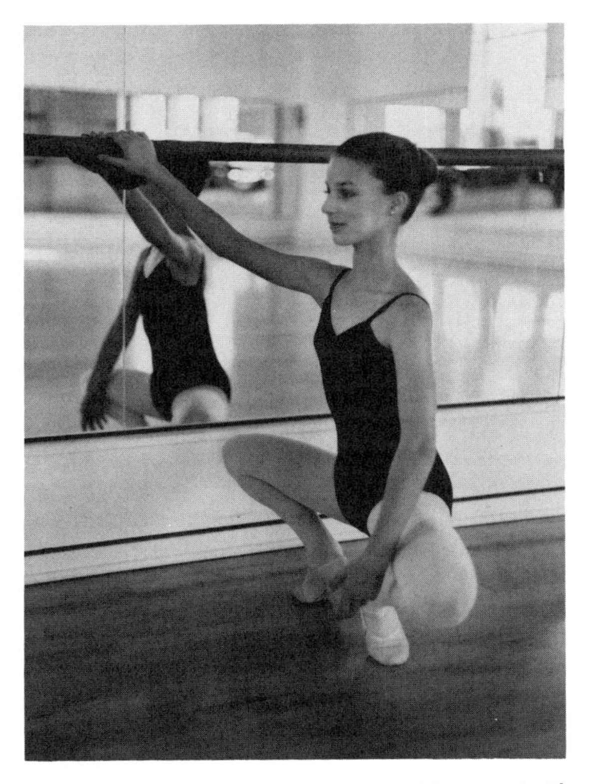

Figure 3-4. When the pelvis is not fully engaged in *grand plié,* weight can drop onto the knees.

of view heightens its aesthetic appeal). The *plié* has the potential for applying tremendous stress to the lower body, especially at the knee. If one understands the role of the pelvis (and especially the psoas) in controlling the weight of the body as it is raised and lowered, rather than allowing that weight to be thrust onto the knee (figure 3-4), then one can greatly reduce the stress. It is our contention that dance teachers are responsible for imparting that kind of understanding with the training.

The *plié* raises yet another issue with regard to the structure of the traditional ballet class. As already noted, such classes usually begin with *pliés,* and, as much of what follows incorporates the *plié,* there would seem to be ample reason for this. However, because *plié* can create a great deal of tension in the lower body, one questions from a physiologic point of view the appropriateness of subjecting the dancer's "cold" body to such stress. The importance of warm-up in preventing injury has been established in many sports. In dance, a total body warm-up to get the blood flowing through the muscles, to lubricate the joints, and especially to get the psoas system engaged *before* attempting a movement like *plié* would also seem important. All of this can be accomplished in as little as 5 minutes by means of floor exercises (figure 3-5). This approach

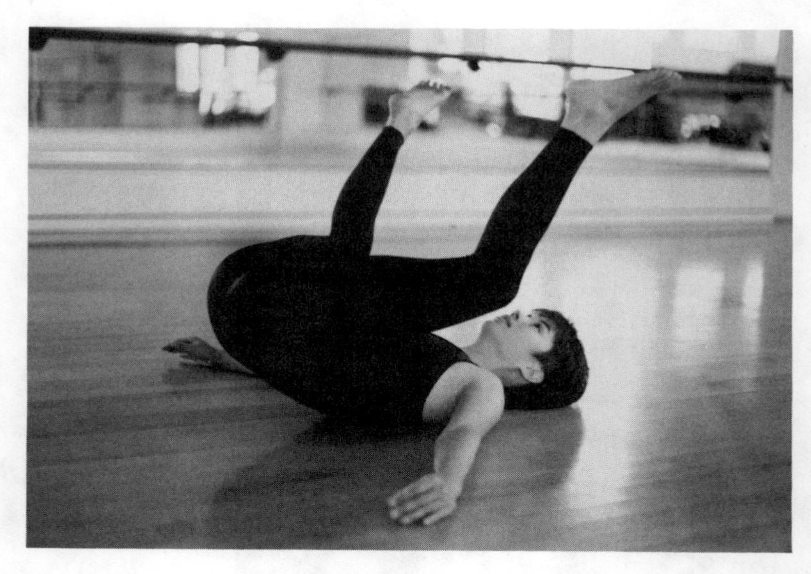

Figure 3-5. Floor exercise to warm up the muscles of the pelvis and lubricate hip and knee joints.

to warming up, which has been explored by many of the styles that comprise modern dance, has the advantage of allowing the dancer to use the spine, pelvis, thigh sockets, knees, ankles, and feet without concern for balance *per se* and without stress on the joints. Some ballet teachers have begun to adapt their training to this way of thinking through the "floor barre"; many others begin class blindly with the *plié,* because that is what tradition dictates.

In focusing on the *plié* as a way of illustrating the need to understand the demands made on the body by ballet technique, we have set aside for the moment the question of how anatomical characteristics influence the body's ability to tolerate those demands. Let us now consider the case of the student who comes to the study of classical dance with a distinct anatomical malalignment —for example, a lordotic spine. Lordosis is virtually always synonymous with a weak psoas major and minor, and the proper performance of a movement like *plié* presupposes a strong psoas. Nor is there anything in the execution of the *plié* itself that is likely to correct the weak-psoas/lordotic condition (figure 3-6). This student is immediately in the insufferable position of being required to perform a movement that an inability to control the hyperextension in the lumbar area places beyond reach. But there is a solution. The informed teacher, seeing the lordotic spine and recognizing its implications for executing *plié,* backtracks from the standard technique and gives *this* student exercises to strengthen both psoas muscles *before* introducing *pliés* (figure 3-7). The problem is addressed through augmenting exercises, and only when the student develops a sense for controlling the anatomical mechanism of movement can there be progression to dance movement *per se.*

If the spine is lordotic when the student stands in first position, and an attempt is made to elevate the leg in second position (to the side), the leg will

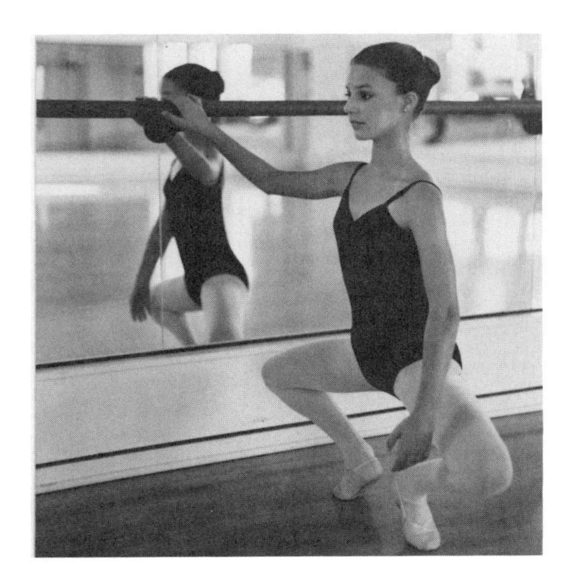

Figure 3-6. Slightly lordotic *grand plié,* with deceptively well aligned lower leg.

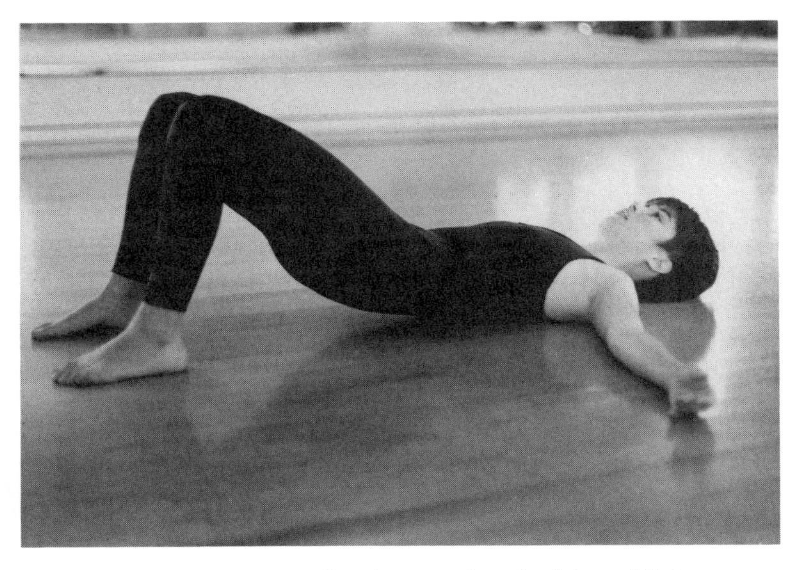

Figure 3-7. Floor exercise ("undercurve," or "pelvic rock") to engage and warm up the psoas.

invariably be placed incorrectly. It is virtually impossible for a person with lordosis to *tendu* in such a way as to prepare the leg properly to extend (elevate) to the side. In this position, it appears that abduction of the externally rotated leg is performed by the gluteus maximus (figure 3-8) rather than both psoas muscles (figure 3-9), which further accentuates lordosis. The *passé (retiré)* move-

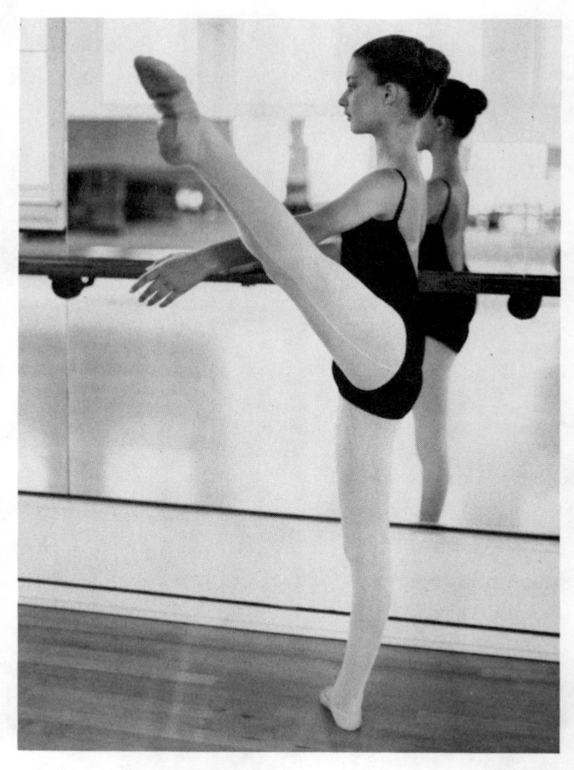

Figure 3-8. Incorrect extension in second position. The gluteus maximus is engaged, causing internal rotation of the extended leg.

ments will also be performed incorrectly because of this malalignment of the pelvis. Again, the solution is to work to get the pelvis placed properly to allow for an accurate *passé* (figure 3-10). The way to do this is to augment the traditional class with exercises that will provide the dancer with a mechanism for overcoming specific anatomic peculiarities.

Dance students too often concern themselves single-mindedly with *results*—with producing what they understand to be the desired shape of a movement. They tend to lack both the inclination and the knowledge to involve themselves meaningfully in the process by which the movement is achieved. As a result, they are prone to fall into movement patterns that are both inefficient and damaging; they substitute idiosyncratic body mechanics to accomplish movements because those that should be used are not available to them. Somewhere down the road of their training, these substitutions come back to haunt them in the form of injuries or simply as inefficient or inhibited movement.

Again, it is the teacher's job to help the student to understand the process by which movement is produced. The teacher must place the end result of technical training—the full realization of movement—in the context of *how* movement is accomplished. This may take more time initially, but it will save the

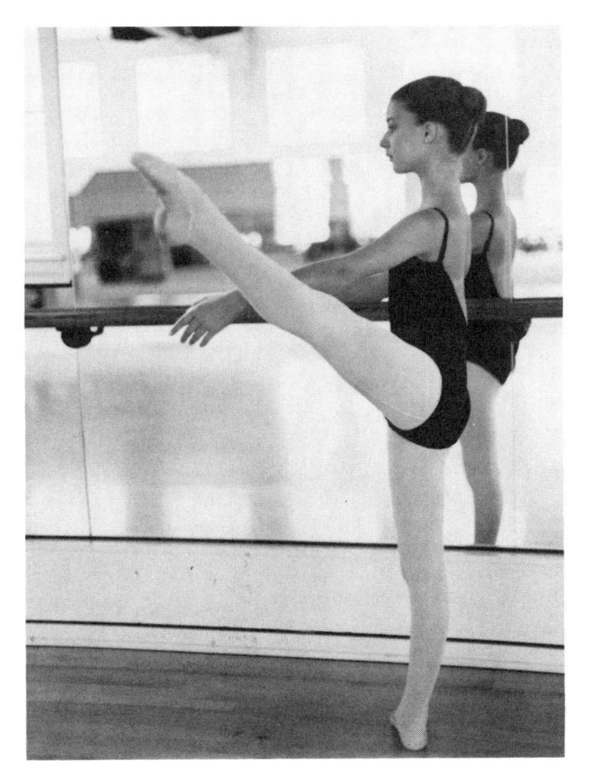

Figure 3-9. Correct extension in second position, with proper placement of the gesturing leg.

student time in the long run in terms of the need to correct bad habits or to sit out injuries.

Anatomy in Teaching

A working knowledge of anatomy as it applies to the body in motion allows the dance teacher to see "beneath the skin"—to see how the muscles, bones, joints, and connective tissue are interacting to produce the desired effect. Just as important, such knowledge will provide the teacher with a vocabulary for use in describing what is needed to the student. Understanding anatomy allows one fully to appreciate the potential in movement and to understand why that potential is not being realized by a given student. Again, an example is in order. One of the main goals of training in dance is to increase the student's "extension" (ability to elevate the leg). Some dancers are naturally endowed with a high extension, but others are not. In the latter case, the enlightened teacher asks, Why doesn't the leg go up any higher in second position, or in a *développé*? What is this student doing to inhibit the desired action? An an-

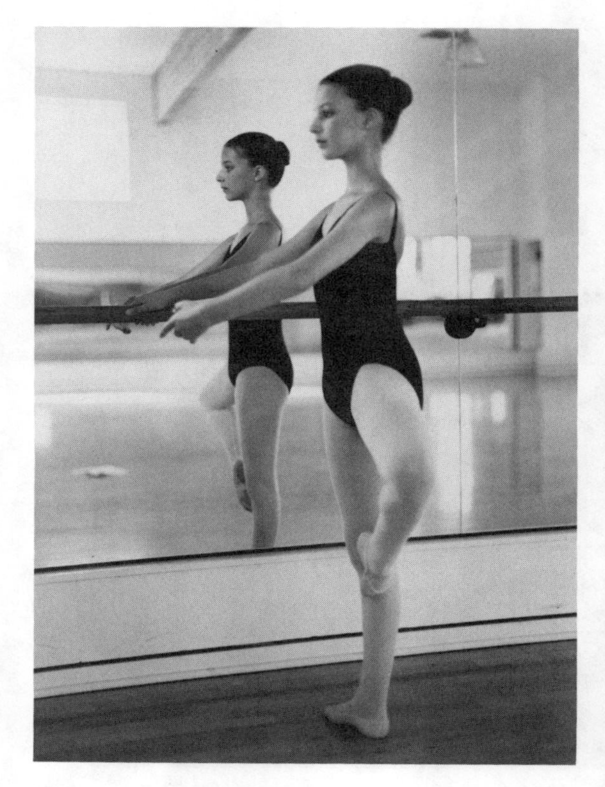

Figure 3-10. Well executed *passé (retiré).*

atomical explanation suggests itself. Perhaps this student is overusing the quadriceps, causing a contraction at the head of the rectus femoris and/or iliacus. If so, how can the student be taught to *release* rather than tighten the rectus or iliacus after the leg reaches 90°? With this kind of approach, based on physiological evidence that can be seen by the experienced eye of the teacher and felt by the student once the student knows what to "listen" for, a solution can be found. A sequence of exercises can be established: sitting on the floor with the legs in second position to allow the student to learn to release the head of the rectus femoris and not overuse the quadriceps, then translating this release to standing for *passés* and *développés,* or into *grands battements* (figures 3-11, 3-12, 3-13, 3-14). This process will help to alleviate the inhibiting factor, which might otherwise have been encouraged by the progression of the standard ballet class.

This problem of the inhibited extension provides another telling illustration of how knowledge of anatomy can be used to prevent injury. The student who is inhibiting extension often develops "clicking" or "popping" at the hip whenever a *grand rond de jambe en l'air* is executed or when the leg is simply raised to the side. This popping usually becomes painful if allowed to continue. Recent studies suggest that it is caused by the sliding of the iliopsoas tendon over the head of the femur when the click is felt medial to the joint. Clicking on

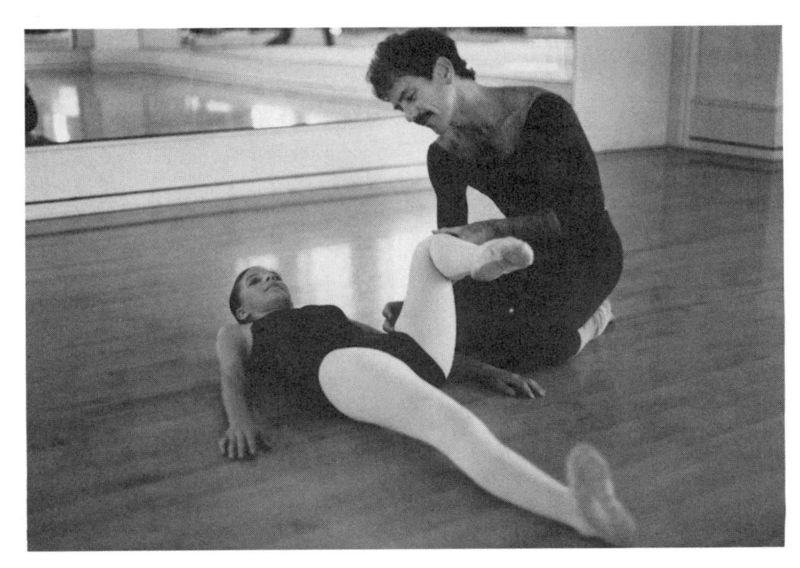

Figure 3-11. Teacher testing for release at the head of the rectus femoris and iliacus.

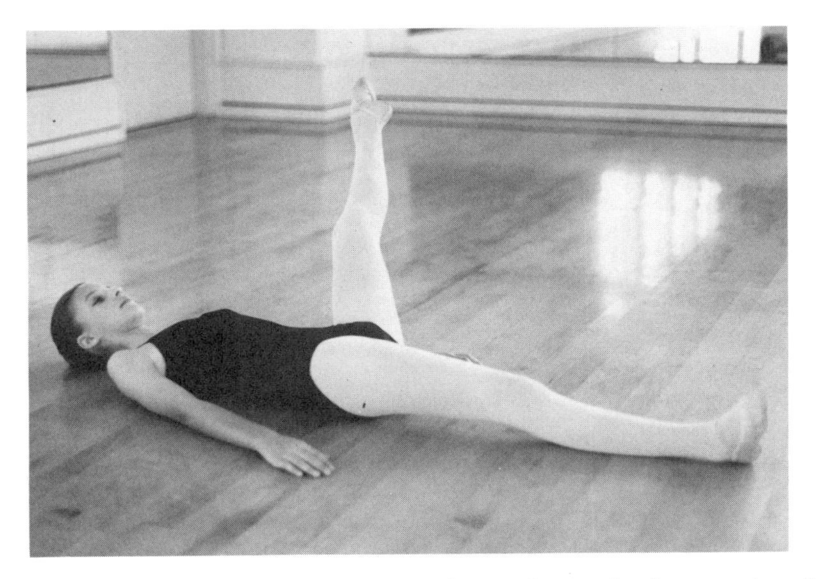

Figure 3-12. Floor work to develop release of extension in second position.

the lateral side of the joint is usually caused by a tight tensor fascia lata.[3,4] The teacher who is willing to take the time to consider exactly how the student is performing the movements that produce the symptom can analyze where the click is occurring—at the head of the rectus, the iliacus, the iliopsoas, or tensor fascia lata—and if it appears to be associated with abnormal alignment or im-

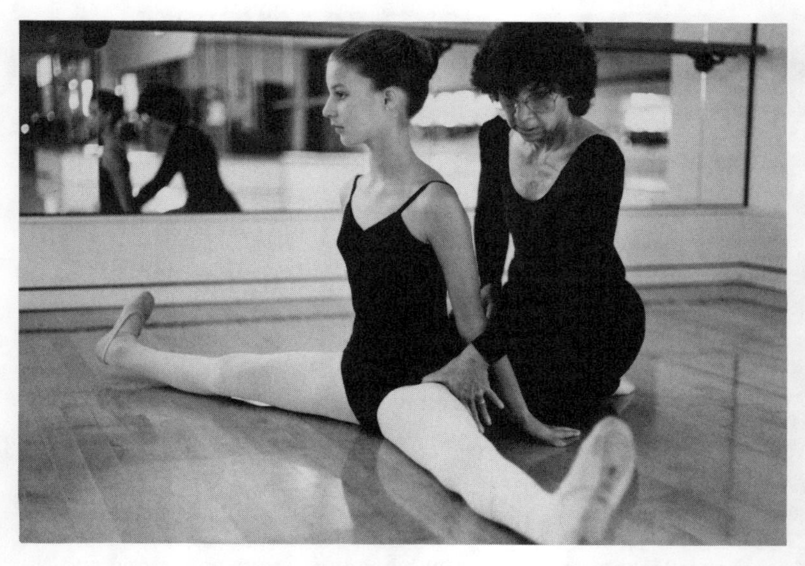

Figure 3-13. Working to correct use of quadriceps and hyperextension of knees in second position (note heels incorrectly lifted off the floor).

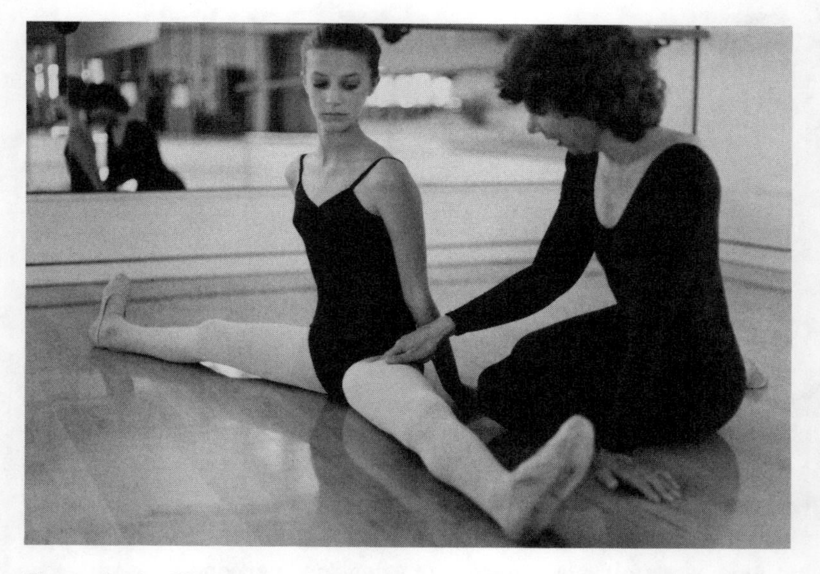

Figure 3-14. With proper release, a correct extension is achieved.

proper mechanics (figure 3-15). Once this has been determined, specific exercises can be prescribed to correct the technique.

The use of exercise for the purpose of correcting anatomical peculiarities and avoiding injuries suggests an analogy of dance training with physical ther-

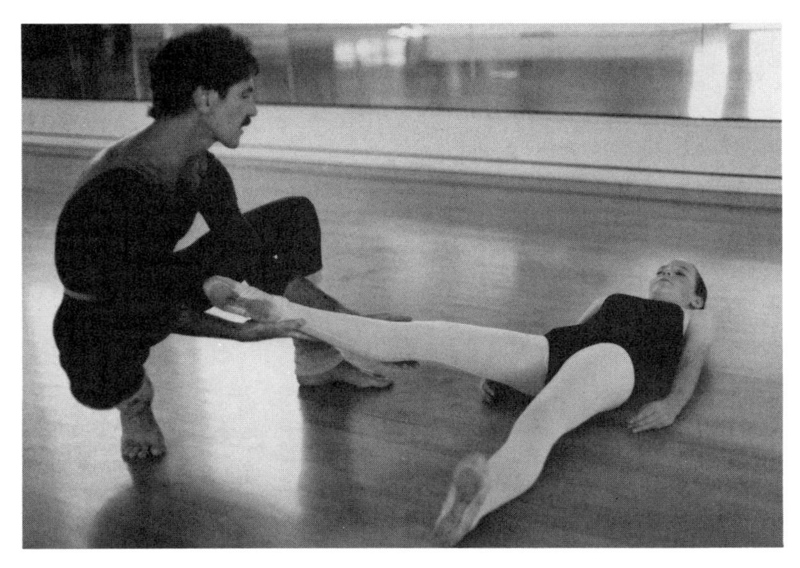

Figure 3-15. Teacher working to eliminate "clicking" around the hip socket.

apy—a comparison that many dance teachers might find inappropriate and unacceptable, since physical therapy is viewed as a clinical discipline, without aesthetic content. In reality, there may be some instructive points of similarity in the two disciplines. For example, both use repetition of prescribed movements as their principal means of stretching and strengthening the body. Indeed, many of the exercises assimilated into various modern techniques (e.g., contractions, or pelvic tilts) are identical to those used in physical therapy for corrective purposes (figure 3-16). Why, then, do we concern ourselves mainly (as we did earlier) with the deleterious effects of repetition when discussing dance training? Our purpose is to emphasize the fact that dance training has two aspects, developing skills *and* minimizing the risk of injury, and to suggest that a proper (i.e., anatomical) understanding of what is involved in the training can turn liabilities into potential assets.

Some Practical Concerns

The same anatomical approach to dance training advocated here opens up the possibility of shedding some scientific light on many practical concerns that to date have been addressed in an essentially haphazard fashion by the teaching profession. For example, how many dance classes per week should a dancer take at any given stage in a career? Should a dancer be allowed to take 5-6 technique classes, plus repertory, plus rehearsals each week, as often happens at summer dance festivals? For ballet students, when is it advisable to start *pointe* training?

One basic answer to all such questions is the one we have already suggested several times—that because all bodies are different, every decision about

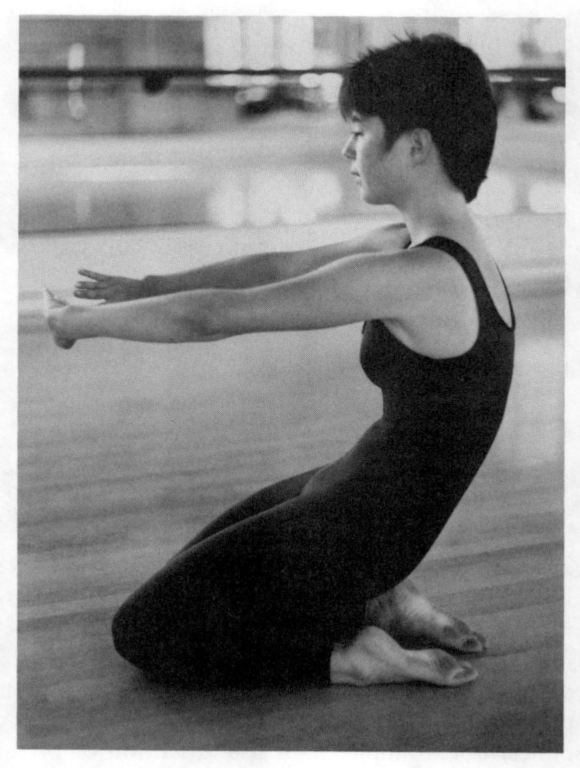

Figure 3-16. "Contraction," used in many modern dance techniques, strengthens the psoas and quadriceps.

how an individual body is to be used must be based on that body's capabilities and needs. This should serve as an antidote to the all-too-common tendency to impose the same regimen (often as dictated by tradition) on all members of a class, day after day. It also suggests the policy of providing adjunctive stretching and strengthening exercises to be used outside class by individual students to address and correct their particular problems. Students who are tight in the hamstrings or quadriceps, for example, can be given exercises to balance those two sets of muscles. Those with tight Achilles tendons can be given exercises to stretch the Achilles and increase dorsiflexion (figures 3-17, 3-18, 3-19). To determine that such imbalances exist and to insist upon the use of corrective measures seems to us entirely within the teacher's area of responsibility.

Beyond this, the field of sports and dance medicine has clearly demonstrated that one of the most important factors in any physical training is to consistently maintain or gradually increase the level of activity. Because sudden or too rapid increases in activity are clearly implicated in many injuries, the beginning student should be introduced slowly to the discipline, with new increments added at regularly spaced intervals. The determining factor in this approach to teaching is the pace at which the body functions most safely, *not* the student's ability to assimilate new material. By the same token, students who have been

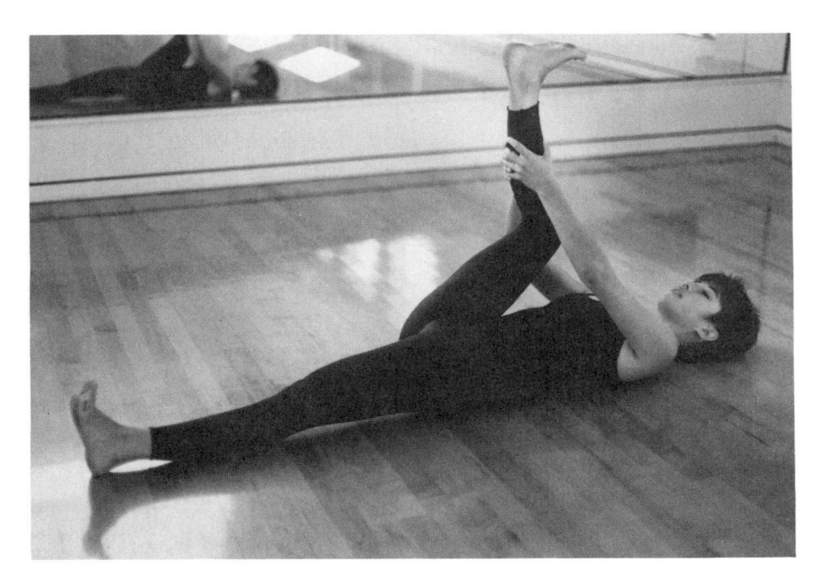

Figure 3-17. The beginning of a series of floor exercises to stretch and strengthen the hamstrings and dorsiflexors.

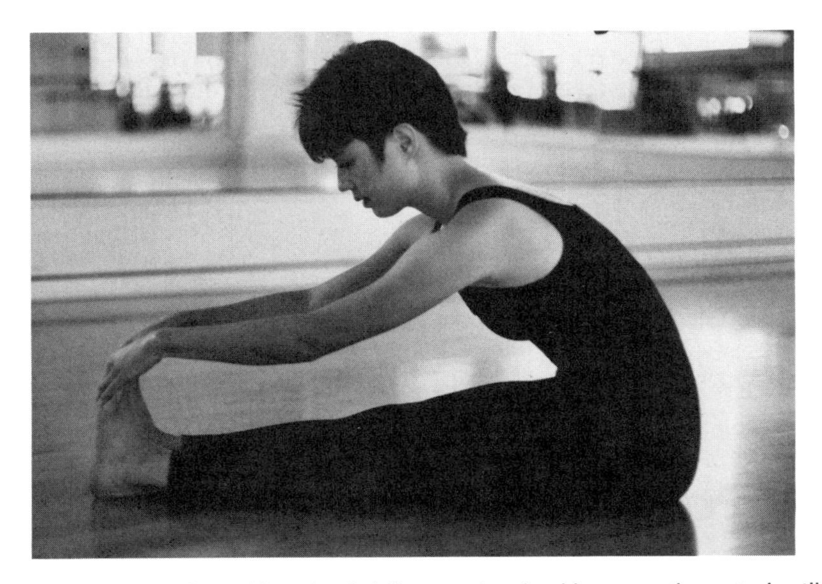

Figure 3-18. Stretching the Achilles tendon (making sure the anterior tibialis tendon is released).

forced for one reason or another to discontinue training must be slowly reintroduced to the discipline, not plunged back into the level of activity they were capable of before the layoff (in this case, recent studies have demonstrated very specifically that 3 weeks after retraining from a layoff has begun there is a falling off of bone density that makes the body far more susceptible to injury).[5]

Finally, this kind of new knowledge has implications for the summer dance festivals that have become so much a part of the dance scene. Even the most dedicated dance student seldom takes more than 5 technique classes per week as a matter of course, yet within days of the start of a summer program, this work load may well be more than doubled. From a health standpoint, such rapid increases are dangerous, and they can be avoided in a number of ways. Those responsible for programming can restrict participation to one technique class per day for the first 2 weeks, with a second class allowed every third day; or, alternately, those students who insist on "getting their money's worth" immediately can be encouraged to increase the amount of work they do in the weeks prior to the festival.

What determines when a dancer is ready to go on toe? By now, our answer should hardly come as a surprise: This determination has almost everything to do with the individual dancer's strength—especially with her alignment—and relatively little to do with how many steps have been mastered in ballet shoes. To impose the added pressure of toe work on a body that has not yet overcome a basic malalignment is to create a situation in which an injury is waiting to happen.

As indicated earlier in this chapter, *growth* is an anatomic factor that imposes very specific concerns on the training of young dancers. We tend to imagine that the young body is infinitely flexible—one thinks, for example, of the 12 to 14-year-olds who have dominated women's world-class gymnastics in recent years—but caution must be the rule. In young children, the growth plates have not closed, and the muscle-tendon units may be under additional tension because of sudden spurts in bone growth. Especially around the hip, in the lower

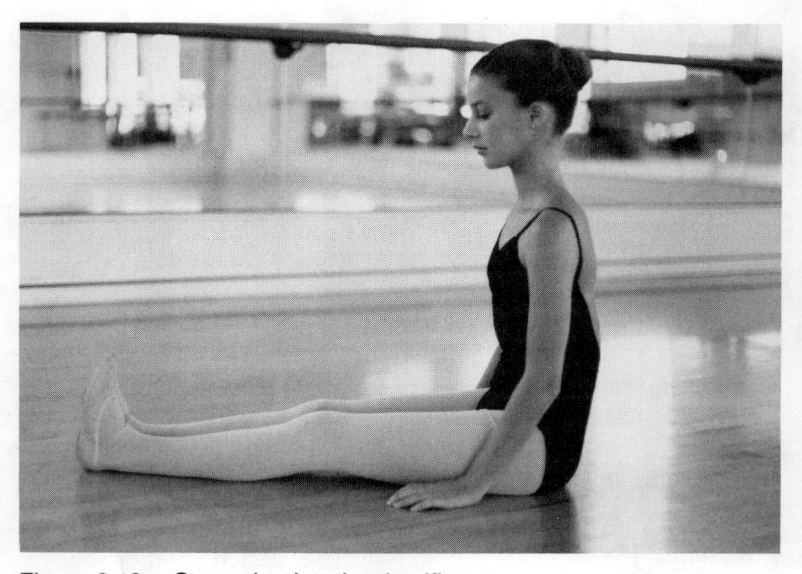

Figure 3-19. Strengthening the dorsiflexors.

back, and at the thigh and knee, the bones can grow quickly enough to stretch muscles and tendons to near capacity, with measurable loss of flexibility occurring. A careful stretching program, practiced regularly, is therefore essential, particularly with the young dancer (figures 3-20, 3-21). Hamstring and quadri-

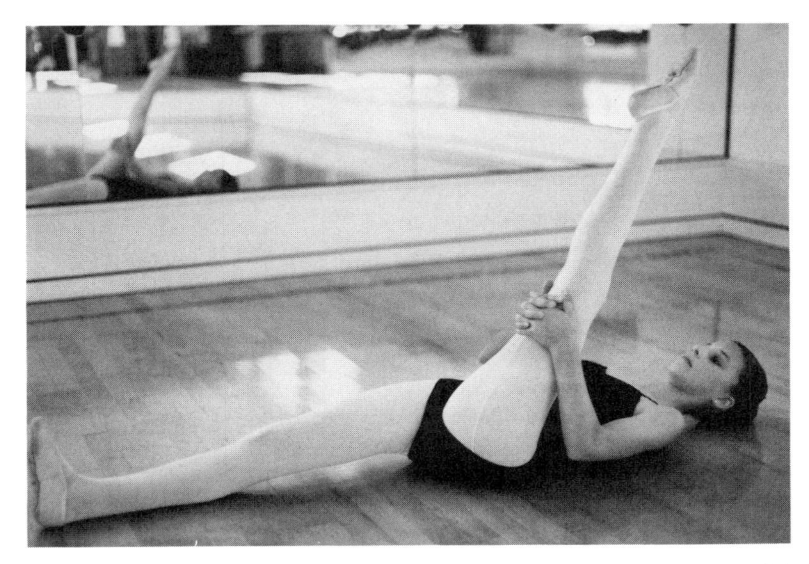

Figure 3-20. Careful stretching of the hamstrings. Floor support minimizes stress on the lower back.

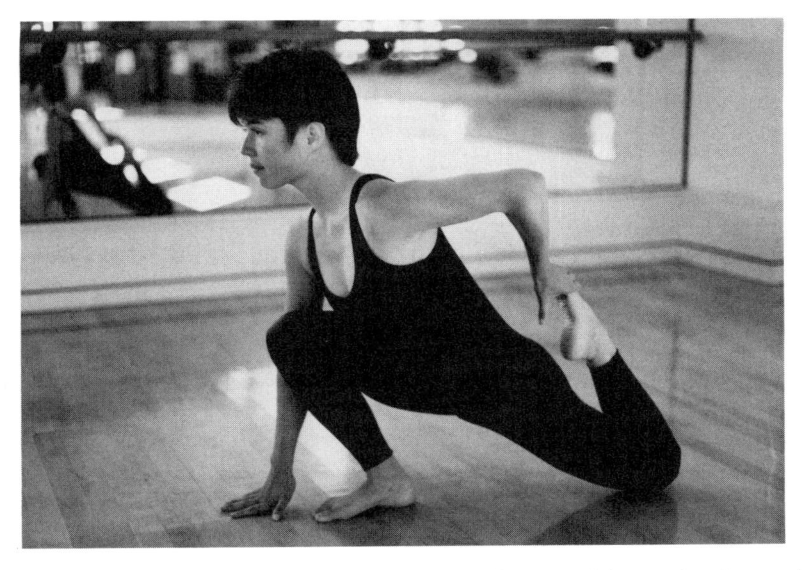

Figure 3-21. Stretch of the quadriceps, being careful to maintain parallel alignment of the hip, knee, and foot of both legs.

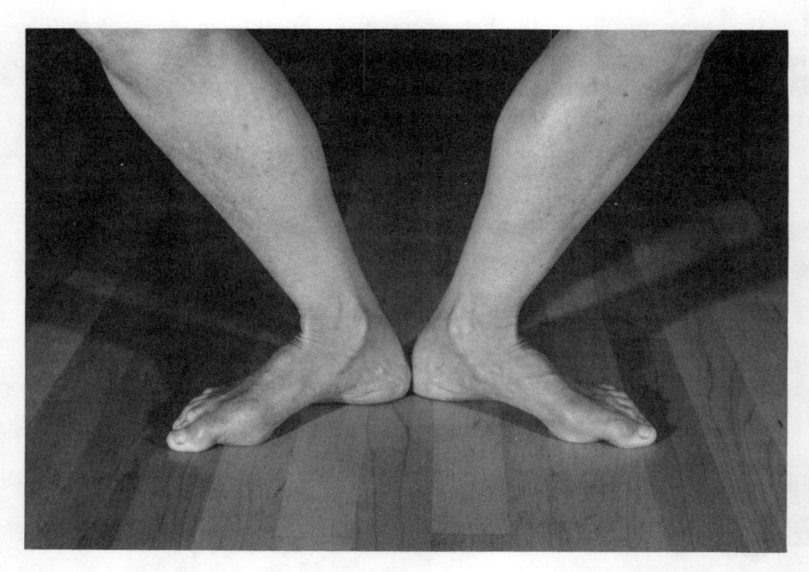

Figure 3-22. Anterior tibialis tendon incorrectly contracted as *demi-plié* is performed in turned-out (first) position.

ceps stretching is very important at this time, as, in extreme cases, the tightness of these muscles can cause avulsion fractures at the sites of insertion of tendon into bone (the apophyses). As previously noted, osteochondritis is another possibility. Young men seem to have a special propensity for lower back tightness. Failure to address this problem can allow the pelvis to align itself in ways that later limit turn-out.

The proper way to maintain (or achieve) flexibility through stretching and thereby reduce the possibility of injury can be illustrated by returning to the *plié* and considering its role in stretching the Achilles tendon, another area of high vulnerability in young dancers. The *plié* can do much of the work required to stretch the Achilles, but only if the tibialis anterior tendon is released. The teacher will, therefore, want to use *pliés* (and, perhaps, some adjunctive exercises) with students who have tight Achilles tendons. In observing how the *plié* is performed, the teacher will pay particular attention to the *front* (anterior) aspect of the ankle, where the desired release in the tibialis anterior tendon can be observed (figures 3-22, 3-23). If this tendon remains contracted during *plié,* especially when landing from jumps and leaps, there is no full stretch of the Achilles, resulting in jarring landings and an increased exposure to possible shin splints and related injuries. The same principle applies to achieving flexibility in the hamstrings: In order to get a full stretch in the hamstrings, the rectus femoris, sartorius, and iliacus all must be released so that a contraction of the quadriceps does not inhibit the stretch of the hamstrings.

The other aspect of growth that needs to be addressed in training young dancers is the problem of muscle-tendon imbalance. Simply put, muscles have two basic functions, to stretch and to contract. When these functions are dis-

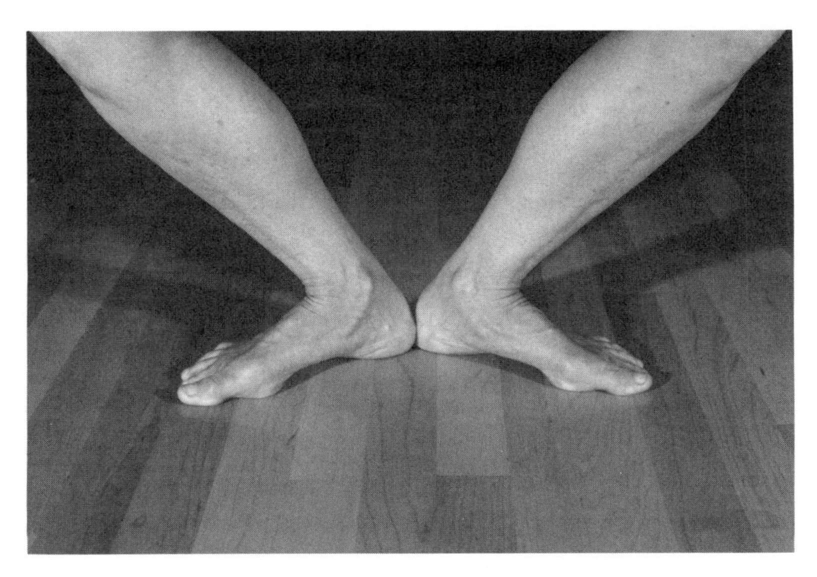

Figure 3-23. *Demi plié* in turned-out (first) position with anterior tibialis tendon released. Note increased flexion and stretch of Achilles tendon.

cussed in relation to any activity, including dance, they are normally defined and measured in terms of flexibility, strength, and endurance. It has already been pointed out that flexibility is a problem for the young dancer because the body parts are developing at different rates. Such is also the problem where strength is concerned: Not all muscle groups develop at the same rate or to the same capacity. This natural imbalance is not an issue for most individuals, but for the young dancer, the training itself can exaggerate it. For example, the quadriceps muscles tend to be stronger than the hamstrings, and ballet training generally contracts the former while stretching the latter, thereby increasing the discrepancy. The dorsiflexor and plantarflexor groups may develop equally in most individuals, but the preponderance of *demi-pointe* and *pointe* work in ballet inevitably causes the dorsiflexors to stretch and the plantarflexors to contract (modern dancers do not usually have this problem because a dorsiflexed foot is used).[2] As we have written elsewhere, activities that encourage muscle imbalance increase the risk of injury; those that promote balance between agonist and antagonist groups reduce it.[6] It is the responsibility of dance teachers, therefore—especially those who deal with young students, where irregular growth spurts are a concern—to structure their approach to training in such a way as to take these anatomical facts into account.

References

1. Solomon R, Micheli LJ. Technique as a consideration in modern dance injuries. Phys Sportsmed 1986; 14(8):83-92.

2. Micheli LJ, Gillespie WJ, Walaszek A. Physiologic profiles of female professional ballerinas. Clin Sports Med 1984; 3:199-209.

3. Sammarco GJ. The dancer's hip. Clin Sports Med 1983; 2(3):485-98.
4. Schaberg JE, Harper MC, Allen WC. The snapping hip syndrome. Am J Sports Med 1984; 12(5):361-65.
5. Scully TJ, Besterman G. Stress fracture—a preventable training injury. Milit Med 1982; 147(4):285-87.
6. Solomon R, Micheli LJ. Concepts in the prevention of dance injuries: a survey and analysis. In: Shell C, ed. The dancer as athlete. Champaign, IL: Human Kinetics Publishers, Inc, 1986; 201-12.

Bibliography

Micheli LJ. Overuse injuries in children: the growth factor. Orthop Clin of N Am 1983; 14(2):337-60.

Micheli LJ. Back injuries in dancers. Clin in Sports Med 2:3 Nov 1983.

Micheli LJ, ed. Pediatric adolescent sports medicine. Boston: Little Brown, 1984.

4

THE CARDIOVASCULAR AND METABOLIC DEMANDS OF CLASSICAL DANCE

Jerald L. Cohen, M.D., F.A.C.P., F.A.C.S.M.

See where she stands! a mortal shape indued
With love and life and light and deity,
And motion which may change but cannot die;
An image of some bright Eternity;
A shadow of some golden dream....

—Percy Bysshe Shelley
"Epipsychidion"

DURING THE RENAISSANCE, GREAT effort was channeled into elucidating the scientific basis of art. It was believed that if art could be analyzed rationally, its secrets revealed and its principles defined, then improvements could be made in its execution. The scientific discoveries of perspective and anatomy made possible the development of modern painting and sculpture. Throughout most of the history of ballet, however, scientific methodology and medical investigation have been largely ignored. Although significant improvements in ballet performance and training have taken place, they have occurred primarily through personal experience and innovations in choreography, without the benefit of scientific discipline. During the past decade, we have begun to witness the application of the scientific method to ballet. This chapter presents some of the findings thus far and describes the physiologic events that occur in response to ballet exercise and their long-term effects on dancers. Knowledge of these aspects of ballet have important implications for the training and care of ballet dancers.

Empirical and Physiologic Study of Ballet Exercise

Before examining the results of physiologic measurements made during ballet exercise, it is necessary to characterize the type of exercise used in ballet from simple empirical observation. One may then compare the results of physiologic testing with these observations and determine whether the experimental measurements are in accord with empiric expectations.

Fundamental to the characterization of ballet exercise is its duration. Most ballet exercise takes place in intervals of 1, 2, or 3 min. followed by varying periods of rest. Although slow tempo dancing and some barre exercises may last somewhat longer, ballet generally is intermittent exercise of brief duration. This fact is a key to understanding the physiology of ballet exercise.

Ballet exercise may be divided into barre and center floor dancing. Whereas the former is used exclusively in the classroom, the latter is employed in class, rehearsal, and stage performance. Ballet may also be classified as slow tempo (adagio) or fast tempo (allegro) dancing.

During barre exercises, the dancer uses the barre as support and works with one leg and arm at a time. The movements at the barre are intricate, require a great deal of balance and control, and are designed to improve strength. Isometric exercise is of great importance in executing these movements, especially in maintaining balance, control, and placement or posture. More dynamic exercise is used in the movements of the working leg.

During center floor dancing, the dancer is unsupported. Through large, broad, traveling steps, the dancer covers the entire dance floor or stage. These movements are more dynamic or isotonic, but some isometric exercise is still needed to maintain balance and support.

The ballet exercise of rehearsal and stage performance may be of three types. Adagio dancing appears to be of lower intensity and is extended over longer periods of time. The single allegro variation from the classical ballet appears to be of high intensity, but lasts only 1 to 3 min. In contemporary ballets, several high-intensity allegro parts may follow in rapid succession.

Ballet exercise may therefore be characterized as either moderate-intensity exercise, with a strong isometric component during adagio dancing, or high-intensity, brief-duration exercise during fast-tempo dancing. In general, the exercise is of the nonendurance type, similar to that seen in gymnastics, wrestling, or sprinting. True, uninterrupted endurance exercise, as observed in long-distance running, is not seen in ballet. One might thus expect that ballet exercise would provide a moderate stimulus to augmenting aerobic capacity.

The complete characterization of the cardiovascular and metabolic demands of ballet exercise would require that physiologic measurements be made during all phases of ballet exercise, including barre work and center floor dancing in class, rehearsal, and stage performance. Direct open-circuit spirometry may be employed during class and rehearsal. Telemetry of heart rate may be used during stage performance. The long-term effects of ballet exercise may be assessed by measuring maximum oxygen uptake and by determining left ventricular dimensions by echocardiography.

Ballet Class and Rehearsal

The first study to use open-circuit spirometry during ballet class work was undertaken by the Veterans Administration Medical Center in East Orange, NJ, and professional dancers from American Ballet Theatre.[1] Ten dancers (4 men, 6 women) representing all ranks in the ballet company (*corps de ballet,* soloist, principal) were monitored during 1-hr. ballet classes. During barre work, cardiorespiratory data were monitored continuously during exercise and rest intervals. Center floor dancing was monitored only during the exercise periods, using portable meteorological balloons.

The results of this study are shown in figure 4-1. During barre exercise, mean $\dot{V}O_2$ averaged 38% $\dot{V}O_2$max for both men and women; center floor exer-

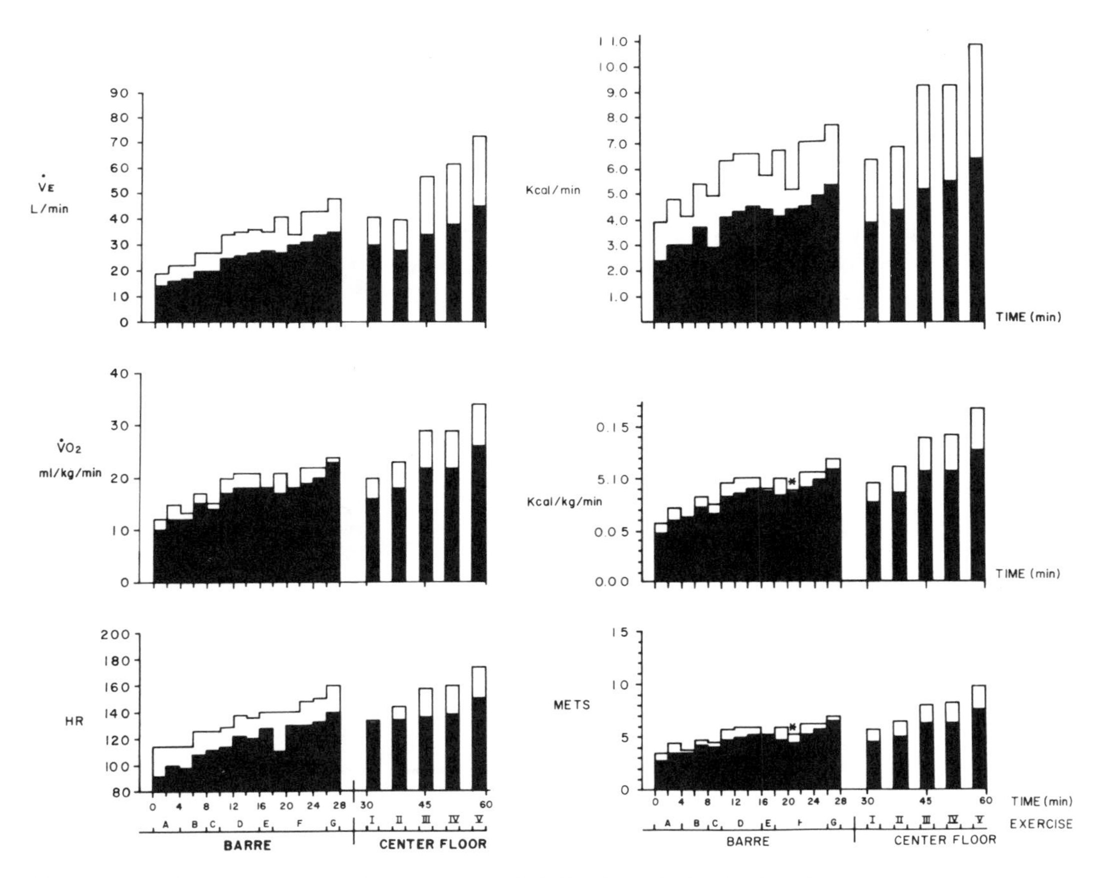

Figure 4-1. Mean cardiorespiratory and metabolic data during ballet class exercise. Separate exercises are labeled A-G and I-V. Open bars = men, filled bars = women. (*means higher for women than men during this interval.) (Reproduced with permission, *Medicine and Science in Sports and Exercise.).*

cise averaged 55% and 46% $\dot{V}O_2max$ for men and women, respectively. Peak $\dot{V}O_2$ during barre exercise averaged 51% $\dot{V}O_2max$ for both sexes; during center floor dancing, peak $\dot{V}O_2$ averaged 71% and 60% $\dot{V}O_2max$ for men and women, respectively. The highest recorded $\dot{V}O_2$ was 77% $\dot{V}O_2max$ for a male principal dancer during an allegro exercise similar to a stage variation. Gross caloric expenditures, derived from $\dot{V}O_2$ measurements, averaged 0.09 and 0.08 kcal/min.$^{-1}$ kg^{-1} for men and women, respectively, during barre work; 0.13 and 0.10 kcal/min.$^{-1}$ kg^{-1} during center floor exercise for men and women, respectively. The highest recorded value was 0.18 kcal/min.$^{-1}$ kg^{-1} for a male dancer during an allegro variation. Heart rates (HR) during barre exercise averaged 134 beats/min.$^{-1}$ (69% HRmax) and 117 (63% HRmax) for men and women respectively; during center floor exercise, 153 (80% HRmax) and 137 (74% HRmax) for men and women, respectively. Peak heart rates during an allegro center floor exercise averaged 178 and 158 beats/min.$^{-1}$ (92% and 85% HRmax) for men and women, respectively, with the highest heart rate recorded at 188 beats/min.$^{-1}$ (98% HRmax). The estimated net caloric expenditure for the entire ballet class averaged 300 kcal h^{-1} for men and 200 kcal h^{-1} for women. Some underestimation of $\dot{V}O_2$ may have occurred during this study, as monitoring included rest intervals during barre work and included the average $\dot{V}O_2$ during nonsteady-state center floor exercises.

Schantz et al conducted another study with dancers of the Royal Swedish Ballet.[2] This study included open-circuit spirometry during barre work, center floor dancing of both moderate and severe intensity, and during a classical solo

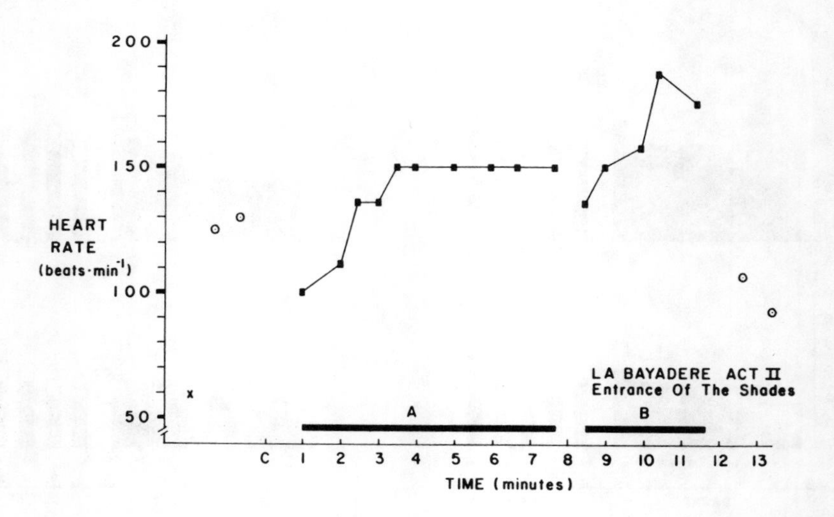

Figure 4-2. Adagio at A, allegro variation at B from the "Entrance of the Shades," *La Bayadère*, Act 2. Horizontal bar = duration of individual dance variation; ■ = heart rate (HR) during dancing; □ = HR between dancing (on stage); ○ = HR between dancing (in wings); × = resting HR. (Figures 4-2 and 4-4 reproduced with permission, *Physician and Sportsmedicine.*)

variation performed as a rehearsal exercise. In addition, blood lactate levels were measured. Measurements from 6 dancers showed an oxygen uptake of 36% $\dot{V}O_2max$ for barre exercise, 43% $\dot{V}O_2max$ for moderate-intensity center floor dancing, and 46% $\dot{V}O_2max$ for high-intensity center floor dancing. During the rehearsal type solo variation, 80% $\dot{V}O_2max$ was reported. These results are similar to those cited above from American Ballet Theatre, but emphasize

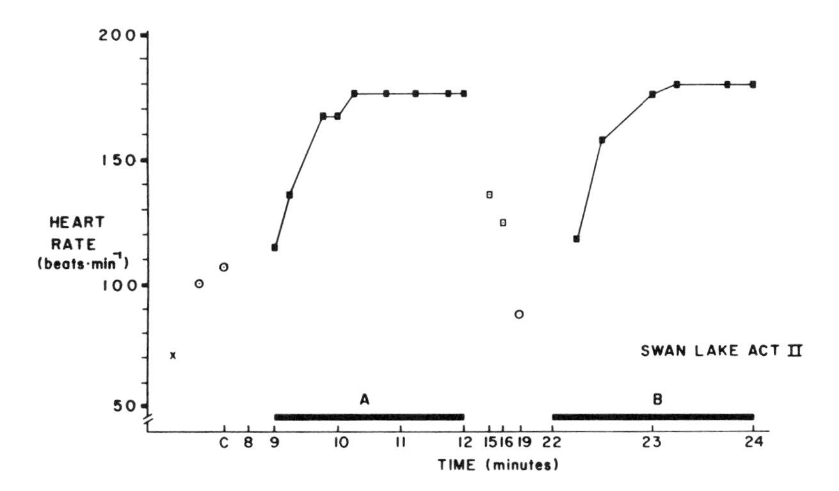

Figure 4-3. Two allegro variations at A and B from *Swan Lake,* Act 2. Same symbols as figure 4-2.

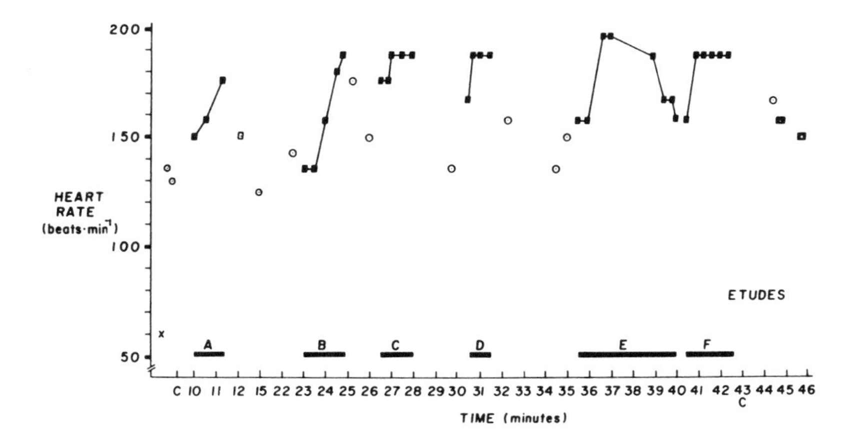

Figure 4-4. Several allegro variations from *Études.* Same symbols as figure 4-2.

the higher $\dot{V}O_2$ during rehearsal dancing. Blood lactate levels average 3mM during each phase of class and 10mM during the solo variation. Lactate levels obtained during maximal cycle or treadmill testing averaged 13mM. The lactate levels recorded during the solo variation were therefore quite high.

Stage Performance

Heart rate telemetry was done by our laboratory with 13 dancers during several live performances of American Ballet Theatre.[3] In general, three types of recordings resulted. The first type, shown in figure 4-2, is a recording made during adagio dancing (a female *corps de ballet* member as a *shade,* in the "Entrance of the Shades" from *La Bayadère.*). The heart rate increased gradually and plateaued at 150 beats/min.$^{-1}$ (77% HRmax). The relatively low-intensity dance lasted a full 8 min. In the second type of recording, seen in figure 4-3, a female soloist performs two brief allegro variations from the classical repertory *(Swan Lake).* The heart rate increases rapidly to 94% HRmax, but each variation lasts only 2-3 min., interrupted by a long rest period. The third type of recording, shown in figure 4-4, was obtained from a principal dancer performing several allegro parts in close succession in a contemporary ballet *(Études).* Here, near maximal heart rates are sustained throughout most of the ballet, with work/rest ratios averaging 1:1.9, similar to those recommended for interval training.[4] Shantz et al[2] also recorded heart rates during performance and obtained similar results.

Experimental Observations of Ballet Exercise

The experimental results obtained above are in agreement with the expectations derived from empirical observations. During barre work, the moderate-intensity exercise registered relatively low $\dot{V}O_2$, heart rate, and blood lactate production. Center floor dancing showed significantly higher $\dot{V}O_2$ levels. Rehearsal variations showed the highest $\dot{V}O_2$ and lactate production. Stage performance also showed high-intensity exercise, with near maximal heart rates during fast-tempo dancing.

Table 4-1. Maximum Oxygen Uptake ($\dot{V}O_2$max) of Professional Ballet Dancers

Study	Ballet Company	Number of Subjects	$\dot{V}O_2$max (ml.min^{-1}.kg^{-1}) Men	Women
Cohen et al (1)*	American Ballet Theatre	4M, 4F	48.20 ± 3.40	43.73 ± 4.32
Kirkendall et al (5)	Cleveland Ballet	14M, 15F	51.97 ± 5.29	39.26 ± 4.57
Schantz et al (2)	Royal Swedish Ballet	6M, 7F	57	51

Data are mean ± S.D.
M = males, F = females
*reference number

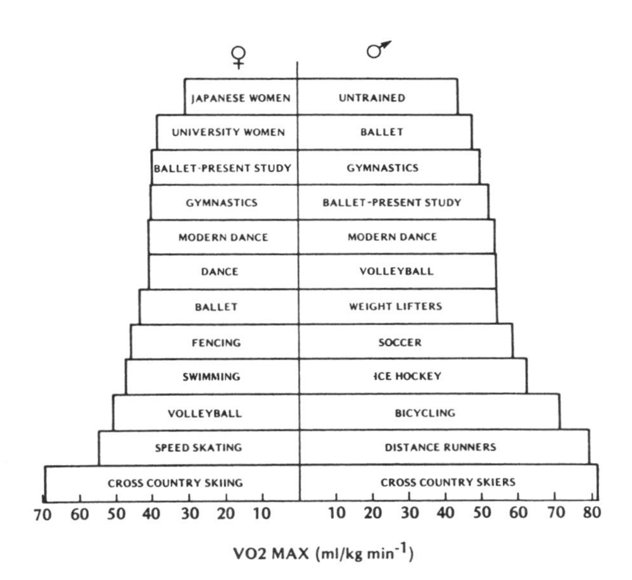

Figure 4-5. Maximum oxygen uptake of ballet dancers and other athletes. (Reproduced with permission, *Clinics in Sports Medicine.)*

Generally, aerobic capacity will improve if exercise is of sufficient intensity to increase the heart rate to 70% of maximum. During class (figure 4-1), this heart rate was reached only during the last half to last third of the barre exercises. Heart rates were higher during center floor dancing and stage performance and were in the training-sensitive zone, but for only brief durations (1-3 min.). It is here that the duration of most ballet exercise becomes important. High-intensity, brief-duration exercise would rely heavily on anaerobic metabolism, as documented above by high lactate production. To the extent that ballet exercise resembles interval training (figure 4-4), an aerobic effect would result. However, the sprintlike, nonendurance nature of ballet exercise would tend to stimulate aerobic capacity only moderately when compared with other more endurance forms of athletic exercise.

Long-Term Training Effects of Ballet Exercise

Maximum oxygen uptake of ballet dancers has been determined in a few major ballet companies.[1,2,5] A summary of these findings is shown in table 4-1. Average $\dot{V}O_2max$ values of these studies are 52 and 44 ml/min.$^{-1}$ kg^{-1} for men and women, respectively. These findings are consistent with values obtained in non-endurance athletes. Kirkendall, et al,[5] using $\dot{V}O_2max$ data, showed the relationship of ballet dancers to other athletes in figure 4-5. As may be seen, dancers are similar to gymnasts and wrestlers.

Kirkendall et al,[5] working with the Cleveland Ballet, studied the effect of

Table 4-2. Echocardiographic Left Ventricular Dimensions of Professional Ballet Dancers

	Men		p Values	Women		p Values
	Dancers N = 14	Controls N = 8		Dancers N = 15	Controls N = 7	
IVS (mm)	11.7 ± 1.4	10.2 ± 0.9	< .05	9.7 ± 1.0	8.0 ± 0.6	< .001
LVWT (mm)	12.9 ± 1.7	10.9 ± 0.8	< .01	10.9 ± 0.9	9.7 ± 0.5	< .01
EDD(mm)	47.8 ± 2.4	45.3 ± 1.5	< .05	43.1 ± 2.3	41.0 ± 1.5	< .05
SF	0.31 ± 0.03	0.31 ± 0.03	NS	0.34 ± 0.03	0.31 ± 0.03	< .05
LVM (g)	285.9 ± 37.5	209.0 ± 12.2	< .001	188.6 ± 28.3	140.5 ± 14.6	< .001

Adapted from Cohen et al (ref 8)
Data are mean ± S.D.
IVS = Interventricular septal wall thickness; LVWT = posterior wall thickness; EDD = end-diastolic dimension; SF = shortening fraction; LVM = left ventricular mass; NS = not significant.
(Reproduced with permission, *American Journal of Cardiology*)

4 months of ballet training on maximum oxygen uptake of the dancers. Preseason $\dot{V}O_2max$ measurements were 37.97 ± 6.64 and 27.74 ± 4.97 for men and women, respectively, and were similar to those in untrained subjects. At peak season, $\dot{V}O_2max$ values increased to 51.97 ± 5.29 and 39.26 ± 4.57 for men and women, respectively. This study showed a very definite aerobic training effect of ballet exercise.

Echocardiographic left ventricular dimensions also provide some evidence of the long-term training effects of different types of exercise.[6,7] Dynamic exercise (endurance running or swimming) produces predominantly increased left ventricular volume secondary to the volume overload (high cardiac output) associated with this type of exercise. Static or isometric exercise (wrestling, shotput) produces mainly increases in wall thickness due to the pressure overload (increased arterial pressure) associated with this type of exercise. Echocardiographic dimensions were determined by our laboratory with American Ballet Theatre dancers (table 4-2).[8] Compared to studies of other athletes, the increases in left ventricular dimensions observed in dancers were relatively small. Dancers showed greater increases in wall thickness than end-diastolic dimension. Although increases in wall thickness may be seen in either dynamically trained (eccentric hypertrophy) or statically trained athletes (concentric hypertrophy), significant increases in left ventricular volume are seen only with dynamic endurance training. The important finding in this study was the absence of marked increases in left ventricular volume, excluding a significant long-term endurance training effect. Again, these findings are consistent with the nonendurance nature of ballet exercise.

Implications

Having measured the caloric expenditure of ballet exercise,[1,2] nutritional guidelines for dancers can be more accurately made. We estimated that in general a dancer's daily caloric intake should fall within the range of 3,000 Cal for men and 2,000-2,200 Cal for women.[9] Based on dietary studies of dancers, male dancers consumed their predicted caloric intake.[9] Female dancers, however, consumed only 1,673 Cal per day in one study[9] and 1,358 Cal in another study.[10] Such caloric restriction in women, a result of conforming to an aesthetic of a lean body type, presents a special challenge to nutritionists.

The lean body type and caloric restriction associated with female dancers may have endocrinologic implications. If the hypothesis that athletic amenorrhea results from an "energy drain" is true,[11] then the caloric deficit of female dancers may help to explain the amenorrhea observed in these individuals.[12]

Ballet dancers may now be categorized as nonendurance athletes. Traditionally, ballet dancers have always trained by doing ballet exercise. This method apparently has stood the test of time. The general level of ballet dancing seems always to be improving. Present training methods for athletes, however, often include exercise that is not directly related to the athletes' own sport: Wrestlers supplement their training with distance running, endurance athletes supplement their training with strength exercises. Whether ballet dancers would benefit from endurance or strength training remains conjectural. Future studies may help to clarify this possibility.

References

1. Cohen JL, Segal KR, Witriol I, McArdle WD. Cardiorespiratory responses to ballet exercise and the $\dot{V}O_2max$ of elite ballet dancers. Med Sci Sports Exerc 1982; 14:212-17.
2. Schantz PG, Astrand PO. Physiological characteristics of classical ballet. Med Sci Sports Exerc 1984; 16:472-76.
3. Cohen JL, Segal KR, McArdle WD. Heart rate response to ballet stage performance. Phys Sportsmed 1982; 10:120-33.
4. Fox E, Mathews D. Interval training: conditioning for sports and general fitness. Philadelphia: W.B. Saunders, 1974.
5. Kirkendall DT, Calabrese LH. Physiological aspects of dance. In: Sammarco GJ, ed. Symposium on injuries to dancers. Clin Sports Med 2: 3. Philadlelphia: W.B. Saunders, 1983; 525-37.
6. Morganroth J, Maron BJ, Henry WL, Epstein SE. Comparative left ventricular dimensions in trained athletes. Ann Intern Med 1975; 82:521-24.
7. Cohen JL, Segal KR. Left ventricular hypertrophy in athletes: an exercise-echocardiographic study. Med Sci Sports Exerc 1985; 17:695-700.
8. Cohen JL, Gupta PK, Lichstein E, Chadda KD. The heart of a dancer: noninvasive cardiac evaluation of professional ballet dancers. Am J Cardiol 1980; 45:959-65.
9. Cohen JL, Potosnak L, Frank O, Baker H. Nutritional and hematologic assessment of elite ballet dancers. Phys Sportsmed 1985; 13:43-54.
10. Calabrese LH, Kirkendall DT, Floyd M et al. Menstrual abnormalities, nutritional patterns and body composition in female classical ballet dancers. Phys Sportsmed 1983; 11:86-98.
11. Warren MP. The effects of exercise on pubertal progression and reproductive function in girls. J Clin Endocrinol Metab 1980; 51:1150-57.
12. Cohen JL, May PB, Kim CS, Ertel NH. Exercise, body weight and amenorrhea in professional ballet dancers. Phys Sportsmed 1982; 10:92-101.

5

DANCE AND MENSTRUAL FUNCTION

Steven Williams, M.D., and Leon Speroff, M.D.

SORANUS, A PHYSICIAN OF Rome (A.D. 98-138), has been acknowledged as a master gynecologist among the ancients. Listing conditions whose chief symptom is amenorrhea, Soranus included "...the youthful, the aged, the pregnant, singers, and those who take much exercise."[1] In the twentieth century, physicians once again are aware of the problem of amenorrhea in the female athlete. Exercise, especially in activity requiring endurance and slenderness, significantly suppresses reproductive functions. Dance requires a combination of endurance and slenderness to achieve a weight that is uniform with the other dancers, can be lifted, and that fits costumes and the vision of the choreographer.[2] Exercise, low body weight, and undernutrition, combined with the emotional stress of competition and performance, all contribute to menstrual dysfunction. Thus, it is not surprising that dancers frequently suffer from menstrual problems. This chapter will discuss menstrual function, then review information on menstrual problems in dancers as well as other athletes. Finally, a program of therapeutic management will be offered.

Basic Principles in Menstrual Function

The presence of menstrual function entails visible external evidence of the menstrual discharge. This requires an intact outflow tract that connects the internal genital source of flow with the outside. As such, the outflow tract requires patency and continuity of the vaginal orifice, the vaginal canal, and the endocervix with the uterine cavity. The presence of menstrual flow depends on the existence and development of the endometrium lining the uterine cavity. This tissue is stimulated and regulated by the proper quantity and sequence of the steroid hormones, estrogen and progesterone; and the gonadotropins, follicle-stimulating hormone (FSH) and luteinizing hormone (LH). Figure 5-1 depicts the blood levels of gonadotropins and gonadal steroids in a normal cycle as measured by radioimmunoassay methods. These hormonal changes can best be described by dividing the cycle into three phases: the follicular phase, ovulation, and the luteal phase.

The Follicular Phase

At 8 weeks of intrauterine life, rapid mitotic multiplication of oocytes begins, reaching a peak of 6-7 million by 20 weeks. Egg depletion by the process known as atresia begins at about 15 weeks of gestation, and by birth the total ovarian content of oogonia has fallen to 1-2 million. By the onset of puberty, the number of eggs has been reduced to 300,000-500,000. It is from this reservoir that the typical cycle of follicle maturation with ovulation and corpus luteum formation will arise. For every follicle that ovulates, close to 1,000 will pursue abortive growth periods of variable length and undergo atresia.

Until age 45-50, when the numbers of oogonia have been exhausted, primordial follicles are continuously undergoing an initial growth and development that in the vast majority of instances is followed rapidly by atresia. During the reproductive years, this pattern is interrupted at the beginning of the menstrual cycle when a group of follicles responds to a hormonal change

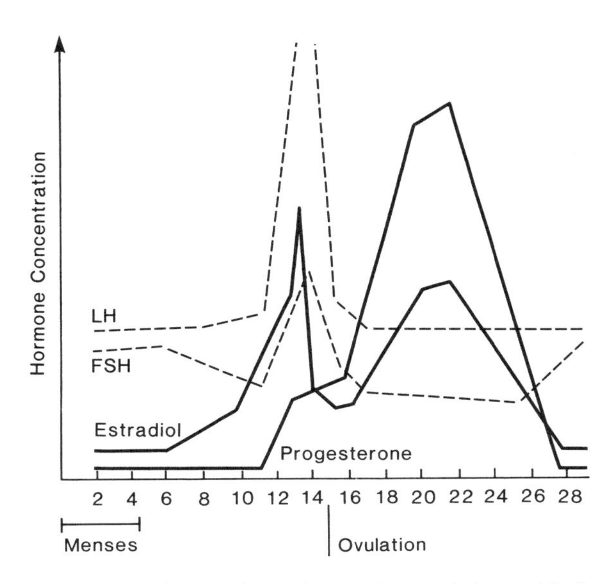

Figure 5-1. Blood levels of gonadotropins and gonadal steroids in a normal cycle as measured by radioimmunoassay methods.

and is propelled to further growth. The most important hormonal event at this time is a rise in FSH, leading to a direct stimulation of follicular growth. During this early period of FSH-stimulated follicular growth, there is little, if any, detectable change in the blood levels of gonadal hormones. A rise in LH also occurs during menses, and the two gonadotropins work together in providing for steroidogenesis in the growing follicle. This cooperative effort of the two gonadotropins is conceptualized in the so-called two-cell explanation of ovarian steroidogenesis.

As the granulosa responds to FSH, continued growth is associated with an increase in FSH receptors. This is a specific effect of FSH itself, but an action that is enhanced very significantly by estradiol. The theca cells are characterized by steroidogenic activity in response to LH, resulting in androgen production. The specific androgens, androstenedione and testosterone, produced in the theca layer, must diffuse into the granulosa layer, where aromatization of the androgens to estrogens is a specific activity induced by FSH. The increased level of estrogen in the peripheral circulation reflects release of the estrogen back toward the theca layer and into the blood vessels.

The estradiol produced by the cooperative effort of the two cells, theca and granulosa, plays an important role in enhancing the activity of FSH and thus promoting the growth and function of its own follicle. As the follicle approaches ovulation, LH receptors begin to appear on the granulosa layer, also induced by FSH in another action enhanced by estradiol. After ovulation, the dominance of the luteinized granulosa layer is dependent upon preovulatory induction of an adequate number of LH receptors and therefore dependent upon adequate FSH action. As LH receptors begin to appear on the granulosa, the granulosa responds with LH-stimulated steroidogenesis, resulting in the release of progesterone and estrogen directly into the bloodstream. The low levels of progesterone in the peripheral circulation are able to reach the pituitary before ovulation. This low level of progesterone takes on an important role in stimulating the FSH midcycle surge.

The rapid growth of the follicle late in the follicular phase when FSH levels are actually decreasing indicates that as the follicle matures it becomes increasingly sensitive to FSH. With follicular growth, the levels of estradiol rise and inhibit FSH secretion; however, the follicle destined to ovulate protects itself from atresia by its own hormone production. High local estradiol concentration increases follicular sensitivity to FSH by promoting the follicular binding of FSH. The decrease in FSH then would be significant in terms of a loss of growth stimulation to the smaller follicles, which are producing less estrogen. A wave of atresia, therefore, is seen to parallel the rise in estrogen, reaching a maximum in the preovulatory period.

The tissue derived from the theca interna of atretic follicles is known as stromal tissue. This tissue is not truly atretic; it continues to secrete steriods, but rather than estrogen, the principal products are androgens, androstenedione, and testosterone. The increase in stromal tissue in the late follicular phase is associated with a rise in androgen levels in peripheral blood. Abnormal accumulation of this tissue, as in anovulation and polycystic ovaries, can give rise to increased androgen production and hirsutism.

Ovulation

In the past, the hypothalamus was viewed as the coordinator of reproductive function. Responding to messages from peripheral organs and from the central nervous system, it exerted its influence through neural transmitters transported to the pituitary by the portal vascular system. However, a more modern concept holds that the complex sequence of events known as the menstrual cycle is controlled by the sex steroids produced within the very follicle destined to ovulate. The hypothalamus plays a permissive role, whereas the qualitative and quantitative changes associated with ovulation are orchestrated by steroid feedback effects on the anterior pituitary (figure 5-2).

The major change in our conceptual thinking has been the movement of the center for the midcycle surge of gonadatropins from the hypothalamus to the pituitary. This surge response is controlled by the ovarian follicle steroid feedback effect on anterior pituitary cells. Experiments in the monkey have demonstrated that gonadotropin-releasing hormone (GnRH) originating in the hypothalamus plays a permissive role. Its administration in hourly bursts need

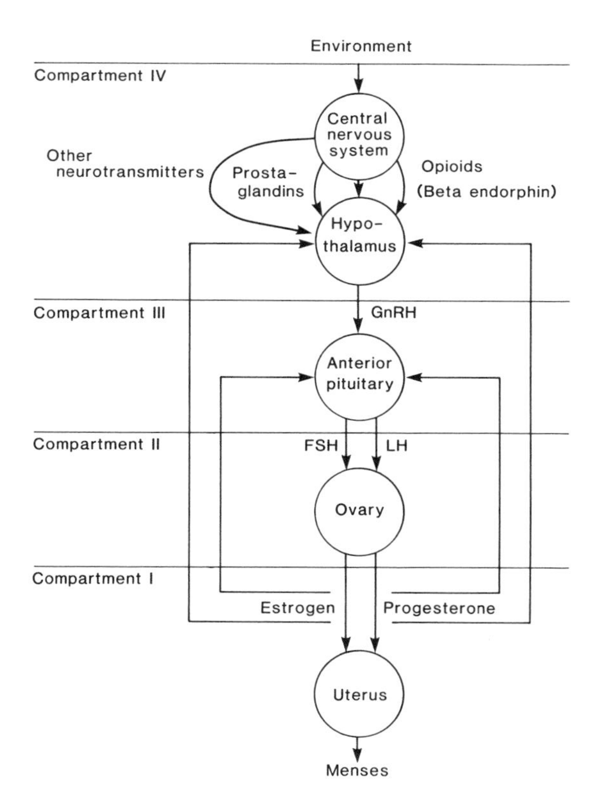

Figure 5-2. Qualitative and quantitative changes associated with ovulation.

only be maintained at a constant rate to produce normal ovulatory cycles in monkeys in which the hypothalamus has been destroyed by a radio frequency technique. In other words, the midcycle surge of gonadotropins is not due primarily to a midcycle surge of GnRH.

GnRH has three principal actions on gonadotropin elaboration: (1) synthesis and storage (reserve); (2) activation (movement of gonadotropins from the reserve pool to a pool ready for direct secretion); and (3) immediate release (direct secretion).

Secretion and storage rates change during the cycle. At the beginning of the cycle, when estrogen levels are low, secretion and storage rates also are low. With increasing levels of estradiol, more gonadotropin is stored in relation to the level secreted. This response to GnRH is governed by the feedback effect of estradiol on the anterior pituitary. Estrogen has a positive effect on the synthesis and storage response, building up the supply of gonadotropins to meet the requirements of the midcycle surge. Premature release of gonadotropins is prevented by the negative effect on estradiol on direct pituitary secretion of gonadotropins.

As the midcycle approaches, responses to GnRH become greater. Each response not only induces release of gonadotropins but also activates the storage pool for the next response. When the estradiol level in the circulation reaches a critical concentration, and this concentration is maintained for a critical length of time, the action on LH secretion in the pituitary changes from inhibitory to stimulatory. The midcycle surge must occur at the right time in the cycle for a mature follicle to ovulate. This extremely precise coordination and timing are accomplished by the follicle itself, through the feedback effects of the sex steroids.

A normal corpus luteum requires an adequate number of LH receptors on the granulosa cells. Induction of these receptors is a specific action of FSH. Therefore, the midcycle surge of FSH is important to ensure adequate LH response and a normal corpus luteum. Emerging progesterone secretion before ovulation is the key influence in this series of events.

Low levels of progesterone in the presence of estrogen augment the pituitary secretion of LH and elicit the FSH surge in response to GnRH at midcycle. As the rising levels of LH produce the morphologic change of luteinization in the follicle destined to ovulate, the granulosa layer begins to secrete progesterone directly into the bloodstream. Because the process of luteinization is inhibited by the presence of the oocyte, progesterone secretion is relatively suppressed, ensuring that only low levels of progesterone reach the pituitary gland. After ovulation, rapid and full luteinization is accompanied by a marked increase in progesterone.

Although GnRH is only permissive, there must exist a necessary and critical range of secretion. Suppression below this critical range probably explains the amenorrhea seen with such conditions as stress, exercise, and anorexia nervosa. The process of puberty represents the rising of GnRH into this critical range. Thus, although the fine tuning of the menstrual cycle is due to an interplay between the follicle and the pituitary, amenorrhea can and does result from suppression of GnRH.

The Luteal Phase

After rupture of the follicle and release of the ovum, the granulosa cells increase in size. They assume a characteristic vacuolated appearance associated with the accumulation of the yellow pigment, lutein, which lends its name to the process of luteinization and the new anatomical subunit, the corpus luteum. During the first 3 days after ovulation, the granulosa cells enlarge and capillaries penetrate into the granulosa layer. By day 8 or 9 after ovulation, a peak of vascularization, associated with peak levels of progesterone and estradiol in the blood, is reached. Steroidogenesis in the corpus luteum is dependent on the low but important quantities of LH available in the luteal phase. Beginning about 10-12 days after ovulation, the corpus luteum enters into a state of regression, which is first marked by a gradual decrease of blood in the capillaries followed by decreasing steroid production.

It is well known that the variability in cycle length among women is due to the varying number of days required for follicular growth and maturation in the follicular phase. In the normal cycle, the time period from the LH surge to menses is consistently close to 14 days. The finite life span of the human corpus luteum may represent a response to the stimulation of the LH surge at midcycle. Degeneration and regression are inevitable unless pregnancy intervenes. With pregnancy, survival of the corpus luteum is prolonged by the emergence of a new stimulus of rapidly increasing intensity, human chorionic gonadotropin (HCG). This new stimulus first appears at the peak of corpus luteum development, just in time to prevent luteal regression. HCG serves to maintain the vital steroidogenesis of the corpus luteum until about the ninth or tenth week of gestation, by which time placental steroidogenesis is well established.

Key Events in the Normal Menstrual Cycle

Several relationships in the regulation of the human menstrual cycle are a key to understanding these events. The first is the rise in gonadotropins that begins at the termination of the preceding cycle and is responsible for the stimulation of a new set of follicles, thus initiating a new cycle. The absence or blunting of this rise in gonadotropins will prevent cycling.

Second, ovulation is due to a surge in LH, which in turn is triggered by rapidly rising levels of estrogen. Inhibition of synchronous timing of the LH surge or inadequate follicular estrogen production will prevent ovulation and possibly create a set of circumstances that will not allow recycling.

Finally, a normal pregnancy will not occur without the concurrent normal life span of the corpus luteum, a life span that depends upon LH maintenance and upon the preovulatory adequacy of gonadotropins to provide full follicular maturation.

The human cycle depends upon essential changes in estradiol levels at key moments. The initial rise in gonadotropins occurs in response to the decline in steroids in the preceding luteal phase. Successful follicular development without premature atresia depends upon adequate estradiol production by the growing follicle. Ovulation is triggered by estradiol at midcycle. The interplay among the follicle, the hypothalamus, and the anterior pituitary depends upon estradiol functioning as a classic hormone to transmit the messages of negative and positive feedback and also upon the local effect of estradiol within the follicle to ensure gonadotropin sensitivity. Events that prevent estrogen production, obstruct the necessary fluctuations in circulating levels, or interfere with target organ estrogen action will result in abnormal or absent menstrual cycles.

Menstrual Dysfunction Among Dancers and Athletes

An increased incidence of many types of menstrual dysfunction has been found in dancers and athletes. In at least two studies, dancers have been reported to have delayed menarche.[3,4] Frisch studied the age of menarche and menstrual periodicity of college swimmers and runners in relation to the age of initiating training. She found that beginning training before menarche delayed menarche, while athletes who began training later had normal menarches. Each year of training before menarche delayed menarche by 5 months. Of the premenarche-trained athletes, 61% had irregular menstrual cycles and 22% were amenorrheic. On the other hand, 60% of postmenarche-trained athletes had regular menstrual cycles and none were amenorrheic.[5] Thus, premenarchal training not only can delay menarche but it is associated with a greater risk of postmenarchal menstrual problems.

Differing types of training have varied effects on menstrual function. When Finnish sportswomen were surveyed, those participating in high-endurance sports such as running and skiing had a much higher incidence of menstrual irregularity (43%) than did volleyball players as compared to controls (27%).[6] The volleyball players reported a 19% incidence, not different from their controls. Another survey found the prevalence of menstrual dysfunction among runners to be twice that among swimmers and cyclists. The survey also showed a correlation between amenorrhea prevalence and training mileage among the long-distance runners (figure 5-3).[7] This correlation was not seen among cyclists and swimmers. The reason for this difference is unclear, but may be related to body weight differences among the groups.

The abnormalities in menstrual function may not be obvious to the athlete. Previously studied basal body temperatures in 14 athletes and up to one-third of "on time" menstrual periods were anovulatory and another third were found to have short luteal phases.[8] Shangold has found luteal phase deficits that appear with an increase in training in an endurance runner.[9] These subtle abnormalities can have an important impact on fertility and risks of breast and endometrial cancer. Their existence implies that we have previously underestimated the prevalence of reproductive problems related to exercise.

In summary, athletes and dancers suffer a high incidence of many menstrual dysfunctions. Up to 61% of dancers and 43% of runners have been reported to have amenorrhea, and if more subtle abnormalities are included, menstrual irregularity becomes a preponderant experience. There is a link to endurance training, which may be explained by considering the role of body fat.

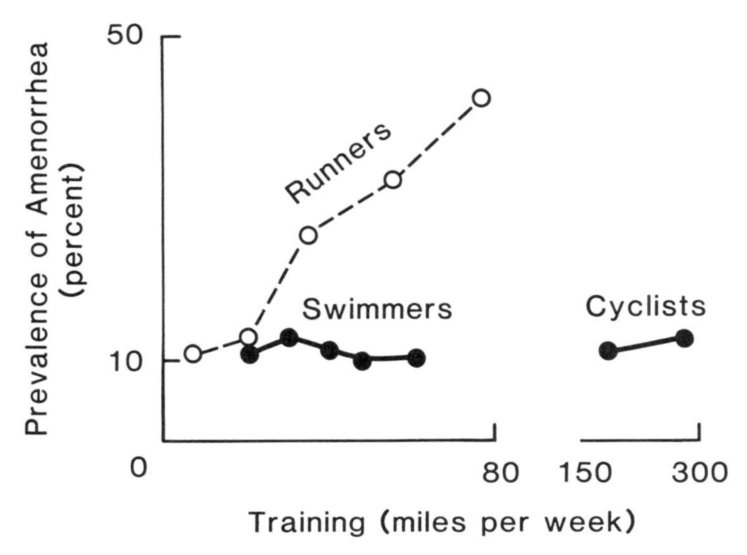

Figure 5-3. Prevalence of menstrual dysfunction among runners, swimmers, and cyclists. (Modified from Sanborn, ref 7.)

The Effect of Body Fat

Body fat and its impact on female reproduction has been extensively studied by Frisch, who theorizes that a critical weight—specifically, a critical amount of body fat—is required for the onset and continued regularity of menstrual function. She pointed out that undernutrition is known to delay sexual maturation in both humans and animals.[10]

Frisch has proposed that about 17% of body weight as fat is required for menarche and 22% of body weight as fat is required for resumption of menses when secondary amenorrhea has resulted from weight loss.[10] This correlation has been observed in a series of studies. Speroff and Redwine found a relationship between body weight and menstrual function in a survey of runners.[11]

Menstrual disorders have been found to correlate with excessive thinness in at least two surveys of ballet dancers.[3,4] Resumption of ovulatory cycles in patients with weight loss amenorrhea was associated with gaining weight, thus lending support to this theory.

A critical amount of body fat to supply energy for reproduction is an attractive theory. It would seem logical that the body would wish to prevent pregnancy during times of undernutrition, but this theory has been challenged. Frisch's calculations of body fat are based on a regression analysis of height and weight. A study employing the more accurate hydrostatic weighing method of determining body fat found no threshold of fatness required for menstruation and no difference in mean body fat between amenorrheic and menstruating athletes.[12]

Twenty-nine dancers entering their first year of professional school had a substantial increase in amenorrhea without any change of weight.[13] Still, there are supportive data, and the Frisch guidelines, although controversial, do give the clinician a method to illustrate this concept to patients (figure 5-4).

When dealing with the low-weight amenorrheic patient, the physician should be aware that another disease, anorexia nervosa, may be disguised by participation in athletics. Anorexia nervosa, a devastating disease of young people, has a mortality rate of 5-15%. The incidence of anorexia nervosa in professional dancers is estimated to be 1 in 20, and 30% in dancers over the age of 20.[15] Diligence in searching for the diagnosis of anorexia is paramount for health care providers interacting with these patients.

The clinical diagnosis of anorexia nervosa is based on the following criteria:

- Onset between age 10 and 30
- Weight loss of 25%, or 15% below normal for age and height
- Specific attitudes of denial and distortion of body image
- At least one of the following: lanugo, bradycardia, overactivity, episodes of overeating, vomiting

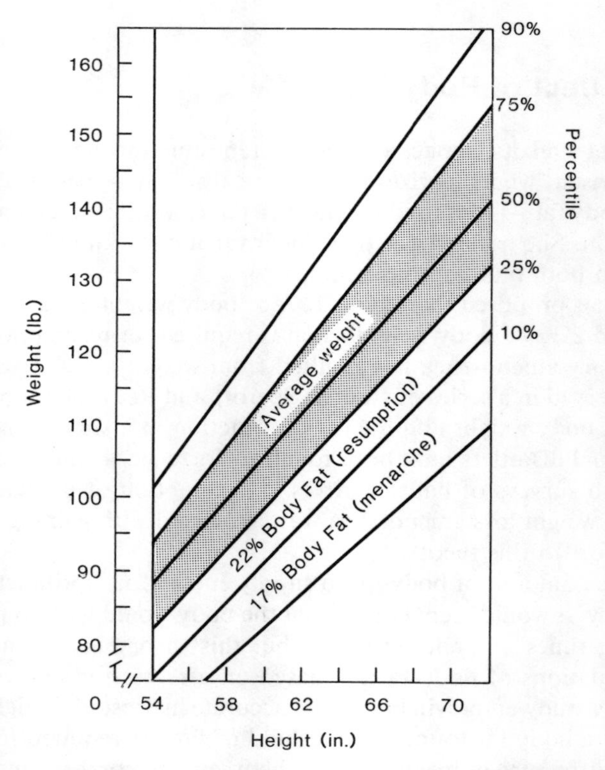

Figure 5-4. Percent of body fat required for menarche and resumption of menses when secondary amenorrhea has resulted from weight loss. (Modified from Frisch, ref 10.)

- Amenorrhea
- No other known illness
- No other psychiatric disorders
- Other characteristics: constipation, low blood pressure, hypothermia, hypercarotenemia, diabetes insipidus

Anorexia nervosa is characterized by an alteration in the hypothalamic-pituitary-ovarian (HPO) axis as well as the hypothalamic-pituitary-adrenal (HPA) axis. The hypothalamic-pituitary-ovarian malfunction centers around a marked reduction in GnRH release. In fact, the anorectic patient may have such a profound decrease in GnRH as to simulate a premenarchal girl. The transition from normal nourishment through malnourishment to the point of amenorrhea is a regression from the adult pattern of GnRH secretion (24-hour episodic secretion) through the pubertal pattern (nighttime only episodic secretion) to one of a prepubertal status (absence of episodic secretion). As weight is regained, the pattern of GnRH secretion gradually returns to normal, beginning with nighttime spikes followed by resumption of ovulation.[16] This evidence supports Frisch's theory on body fat in that as weight is lost, a gradual alteration of GnRH secretion progresses to absence of GnRH and loss of menstrual function. Weight gain reverses this process, and resumption of menses occurs.

Hypercortisolism is the reflection of adrenal malfunction in anorexia nervosa. The defect appears to be at or above the hypothalamus. Recently, the response of serum ACTH to a corticotropin releasing hormone (CRH) challenge was studied in anorectics before and after correction of weight loss.[17] While they were underweight, hypercortisolism and a blunted ACTH response to CRH were present, suggesting appropriate pituitary function in the face of elevated cortisol. Correction of weight loss is associated with a return to normal cortisol levels and normalization of the CRH test. Thus, the hypercortisolism of anorexia may reflect alterations of the hypothalamic set point for cortisol, with the pituitary and adrenal responding appropriately to these higher commands.

Successful therapy for anorexia nervosa depends on early diagnosis. Behavioral modification, psychotherapy, force feeding, or a combination of these therapies have been employed. Most important, health care providers as well as coaches, instructors, and fellow dancers should be sensitive to the high prevalence of this deadly disease and direct patients to proper therapy.

The Effect of Stress on Menstrual Function

Yet another variable that is involved in exercise-related menstrual dysfunction, and in anorexia nervosa, is stress. Quantitative measurement of stress is difficult, and various stressors have differing impacts. For example, the emotional stress of a final exam may be hard to compare to the physical stress of a marathon. This variation in what causes stress, either emotional or physical, makes research on its relationship to reproduction difficult. A dramatic example of the impact of stress on reproduction is found in a review published by

Drew in 1961 in which menstrual experience of women in World War II concentration camps was summarized.[17] Women separated from their families had higher incidences of amenorrhea despite the same diet and threat of death. Drew cited a remarkable study in 1940 showing that 100% of men and women sentenced to death for severe crimes developed total gonadal atrophy. Without exception, women became amenorrheic immediately after sentencing. Extreme stress appears to have a dramatic impact on gonadal function, but do lesser degrees of stress cause difficulties in reproduction? In Warren's 1980 study of pubertal ballet dancers, the progression of sexual development and the onset of menarche correlated in 10 of 15 subjects with a decrease in exercise or injury causing forced rest of at least 2 months' duration.[4] This occurred without changes in weight, strongly suggesting an independent role for the physical and emotional stress of training.

Stress combined with weight loss may have an even greater impact. Twenty-eight untrained college women were divided into two groups, one on a weight-maintenance and the other on a weight-loss diet, and all were placed on a strenuous exercise program.[18] Menstrual function was studied by clinical and hormonal criteria during the 2-month program. Only four subjects (three in the weight maintenance group) had normal menstrual bleeding during the observation period. The weight loss group more frequently had delayed menses and loss of LH surge (table 5-1). Six months later, no longer on the program, all of the women were cycling normally. Exercise alone, then, seems able to induce menstrual dysfunction, but when combined with weight loss, the effect is amplified.

If physical and emotional stress do have a role in menstrual dysfunctions, can we identify specific tests to predict dysfunctions? Loucks and Horvath compared blood levels of hormones associated with stress in groups of eumenorrheic and amenorrheic runners.[19] These metabolic indexes of stress were not significantly different in the two groups. Similarly, psychologic testing found no difference in eumenorrheic and amenorrheic runners. Thus, these

Table 5-1. Effects of Exercise on Menstrual Function in Two Groups of Subjects

Abnormality	Group: Weight Maintenance (N = 12), No. of Subjects (%)	Group: Weight Loss (N = 16), No. of Subjects (%)	p Value
None	3	1	NS
Clinical disorders			
Abnormal bleeding	7	7	NS
Delayed menses	1	12	<0.005
Hormonal disturbance			
Abnormal luteal function	8	10	NS
Loss of LH surge	5	13	<0.050

Modified from Bullen BA et al (ref 18)

metabolic and psychologic indicators did not reveal a quantitative measurement by which stress causes menstrual problems in some but not in others.

In summary, stress has been shown to be related to menstrual disturbance in several studies, and weight loss appears to amplify the effect. However, hormonal and psychologic testing have not been able to predict those women who will or will not develop menstrual dysfunction. As more information is gathered on the mechanisms of amenorrhea, perhaps the link to stress and reproduction will be discovered.

The Mechanisms of Weight Loss and Stress-Related Amenorrhea

The specific mechanisms by which weight loss and exercise cause menstrual dysfunction have not been defined. Large amounts of clinical data have been collected and many theories presented. First, let us review theories on the impact of weight loss.

Frisch has presented four mechanisms through which adipose tissue is involved in the metabolism of estrogens.[10] First, adipose tissue (i.e., breast, abdominal, omental, and fatty marrow of long bones) has the capability of aromatizing androgens to estrogens, thus becoming a significant source of extragonadal estrogen. Second, body weight has been shown to influence the direction of peripheral estrogen metabolism to more or less potent estrogen forms. Third, the level of the important sex hormone binding globulin, which directs transport of estrogens throughout the body, can be altered by changes in weight. Finally, fat tissue has the ability to store estrogen. Certainly these mechanisms exist, but their ability to affect menstrual performance has not been clearly established. The amenorrhea associated with stress and exercise is at least hypothalamic, and there is no evidence to suggest that these alterations in peripheral metabolism can affect central function. Perhaps there is another messenger to the hypothalamus that is affected by caloric deprivation, but at this writing no such substance has been found.

Many hormone levels fluctuate with exercise. Increases in cortisol, adrenal androgens, testosterone, prolactin, and growth hormone have been reported. Even the anticipation of exercise was found to increase LH levels.[21] The hypercortisolism seen in runners appears to be a result of increased production of cortisol. When ACTH stimulation tests were performed on runners, their cortisol response was no different from nonrunners'.[22] Thus, the abnormality leading to increased cortisol in runners must be at or above the pituitary. Testing with CRH to further evaluate this axis has not been reported. The impact of this hypercortisolism on amenorrhea is unknown, but this study found no difference in 24-hour cortisol production between amenorrheic and eumenorrheic runners, leading one to suspect that hypercortisolism is not the cause of amenorrhea in this group of women.

Chang et al studied the acute effects of exercise on prolactin and growth hormone secretion.[22] No differences were found in prolactin and growth hormone responses to exercise among eumenorrheic, oligomenorrheic, and amenorrheic women. Thus, prolactin and growth hormone do not appear to be responsible for athletic menstrual dysfunction. Thyroid metabolism has been reported to be mildly impaired during endurance training. These changes include decreased levels of the active T_3 and increases in T_4 and the relatively inactive rT_3.[23] Gonadal function is very sensitive to thyroid dysfunction, but these changes are transient and within the range of normal.

The most interesting theory links exercise to the HPO axis via the endogenous opiate neurotransmitter, beta-endorphin. The site of GnRH secretion, the arcuate nucleus in the hypothalamus, has a very high rate of endorphin production, and there is reason to believe these endorphins can affect GnRH release. Beta-endorphin has been shown to exert an inhibitory influence on GnRH pulses, and administration of naloxone (an opiate receptor antagonist) elicits a rise in LH levels.[24] Thus, we know that beta-endorphins suppress GnRH secretion, but does exercise or stress influence beta-endorphin? Carr et al reported that exercise increases plasma beta-endorphin and that training augments this effect.[25] Subsequent work failed to confirm the augmentation of beta-endorphin release by training, but did confirm elevation of the neurotransmitter during exercise.[26]

The theory that beta-endorphin is responsible for menstrual dysfunction in athletes is attractive. Although elevation of beta-endorphin and knowledge of its involvement in the HPO axis does not prove it to be the major pathway of menstrual dysfunction in these patients, the available information represents a logical explanation consistent with many of the reported facts. The manifestation of such a mechanism would be a decrease in GnRH release, and a decrease in GnRH pulse frequency from 90-100 min. to >6 hours is noted to follow exercise.[20] In addition, Cumming et al have found a decrease in pulsatile release of LH (which reflects GnRH secretion) in normal menstruating runners.[27] Although the relationship between beta-endorphin and this decreased LH activity is yet to be proven, a variety of defects in GnRH secretion from none to profound can lead to the previously described spectrum of eumenorrhea through defective luteal phases to amenorrhea.

Therapy

Management of athletic menstrual dysfunction depends on precise diagnosis of the problem and, if required, hormonal replacement therapy. It must be remembered that athletic menstrual dysfunction is a diagnosis of exclusion. The protocol for evaluating amenorrhea is the same regardless of the patient's occupation or recreation. Abnormalities in thyroid and prolactin metabolism frequently cause menstrual dysfunction, and screening for these problems by obtaining serum TSH and prolactin levels is necessary. The use of a "progestin challenge" is very helpful. This test involves prescribing a 5-day course in progestin therapy. If the endometrium has been exposed to estrogens recently, menstrual bleeding will follow. Absence of bleeding to a progestin challenge indicates hypoestrogenic amenorrhea or problems with the endometrium itself (end organ problem). To differentiate these conditions, an estrogen progestin challenge is used. This provides estrogen to the endometrium; thus, absence of menstrual bleeding following this challenge indicates end organ problems. Bleeding indicates hypoestrogenic hypogonadotropin amenorrhea, which must be confirmed by measuring the serum levels of the gonadotropins. By following this simple protocol, patients with menstrual dysfunction can be quickly placed into several diagnostic categories, including hyperprolactinemia thyroid dysfunction, end organ problems, and anovulatory or hypothalamic amenorrhea[28] (figure 5-5). All of these diagnoses have an impact on the patient's current and future well-being as well as her fertility.

Anovulation

Anovulation is associated with estrogen production alone, unopposed by progesterone. Long-standing estrogen stimulation is associated with endometrial hyperplasia, a premalignant change in the endometrium.[3] In addition, the risk of premenopausal breast cancer is increased among anovulatory women.[30] Thus, anovulatory women are placed at risk for two important malignancies. For this reason, regular therapy with progestational agents is strongly recommended; for example, 10 mg medroxyprogesterone daily for the first 10 days of each month. This clearly prevents endometrial cancer and may reduce the risk of breast cancer.[31]

Hypothalamic Amenorrhea

Hypothalamic amenorrhea is the classic presentation of athletic menstrual dysfunction. This condition is associated with low levels of estrogen,

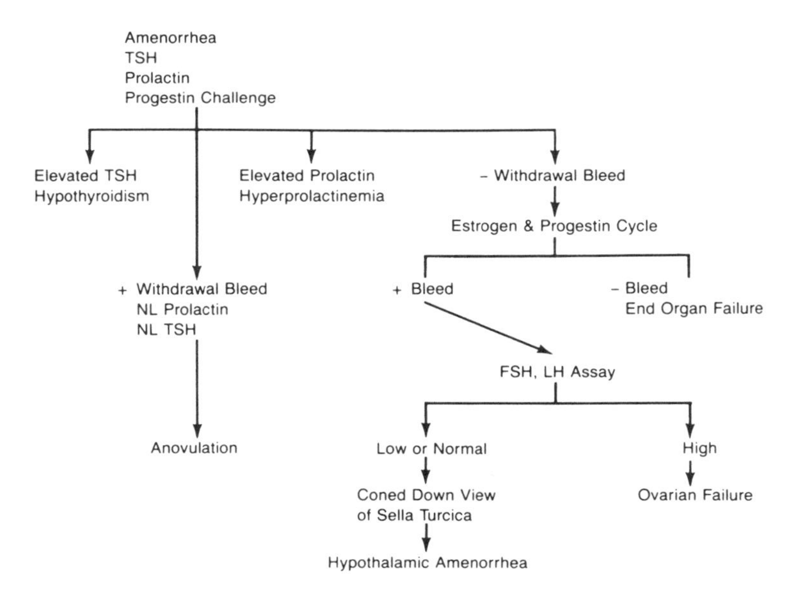

Figure 5-5. Placement of patients with menstrual dysfunction into diagnostic categories. (Modified from Speroff, Glass, Kase, ref 28.)

placing the patient at risk for problems associated with low estrogen, osteoporosis, and cardiovascular disease. The most common clinical presentation of hypoestrogenism is the menopause, and osteoporosis and cardiovascular disease have certainly been studied more in postmenopausal women than in athletes. The concepts remain the same; however, data in hypothalamic amenorrhea of athletes have indicated that the process is similar.

Osteoporosis has many causes, but the most common is associated with the menopause and loss of estrogen. Postmenopausal osteoporosis, a major health problem in this country, is frequently responsible for spinal compression fractures and hip fractures in the postmenopausal population. Although the long-term impact of hypoestrogenism on osteoporosis in postmenopausal women is known, the effects of hypoestrogenism in athletes and dancers are just beginning to be understood.

At least two forces are involved in the bone metabolism of the athlete. Exercise is known to improve bone density, whereas hypoestrogenism is known to decrease it. Which force is stronger in the young athlete? The bone density of eumenorrheic athletes has been found to be no different from normal, but amenorrheic athletes' bones have significantly reduced bone densities.[32] Thus, of the two forces described, hypoestrogenism appears to be the most powerful. A recent clinical survey confirms this prediction. A survey of 75 dancers showed a high incidence of scoliosis and stress fractures, which correlated with increased age of menarche, incidence of secondary amenorrhea, and duration of amenorrhea.[34]

This is a very serious point, as these young women are clearly suffering from injuries and pain of hypoestrogenic bone loss. Fortunately, these osteopenic changes are probably reversible. Drinkwater et al studied lumbar bone density in seven athletes while amenorrheic and after resumption of menses.[35] The resumption in menstrual function was associated with a 10% reduction in running mileage and a 1.9 kg increase in weight. A significant improvement in bone density was found, although it was not yet to the level of normally cycling women.

Because estrogen replacement protects the bones of postmenopausal patients from osteoporosis, the authors believe strongly that hypoestrogenic dancers should be treated with estrogen-progestin replacement therapy. Calcium supplementation of 500 mg elemental calcium per day should also be included in the patient's treatment plan. If the patient does not take estrogen replacement, then calcium supplements of 1,000-1,500 mg per day should be prescribed. With this regimen, we can expect to see improvement in bone metabolism and less risk of injury.

The long-term risk of cardiovascular disease in the hypoestrogenic athlete has not been evaluated. Again referring to the postmenopause model of hypoestrogenic patients, estrogen replacement therapy reduces the risk of heart attack as compared to menopausal nonestrogen users.[36] The mechanism of this reduced risk is thought to be estrogen elevation of the protective HDL cholesterol in the blood, one of the proteins involved in transport of cholesterol. This argument can also be applied to the hypoestrogenic athlete, and we can assume a similar protection is provided hypoestrogenic athletes treated with estrogen replacement therapy.

Method of Treatment

Estrogen replacement may consist of conjugated equine estrogen, 0.625 mg daily (or its equivalent) for the first 25 days of each month and medroxy-progesterone acetate 10 mg per day on days 16 through 25. This dose is enough to protect the bones, the endometrium, and probably the cardiovascular system, and usually is enough to restore menstruation. However, this dose is not enough to protect against pregnancy. Occasional ovulations may occur and pregnancy can result. If the patient needs hormone replacement and is sexually active, the new low-dose oral contraceptives provide all the advantages of hormone replacement as well as protection against pregnancy. Of course, when the athlete discontinues the oral contraceptive in the future, she may well find herself amenorrheic again. This "postpill amenorrhea" is to be expected; it is not due to the oral contraceptive itself. Many forms of calcium supplementation are available. The patient should choose the least expensive form of supplementation that is tolerated by her digestive system and provides 500 mg of elemental calcium per day.

Summary

Although extensively studied, little has been clearly proven regarding the etiology of menstrual dysfunction in dancers and athletes. The dysfunction is varied, and the physician must remember that athletic menstrual dysfunction is a diagnosis of exclusion. When needed, a program of hormone replacement, either progestin alone or estrogen plus progestin should be used along with calcium supplements. Physicians and other participants in dance (coaches, parents, fellow dancers), should note the impact of stress and weight loss on reproductive functions and be alert for signs of the dangerous anorexia nervosa.

References

1. McKay WJS, Wood W. The history of ancient gynaecology. Bailliere, Pendall, and Cox, 1901.
2. Vincent LM. Competing with the sylph. Kansas City KS: Andrews and McMeel, 1979.
3. Frisch RE, Wyshak G, Vincent L. Delayed menarche and amenorrhea in ballet dancers. N Engl J Med 1980; 303:17.
4. Warren MP. The effects of exercise on pubertal progression and reproductive function in girls. J Clin Endocrinol Metab 1980; 51:1150.
5. Frisch RE, Gotz-Welbergen AV, McArthur JW et al. Delayed menarche and amenorrhea of college athletes in relation to age of onset of training. JAMA 1981; 246:1559.
6. Ronkainen H, Pakarinen A, Kauppila A. Pubertal and menstrual disorders of female runners, skiers, and volleyball players. Gynecol Obstet Invest 1984; 18:183.
7. Sanborn CF, Martin BJ, Wagner WW. Is athletic amenorrhea specific to runners? Am J Obstet Gynecol 1982; 143:859.
8. Prior JC, Cameron K, Yuen BH, Thomas J. Menstrual cycle changes with marathon training: anovulation and short luteal phase. Can J Appl Sport Sci 1982; 7:173.
9. Shangold M. The relationship between long-distance running, plasma progesterone, and luteal phase length. Fertil Steril 1979; 31:130.

10. Frisch RE. Body fat, puberty and fertility. Biol Rev 1984; 59:161.

11. Speroff L, Redwine DM. Exercise and menstrual function. Phys Sportsmed 1980; 8:42.

12. Loucks AB, Horvath SM, Freedson PS. Menstrual status and validation of body fat prediction in athletes. Hum Biol 1984; 56:383.

13. Abraham SF, Beumont PJV, Fraser IS, Llewellyn-Jones D. Body weight, exercise and menstrual status among ballet dancers in training. Br J Obstet Gynecol 1982; 89:507.

14. Warren M. Effect of exercise and physical training on menarche. Semin Reprod Endocrinol 1985; 3:17.

15. Boyar RM, Katz MJ, Finkelstein JW et al. Anorexia nervosa immaturity of the 24-hour luteinizing hormone secretory pattern. N Engl J Med 1974; 291:861.

16. Gold PN, Gwirtsman H, Avgerinos PC et al. Abnormal hypothalamic-pituitary-adrenal function in anorexia nervosa. N Engl J Med 1986; 314:1335.

17. Drew FL. The epidemology of secondary amenorrhea. J Chron Dis 1961; 14:396.

18. Bullen BA, Skrinar GS, Beitins IZ, Von Mering G, Turnbull BA, McArthur JW. Induction of menstrual disorders by strenuous exercise in untrained women. N Engl J Med 1985; 312:1349.

19. Loucks AB, Horvath SM. Exercise-induced stress responses of amenorrheic and eumenorrheic runners. J Clin Endocrinol Metab 1984; 59:1109.

20. Cumming DC, Rebar RW. Hormonal changes with acute exercise and with training in women. Semin Reprod Endocrinol 1985; 3:55.

21. Villaneuva AL, Schlosser C, Hopper B, Liu JH, Hoffman DI, Rebar RW. Increased cortisol production in women runners. J Clin Endocrinol Metab 1986; 63:133.

22. Chang FE, Dodds WG, Sullivan M, Kim MH, Malarkey WB. The acute effects of exercise on prolactin and growth hormone secretion: comparison between sedentary women and women runners with normal and abnormal menstrual cycles. J Clin Endocrinol Metab 1986; 62:551.

23. Boyden TW, Pamenter RW, Rotkis TC, Stanforth P, Wilmore JH. Thyroidal changes associated with endurance training in women. Med Sci in Sports and Exerc 1984; 16:243.

24. Yen, SSC. Opiates and reproduction: studies in women. In: Delitala G, ed. Opioid modulation of endocrine function. New York: Raven Press, 1984.

25. Carr DB, Bullen BA, Skrinar GS et al. Physical conditioning facilitates the exercise induced secretion of beta endorphin and beta-lipotropin in women. N Engl J Med 1981; 305:560.

26. Howlett TA, Tomlin S, Ngahfoong L et al. Release of b-endorphin and met-enkephlin during exercise in normal women: response to training. Br Med J 1984; 288:1950.

27. Cumming DC, Vickovic MA, Wall SR, Fluker MR, Belcastro AN. The effect of acute exercise on pulsatile release of luteinizing hormone in women runners. Am J Obstet Gynecol 1985; 153:482.

28. Speroff L, Glass RH, Kase NG. Clinical gynecologic endocrinology and infertility. Baltimore: Williams and Wilkins, 1983; 141.

29. Benirschke K. The endometrium. In: Yen SSC, Jaffe RB. Reproductive endocrinology. Philadelphia: WB Saunders, 1986; 385.

30. Cowan LD, Gordis L, Tonascia JA, Jones GS. Breast cancer incidence in women with a history of progesterone deficiency. Am J Epidemiol 1981; 114:209.

31. Gambrell RD Jr. The menopause: benefits and risks of estrogen-(progestogen) replacement therapy. Fertil Steril 1982; 37:457.

32. Drinkwater BL, Nilson K, Chesnut CH III. Bone mineral content of amenorrheic and eumenorrheic athletes. N Engl J Med 1984; 311:277.

33. Lindsay R, Aitken JM, Anderson JB, Hart DM, MacDonald EB, Clarke AC. Long-term prevention of postmenopausal osteoporosis by estrogen. Lancet 1976; 1:1038.

34. Marcus R, Cann C, Madvig P et al. Menstrual function and bone mass in elite women distance runners. Ann Intern Med 1985; 102:158.

35. Warren MP, Brooks-Gunn J, Hamilton LH, Warren LF, Hamilton WG. Scoliosis and fractures in young ballet dancers. N Engl J Med 1986; 314:1348.

36. Drinkwater BL, Nilson K, Ott S, Chestnut CH. Bone mineral density after resumption of menses in amenorrheic athlete. JAMA 1986; 256:380.

37. Henderson BE, Ross RK, Paganini-Hill A, Mack TM. Estrogen use and cardiovascular disease. Am J Obstet Gynecol 1986; 154:1181.

6

NUTRITION AND THE DANCER

Alvin R. Loosli, M.D., Joan Benson, R.D., and Donna M. Gillien, M.S.

THE THIN, WISPY BODY has been the artistic standard for the female ballet dancer for the past 100 years. The classical dancers of the nineteenth century romantic period were like ghosts blowing weightlessly across the stage. In the 1920s, George Balanchine arrived from Russia to begin leadership of the New York City Ballet. He further refined the romantic period image of the ballet dancer to the thin, sylphlike ballerina she is today. The long, thin woman became the aesthetic standard. Uniformity and a pleasing line with "the look" are the ultimate goals. It is no wonder that female ballet dancers are therefore preoccupied with their weight.[1,2]

Today, thinness is a standard by which not only dancers are judged but by which all women are judged. The pursuit of the ideal body form has led dancers to try to manipulate their weight in inappropriate and frequently pathologic fashion.

Studies of Dancers' Nutritional Status

Little scientific evidence confirmed the abnormal eating patterns until Garner and Garfinkel in 1978 documented the high incidence of anorexia nervosa associated with female ballet dancers.[3] Using their eating attitude test, they discovered an astounding 5 percent incidence of anorexia nervosa, a condition characterized by self-induced starvation. In ballet dancers, the physiological consequences of anorexia nervosa include ketonemia, loss of muscle tissue, reduced blood volume, hypotension, weakness, and fainting. Recent research has shown the bone density of anorexic women to be equivalent to that of 60-year-old women.[4]

Shortly after the Garner and Garfinkel research was published, Vincent published his book *Competing with the Sylph.*[1] Vincent, a dancer himself and a radiologist, studied the nutrition habits of the New York City Ballet students by means of interviews. This work seemed to bridge the gap between the ballet and scientific community regarding dance nutrition. In his book, Vincent describes the ballet world of dieting, dehydration, diuretics, and anorexia nervosa: "If one didn't know any better, one might get the impression that certain dancers are intentionally bent on dehydrating themselves... Worse yet, some will pursue sweat sessions while simultaneously restricting water and salt, an outlandishly stupid and dangerous practice." As little as 2 percent dehydration will impair thermoregulatory function, and 3 percent reduces muscle endurance.[5]

Dancers are not the only athletes to intentionally dehydrate. Wrestlers, jockeys, and Little League football players may participate in intentional dehydration as they try to meet weight restrictions. Most of these athletes rehydrate prior to their athletic performance, however. The dancer is in the chronic state of dehydration much of the time, a condition that induces fatigue, poor performance, and increased risk of injury.

Scientific evaluation of the female ballet dancer's nutrition practices has been documented by two recent research projects. Calabrese et al evaluated the nutrition patterns and body compositions of professional female classical ballet dancers.[6] Benson et al documented the nutritional practices of serious female adolescent ballet dancers.[7] Although the two groups are quite different, one being adult professionals and the other adolescent amateurs, findings in both groups are similar. Tables 6-1 and 6-2 summarize these two research projects. It should be noted that slightly different standards of nutritional inadequacy were used for each group.

Calories, the most basic nutrient, appeared inadequate in both professional and amateur. Special concern should be given to inadequate calorie intake in the adolescent population. Pugilese has demonstrated growth retardation in the chronically dieting teenager.[8]

Severe deficiencies in folic acid and Vitamin B_6 intake occurred in both groups. Because these vitamins are concerned with energy, metabolism, and hemoglobin production, deficiencies may manifest themselves in poor performance.

Of most importance seemed to be the mineral content of these dancers' diets. Calcium, the important mineral in bone strength, was seriously deficient in 60 percent of the professionals and 40 percent of the adolescent dancers. With the recent implication of low calcium intake, amenorrhea, and osteoporo-

Table 6-1. Three-Day Nutritional Survey of Female Ballet Dancer

	Professional[1] (mean day)	Adolescent[2] (mean day)
Kilocalories	1,358 Cal	1,890 Cal
Total protein	47.4 gm	72 gm
Total fat	52.3 gm	75 gm
Total carbohydrate	168.3 gm	235 gm

Table 6-2. Vitamin and Mineral Intake of Female Ballet Dancers

	Professional (% dancers with less than 85% RDA, including supplements)	Adolescent (% dancers with less than 66% RDA, including supplements)
Vitamin A	40	10
Folic acid	80	58
Vitamin B_6	65	42
Vitamin B_{12}	55	16
Vitamin C	12	8
Iron	78	50
Calcium	60	40
Zinc	100	75

sis, these low levels of calcium ingestion seem ominous.[9] Iron intake was inadequate in 50 percent of the adolescents. Although frank iron deficiency in dancers is unusual, subclinical iron deficiency manifested by decreased total body stores, when combined with dehydration may further compound the risk of fatigue, poor performance, and injury. Eighty percent of all dancers had inadequate zinc intake. Once again, frank zinc deficiency states are rare, but chronic tendinitis or poor wound healing after surgery may result from inadequate zinc intake.

The scientific evaluation of the use of vitamin and mineral supplements is interesting. Calabrese and Benson both show that female ballet dancers, although they use supplements regularly, more often than not use them inappropriately. They rarely make up for nutritional deficiencies with their supplements. For instance, the dancer who is low in iron intake in her food infrequently takes iron pills.

Nutritional surveys of the type Calabrese and Benson completed must be interpreted with caution. Some errors in method and data collection are inevitable. However, these studies should provide a sound basis for nutritional counseling of the female ballet dancer.

Even fewer scientific data are available for male ballet dancers. Because male dancers do not have the strict weight requirements and naturally are able to eat more calories, nutrition problems, dehydration, nutritional deficiencies, and eating disorders occur less frequently. Sound nutritional practices in the male dancers must be encouraged, however.

What about the modern or less traditional female dancer? Any female dancer who is pursuing the ideal body form or "the look" will have all the risks inherent in that pursuit—that is, dehydration, nutritional inadequacies, and eating disorders. These female dancers must also have sound nutrition counseling and advice.

Counseling the Dancer

Advising the ballet dancer about nutrition and weight loss poses a unique challenge to the counselor. First, a dancer who is anxious about body size may be far from having the appearance of one in need of weight loss counseling. Dancers who are at ideal body weight by medical standards, however, are likely to be considered obese by the artistic directors' more stringent weight standards. Therefore, the counselor must relinquish any previous notions of ideal body weights generally applicable to the nondance population.

Second, because of the prevalence of distorted body image,[2] amenorrhea,[6] and episodes of binging often followed by vomiting or purging[1] behavior among dancers, one may be tempted to suspect that frank eating disorders are ubiquitous in the dance population. The difficulty of diagnosing anorexia nervosa accurately in a ballerina who is required to be exceedingly thin and is therefore highly preoccupied with her weight cannot be overemphasized. Garner et al have shown that women who are highly preoccupied with their weight often display psychopathy similar to anorexia nervosa, yet fail to meet the rigorous diagnostic standards for that diagnosis.[3]

Third, training activities for ballerinas, which feature short periods of high-intensity dance, require that they severely restrict their calorie intake in order to maintain the required body size. To lose weight, dancers may actually restrict their calorie intake to levels below that regarded as safe by clinicians.

Fourth, the reported nutrition beliefs and practices among dancers are problematic. Several studies have suggested that dancers consume inadequate amounts of macro and micro nutrients.[6,7] In addition, dancers may not be receptive to scientifically accepted nutrition information. They often get advice on diet and weight control from other dancers or dance instructors and may lack confidence in more orthodox approaches.

Finally, the dancer's hectic schedule and beliefs regarding the ergogenic benefits of consuming specific foods only at specific times creates many restrictions upon the scheduling of meals.

The Treatment

Obviously, many factors must be considered when advising a dancer about diet and weight control. One first needs to gather information about the individual. Is the dancer in a growth spurt? Is the addition of routine aerobic exercise a possibility? What is the dancer's impression of her own body size, and how much weight loss is desired? A reasonable dance weight, based on a target body composition (percent body fat) and appearance, can be arrived at by taking skinfold measurements at four sites (triceps, biceps, subscapular, and iliac crest) and by comparing the individual's height to the weights listed for the lowest weight for frame size on the Metropolitan Life Insurance tables. Frame size is estimated by taking wrist circumference. Body fat of 12–17 percent is usually considered acceptable for ballet.

If the dancer agrees with the proposed goal weight, then a calorie level that may offer a reasonable rate of weight loss can be determined. Intensive training and optimal performance require sufficient calories to maintain body protein and glycogen stores. Adequate calories are especially important for the adolescent dancer in meeting the increased needs of pubertal growth and development.

To design an appropriate diet, one needs next to examine actual dietary practices. A thorough diet history should include when, where, and what the dancer eats. Types of supplements, foods allergies or aversions, budget, and binge-associated foods should be noted. From this history, the usual daily calorie intake can be calculated. A deficit of about 600 calories below this amount will result in a loss of 2–2½ lb. per week. Caloric needs can also be estimated by multiplying ideal weight in pounds by 15 (by 30 during a growth spurt). Subtracting 500 calories from this amount would provide an energy level resulting in similar weight loss. If the diet history reveals that a dancer is maintaining an undesirably high weight on an intake of less than 1,200 calories, then increasing aerobic activity is preferred to any further reduction in diet. Because the typical dance routine is a series of starts and stops, where time spent actively exercising is relatively short compared to the amount of time at rest, calorie expenditure in class is limited. The addition of aerobic exercise, such as swimming or cycling, would shift the balance of calories expended to calories consumed in the direction of weight loss without further risking nutritional deficits. However, dancers should be cautioned against running or jogging because of the high risk of joint injuries associated with this activity.

Studies have reported that dancers engage in binge behavior more frequently than age-matched controls.[3] Boredom, depression, anxiety, and loneliness are the most commonly reported nonhunger cues triggering binge eating. Behavioral or psychological counseling may be useful to an individual plagued with such problems. In addition, the dancer can be cautioned to pay attention to those foods that trigger binge behavior. Rather than buying a binge-associated food, such as a whole chocolate cake, the dancer could satisfy an urge by ordering a piece of cake at a restaurant, where the ability to go back for seconds or thirds is curtailed.

In devising a diet plan, one will need to consider that the dancer's eating habits are dictated by a hectic schedule of class, performance, and rehearsal. On the eve of a performance, the main meal is delayed until late at night. During the day, dancers tend to skip meals, grab quick snacks or sodas from vending machines, and eat outside of the home. Fluid intake may be neglected. Therefore, it may be useful to construct several specific menus tailored to the calorie needs, schedules, and food preferences of the individual. The difficulties in making food more portable, varied, and consistent with life "on the road" are unavoidable. Nevertheless, the eventual diet ideally should be composed of at least 60% carbohydrate calories, 15–20% protein, and 15–20% fat. Nutritional adequacy is achieved by including the following foods:

Low-fat milk group—Two servings for adults, 4 for adolescents. One serving equals: 8 oz. skim milk, 8 oz. nonfat yogurt, 1½ oz. low-fat cheese (light cheese or mozzarella), ½ cup cottage cheese. These foods provide protein, calcium, and riboflavin.

Low-fat meat group—Two servings. One serving is equal to 2 oz. of cooked lean beef, poultry, pork or fish, or 1 cup cooked beans or ½ cup of tofu. These foods are excellent sources of iron, zinc, B vitamins, and high quality protein.

Fruits and vegetables—Four servings. One cup raw or ½ cooked vegetables, or 1/2 cup juice, or one piece of fresh fruit is one serving. Dark, leafy, green, or orange vegetables are high in vitamin A and are recommended 3–4 times a week. Citrus fruits are rich in vitamin C and are recommended daily. All of these foods are good sources of carbohydrates and fiber.

Grain group—Four servings. One slice of bread, 1 cup of dry cereal or 1/2 cup of cooked cereal or cooked pasta, rice, mashed potatoes, or corn, or one small baked potato equals one serving. Whole-grain foods are preferable. All are excellent sources of complex carbohydrates and B vitamins and fiber.

When and in what form these foods are consumed are issues decided upon by the dancer and the nutritionist. The above recommendations provide <1,200 calories a day, and represent a minimum intake for weight loss. The challenge is to prepare these foods with a minimum of fat. Additional fat is not essential for good health or performance and will increase calories dramatically. To cut the fat intake:

1. Meats should be trimmed of visible fat and, rather than being fried, should be roasted, stir fried in a Teflon pan or with a nonfat cooking spray, or stewed with spices, bouillon, or wine.
2. Vegetables can be steamed with herbs, boiled in bouillon, or flavored with soy sauce.
3. Pasta can be mixed with nonfat yogurt and herbs or sprinkled with low-fat cheese, garlic, or tomato bits. Tomato-based sauces are lower in fat than cream-based sauces.
4. Potatoes may be topped with buttermilk or buttermilk-based dressing made with diet mayonnaise.
5. Diet margarine spread thinly on bread provides considerably less fat than butter or margarine.
6. Tuna can be mixed with a combination of nonfat yogurt or sour half-and-half and diet mayonnaise.
7. Low-calorie salad dressings often contain negligible fat, but amounts vary, and labels should be examined.
8. Restaurants are now catering to a diet-conscious clientele. Salads may be ordered with dressing on the side, and broiled or grilled chicken and fish are usually available. The fat content of mixed dishes such as stroganoff or lasagna is inconsistent, and these foods are best avoided. Starches and vegetables can be requested without additional butter.

Unquestionably, the time spent planning a nutritious low-fat and convenient diet is well worthwhile to a dancer whose career success depends upon a healthy, injury-free, and well-nourished body. It is advisable for dancers who must restrict their calorie intake to include a daily vitamin and mineral supplement, providing 100% of the RDA for these nutrients. In addition, food supplements such as Instant Breakfast, which can be mixed with skim milk and is available sugar-free, and Ensure provide one-fourth of the RDA for nutrients and are acceptable meal replacements.

In few disciplines is food such an emotional issue as in ballet. Helping the dancer plan a diet that is nutritionally complete, provides adequate energy for dance, and yet maintains a trim body cannot be done in one visit. Follow-up and continuous support are essential to success, but the rewards of such efforts can be great.

References

1. Vincent LM. Competing with the sylph. Kansas City, KS: Andrews and McMeel, 1979.
2. Gordon S. Off balance. New York: McGraw-Hill, 1983.
3. Garner DM, Garfinkel PE. Sociocultural factors in anorexia nervosa. Lancet, 1978; 2 (8091): 674.
4. Crosby L, Kaplan F, Pertschuk MJ, Mullen JL. The effect of anorexia nervosa on bone morphometry in young women. Clin Orthop & Rel Res, 1985; 201:271–277.
5. McArdle WD, Katch FI, Katch VL. Exercise physiology. Philadelphia: Lea & Febiger, 1986; 451–453.
6. Calabrese LH, Kirkendall DT, Floyd M et al. Menstrual abnormalities, nutritional patterns and body composition in female classical ballet dancers. Phys Sportsmed 1983; 11:86–98.
7. Benson J. Gillien DM, Bourdet K, Loosli AR. Inadequate nutrition and chronic calorie restriction in adolescent ballerinas. Phys Sportsmed 1985; 13:79–90.
8. Pugliese HT, Lifschitz F, Grad G et al. Fear of obesity: a cause of short stature and delayed puberty. N Engl J Med 1983; 309:513–518.
9. Cann CE, Martin MC, Genant HK. Detection of premenopausal women at risk of the development of osteoporosis. 64th Annu Meeting of Endrocrine Soc, San Francisco, 1982.

7

THE YOUNG BALLET DANCER

A. J. G. Howse, F.R.C.S.

UNFORTUNATELY, THE YOUNG BALLET dancer is often the subject of mishandling, normally through ignorance and poor teaching. Much of the trouble arises because the teachers set goals for their young students that are physically impossible for them to attain. Some of the results of poor training will be considered in this chapter.

The Age to Start Dancing

Although a keen student can start learning to dance at any age, even as late as early adult life, there is no doubt that those who start early have a distinct physical advantage over those who do not start until their teens. Children should, therefore, start to dance as early as possible. Initially, this should be confined to rhythm, coordination, development of musicality, and generally enjoyable activity. Without making too much of a chore of it and thus discouraging the child, great concentration should be placed on strengthening all the muscle groups. During these early years, there should be no particular effort to get the child to turn out and no concentration on ballet technique as such until about the age of 10. The child's own image is, of course, with the feet turned out as far as they will go, but this should be discouraged. Unfortunately, it is in the very young child that the greatest damage can be done by stressing turnout. For the child who is starting early, a sympathetic, knowledgeable, and understanding teacher is essential. We have found that with such a teacher, the children gain far more than they would if attempting complex ballet techniques at an early age. They soon assimilate these techniques at the age of 9 or 10, and when they start to do so they are very much stronger as a result of the concentration on general exercise and strengthening; also, they have far better balance and coordination.

Stretching certainly should not take place until the children are about 10 years old, unless they are unusually mature. When active stretching does start, it should be by the hold/relax technique so that it is under full control. Passive stretching by a third party is highly undesirable because it pushes the child down into splits, forcing the foot passively into excessive *pointe* and forcibly stretching the hamstrings. Time spent on teaching the exercises for the isolation of various muscle groups is also well worthwhile. This can be helpful when the youngsters are doing exercise patterns.

It must always be remembered that most children who attend dance classes are merely going to pursue dance as a hobby and for pleasure; only a very small minority will eventually progress to a professional dancing school.

Selection and Body Types

Probably the only body type that can be definitely ruled out for dancing is the large, heavy-framed body. This is, of course, particularly applicable to the female, but even a large, heavy-framed male dancer would be unsuitable for many parts. At present, as far as the females are concerned, the image is that of a dancer who is slender, relatively light-boned, and not very tall. However, as various paintings and photographs over the years have shown, fashions in shape do tend to vary. Later in life, when the student is approaching the time for entering a dance company, the selection for classical ballet is more rigid than for contemporary or modern dance, where wider variation in body type is acceptable.

Joint mobility is one of the paramount considerations in the selection of students, a process which for most professional schools in the United Kingdom, generally takes place when the dancer is about 10 years old. Although with good training, the mobility of the joints can be increased and tight areas can be stretched to a certain extent, this improvement is not exceptionally great. In other words, a child who is stiff at the age of 10 will not, even with the best of training, become very mobile by the time growth is complete. Therefore, general stiffness is certainly a contraindication to dancing. The student would not be able to attain the required positions of turn-out, back bends, *arabesques,* and *grands battements* and would, as a result, be prone to recurrent injury.

Not nearly so well recognized, however, is the opposite situation, the student who is extremely mobile. Hypermobile dancers have far greater problems and are certainly much more prone to injury than those who are on the slightly stiff side of the desirable range of joint mobility. In the very mobile dancer, strength is extremely important in controlling hypermobility. Hypermobility, accompanied by even relative muscle weakness, is absolutely certain to lead to recurrent injuries, frequently more severe than those sustained by the average dancer. These injuries tend to multiply, with one injury producing a further injury at a different site or recurring at the same site, and can lead to early termination of a dance career. Unfortunately, the hypermobile dancer can have great difficulty in building up sufficient strength to control the very mobile joints. Unfortunately, hypermobile students are often welcomed as being excellent material for ballet. But they should not be accepted unless they display considerable potential dance talent, just as a slightly stiff student should not be considered unless apparently talented.

Good mobility (not hypermobility) is essential in the spine, where one would wish to specifically exclude a stiff lower lumbar segment. The natural turn-out with the hips extended must be in excess of 45-50° on each side. Less than this will tend to lead to problems, particularly with the knees and feet. This is because the student will tend to force the turn-out, turning the feet excessively and producing a rotational strain at the knees. Relatively loose hamstrings, calf muscles, and Achilles tendons are desirable. Of course, a well-pointed foot is an essential for classical ballet.

Restriction of extension of the great toe joint (i.e., an early hallux rigidus) is a contraindication to any form of dancing, as the restricted movement will gradually increase over time and will interfere with *demi-pointe* work, also an essential requirement in any form of dance.

The selection panel should not be misled into thinking that genuine tightness in any area is going to improve significantly, no matter how careful the training might be. However, the extremely talented child will probably be able to cope with a multitude of physical difficulties that would prove the downfall of the average dancer. Additionally, the various different dance forms can accommodate a variety of body types that might be unsuitable for classical ballet.

The Age to Start *Pointe* Work

There is no particular age to start *pointe* work. It has always been considered that about 12 is correct, but this broad statement does not take into account the state of development of the child. *Pointe* work certainly should not commence until growth has been completed in the feet and strength has been gained in the feet, ankles, legs, and trunk. Many well-known dancers have achieved great success in their professional careers even though they were physically unable to start their *pointe* work until they were into their mid-teens.

The child must be able to hold the turn-out at the hips, be generally stable around the hips on one or both legs, and be strong and stable in the trunk. Should there be any weakness or instability in any of these areas, the child will be extremely unstable and unsafe when coming up on *pointe.* Far better long-term results are obtained if *pointe* work is deferred until the child is ready physically and not begun just because a certain calendar age has been reached.

Pointe work must be avoided when the feet and body are still soft and mobile because considerable damage can be done. Also, a word of caution about children with hypermobile feet and ankles: It is at this time that if they come up onto the overpointed foot they can sustain damage along the dorsum of the foot and the front of the ankle. As with other areas of hypermobility, students with hypermobile feet must work so that they have extra-strong muscles that will control the pointed foot in the optimum position and prevent it from overpointing when they are on full *pointe.*

Growth Spurts

Many of the problems facing the teacher who instructs classes rather than individual students are associated with the different rates of growth and stages of maturity of children who are about the same age. Nearly all children tend to have one or more growth spurts in adolescence during which they grow very rapidly in a short period. However conscientious the teacher has been in working for and attaining a satisfactory level of strength, when a growth spurt occurs the strength can seem to disappear completely, and children can become relatively uncontrolled in their movements. This is a time for extra care on the part of the teacher and a restraining hand on the activities of the children. During a growth spurt, students must work carefully. They will need encouragement, as they often feel that they are falling behind their contemporaries, and will need reassurance that once growth at this rate has stopped, their strength and control will return.

Also associated with a growth spurt is the relative stiffening of various areas. In a growth spurt, the long bones grow faster than the soft tissues, and apparent tightening can result. This is particularly apparent in the hamstrings and the gastrocnemius-soleus tendon complex. When the growth spurt ceases, the soft tissues catch up in growth and the previous mobility is restored. It is extremely important that the child be actively discouraged from any excessive stretching during these periods, as stretching muscles that have weakened during the growth spurt can cause damage.

Diseases and Injuries in the Young Dancer

Children are prone to a variety of childhood ailments during the course of which they normally should not dance. In the active child, probably the most significant of these conditions is mononucleosis, a disorder that can be extremely debilitating. If the infection has been anything more than slight, it may be as long as a whole term before the child can return to full dance training. Should the return be too soon, the child will be highly vulnerable to injuries.

Development of scoliosis in adolescence is not uncommon, but most cases fortunately remain mild. Treatment, if required, should be undertaken by an orthopedic surgeon, and certainly an opinion should be sought early. Most scolioses occur in the dorsal region, where movement normally is relatively limited. The area of the spine affected by the scoliosis tends to become very stiff. If the lumbar region is affected, this stiffness can seriously interfere with the range of movement required by dance. Apart from that factor, scoliosis per se is not a contraindication to continued dance training. Indeed, the exercise of dancing may act as an adjunct to that specifically prescribed by the orthopedic surgeon. It should be realized that unless the scoliosis is minimal, the resulting deformity will almost certainly rule out acceptance of the student by a professional company when training has been completed. Once marked scoliosis has developed, therefore, it should be emphasized to the student and to the parents that continuation of dancing should be for pleasure rather than with the thought of a professional career.

As far as injuries are concerned, there is no significant difference between those sustained by adolescents and those sustained by adults. There are, however, some conditions in the young dancer that are worthy of special mention, the most important being anterior knee pain. This is probably the complaint that most frequently brings a young dance student to the orthopedic surgeon. Anterior knee pain can be divided into two categories; in the first, the pain is associated with the patella, and in the second, it is associated with the tibial tubercle.

Pain around the patella is frequently mislabeled chondromalacia patellae, a relatively rare condition. Although there are usually no actual changes of chondromalacia in the patellar articular cartilage in the child with knee pain, the symptoms are most frequently associated with the patellofemoral joint. The pain is sometimes confined to the inferior pole of the patella and the proximal portion of the patellar tendon. In this age group, pain at all these sites is almost invariably associated with muscle weakness and imbalance. In particular, this imbalance is between the lateral part of the quadriceps muscle (the vastus lateralis) and the medial part of the muscle (the vastus medialis). The medial weakness often will include the adductors, with weakness in these latter two frequently occurring together in a variety of conditions. An imbalance between the vastus lateralis and the vastus medialis will produce lateral tracking of the patella, as in this situation the vastus lateralis is always stronger than the medialis. As a result of this lateral tracking, patellofemoral pain develops, and this is labeled chondromalacia patellae. At the same time, an oblique pull is applied to the patellar tendon. This may result in pain at the inferior pole of the patella and in the upper fibers of the patellar tendon.

The muscle imbalance is frequently associated with rolling at the feet, forcing the turn-out and excessive turn-out of the feet, or having the body weight too far back from any cause. The presence of hyperextended knees tends to aggravate the situation because the weight is pushed back and because such knees discourage an adequate quadriceps contraction (the dancer tends to relax onto the posterior capsule and not pull the quadriceps up properly when working).

Pain at the tibial tubercle is usually due to Osgood Schlatter disease, which is an osteochondritis of the tibial tubercle apophysis. This condition is very common in active and athletic adolescents and not just in dance students. It is probably most commonly produced by a relative weakness of the quadriceps muscle, frequently associated with a period of rapid growth. This relative weakness of the quadriceps causes a jerking pull on the lower tendon attachment rather than an even, controlled pull.

Both patella-type pain and tibial tubercle pain are best treated by rest from activity if the condition is very painful, followed by a gradual buildup in muscle strength. In particular, much attention must be given to the correct lateral/medial balance of the quadriceps so that by the time the treatment program has been completed, any tendency for lateral tracking of the patella will have been overcome. Additionally, technical help will be required to correct a situation in which the body weight is too far back. This help is particularly appropriate if there are hyperextended knees so that the child can be taught to pull up with the quadriceps and hold the knees straight instead of pushing back on them.

In the feet, the commonest condition commencing in adolescence is hallux rigidus, a degenerative arthritis of the first metatarsophalangeal joints. This progressive disease, which gradually decreases the range of movement of the great toe, cannot be halted, and its presence is a contraindication to an attempted dance career.

Adolescent hallux valgus, a familial condition, starts as a metatarsus primus varus. If severe, the condition is best treated by an osteotomy of the first metatarsal. This should be carried out in the mid-teens, when growth of the feet has stopped. Care must be taken to ensure that the surgery does not result in any stiffness developing in the first metatarsophalangeal joints.

Osteochondritis of the head of the second or third metatarsal (Freiberg infraction) occurs in adolescence, although it is not particularly common. If detected early, it can be treated by surgery. The neck of the metatarsal can be opened, the flattened metatarsal head can be pushed back up into shape, and the head of the metatarsal then can be packed with cancellous bone obtained from the shaft of the metatarsal. Dancing should be avoided, along with any other athletic activity, until the bone has consolidated and the head of the metatarsal can be seen by x-ray as having regained its normal shape and texture. Unfortunately, the condition is usually not detected until considerable collapse of the metatarsal head and some necrosis of the bone have taken place. At this stage, it is far too late to attempt any reconstruction of the metatarsal head. By this time, the condition will have resulted in some stiffness of the affected metatarsophalangeal joint. If the stiffness is sufficient to cause pain and disability, it can be relieved surgically by excision of the proximal half of the proximal phalanx and any prominent osteophytes of the metatarsal head. If this is followed by intensive physical therapy to help regain full movement of the metatarsophalangeal joint, the result is entirely satisfactory, and there will be no interference with future dancing, even though the affected toe will be slightly shortened.

Most other injuries sustained by the young ballet dancer can be treated in the same way as if the same injuries occurred in an adult. Because of the importance of early detection, one other condition is worthy of mention even though its treatment is not different in the adolescent. This condition is a stress fracture of the pars interarticularis, usually of the fifth lumbar vertebra but sometimes of the fourth. This stress fracture commonly occurs when the child is inappropriately encouraged or allowed to turn out the feet excessively. If the turn-out is forced at the feet and cannot be matched by comparable turn-out at the hips, then the dancer, whether child or adult, will drop into a lordotic posture. If continued for an appreciable length of time, this posture leads to a gradual weakening of the trunk muscles in children. They may never be able to develop any strength in the trunk muscles. This in turn places considerable stress on the fourth and fifth lumbar vertebrae, particularly when landing from jumps, and in due course a stress fracture of one or both partes interarticulares will occur.

Any young ballet dancer who complains of persistent lower back pain that does not respond to conservative measures should be suspected of having a stress fracture, particularly if the turn-out is rather tight and if a lordotic posture is assumed during work. Oblique x-rays of the lumbar spine may show the stress fracture, but frequently this will not become radiologically apparent for some months after the onset of symptoms. If there is any doubt at all, a bone scan will demonstrate a hot spot indicative of a developing stress fracture. It is the author's opinion that the correct treatment of a stress fracture following early detection is 4 months in a plaster cast in order to give the fracture a chance to heal. This should be followed by a graduated and intensive course of strengthening exercises for the trunk muscles. Associated with this should be technical help in order to correct any lordosis tendency and any tendency toward excessive turn-out. If—and only if—the child is really well disciplined and is under the constant supervision of the physical therapist or medical attendant can the plaster very occasionally be omitted and treatment with rest from dancing, isometric trunk exercises, and use of a temporary corset by day be substituted. The latter course of treatment calls for complete reliability on the part of the dancer, who must avoid doing anything stressful for the back during the healing period.

Results of Poor Training

Ballet technique, like any other skill, is learned by constant repetition, which produces engrams, or subconscious movement patterns. Accuracy is of prime importance in the development of the engram, as any variation will prevent its proper development. If the teaching is poor, incorrect engrams will be learned, and these will be difficult or impossible to change later in life.

Among the results of poor training are many of the conditions already mentioned. Probably the most serious is forcing the feet to turn out farther than the hips will allow. This results in lordosis and possible spinal injury. Also associated with excessive turn-out are knee and foot injuries. The excessive turn-out and the weak trunk will prevent the dancer from placing the weight correctly, and this itself will aggravate the general weakness. Excessive turn-out and lordosis may result in the development of tightness in the fronts of the hips, which can then prevent adequate correction of the lordosis at a later stage unless the tightness is first eliminated.

Frequently associated with excessive turn-out and the tightening at the front of the hips as a result of the incorrect weight transmission is general weakness of the quadriceps and the adductors. The situation is greatly aggravated by the presence of uncontrolled hyperextended knees.

Even in the absence of any of the above problems, hyperextended knees can, if uncontrolled, lead to weakening of the quadriceps and the inner side of the thigh muscles. This is associated with the development of the anterior knee pain mentioned earlier. From the first, the skillful teacher will help young dancers to control hyperextended knees, teaching them to pull up with their thighs and to avoid pushing back.

If the child has been allowed to turn out the feet excessively from an early age, a genuine tibial torsion can develop so that the feet are, in fact, more turned out than the knee. The feet may also roll when there is excessive turn-out, although rolling may merely be associated with weakness of the feet and incorrect weight placement.

Failure to teach a proper *battement tendu* will prevent the forefoot muscles from becoming strong, as the intrinsic muscles do not work in an incorrect *tendu*. As the child tries to point the foot better, she will reinforce the effort with the long toe flexors which, if unopposed by an effective intrinsic muscle combination, will lead to flexion of the toes. A correct *tendu*, in which the stretch extends out to the tips of the toes, will encourage the intrinsics to work strongly. A great aid to a correct *tendu* is work without shoes.

There are many other unfortunate results of improper training; indeed, no portion of the body can be considered exempt from trouble produced by an inept teacher. The greatest service a teacher can provide for the young ballet dancer is to help in the development of proper strength, correct technique, and correct posture of the body and limbs, with correct centering and weight transmission. Without this grounding, young dancers have no sound basis on which to build their complicated dance techniques as their studies advance.

8

FOOT AND ANKLE INJURIES IN DANCERS

Barnard Kleiger, M.D.

DANCERS ARE SUBJECT TO the same foot problems that afflict the general population, and it would take more than a single chapter to describe them all. However, because of the nature of their work, special difficulties do appear earlier and more frequently in dancers,[1] and this chapter is focused on these problems.

The biomechanics of the foot are modified by differences in size, shape, flexibility, and strength. This is best demonstrated by the dancer who develops hypertrophy of the second metatarsal because the big toe is shorter than the second toe.

Dance Technique

Creating aesthetic movement for professional performance requires that assymetrical functional axes in the lower limb be synchronized. The hip axis is anteverted (rotated laterally) 12°, the knee axis is transverse, and the ankle axis is rotated laterally about 12°, aligning with the hip axis.[2] To synchronize these axes, the thigh and leg rotate around vertical axes. Malalignment of any axis disturbs this synchronization. This can be recognized in the performance of a *plié,* which requires flexion at the knee and hip, with the thigh in maximal lateral rotation.[3,4] Dancers turn out the feet as close to 90° as possible, but this turn-out cannot be reached unless the hip rotates laterally at least 50°. Lacking that range, some dancers compensate by forcing the range of lateral leg rotation beyond the normal.[4] A forced turn-out stresses the lower limb joints and creates a functional valgus position, with most of the abnormal stresses dissipated at the knee. Dancers know that forcing the turn-out is risky, but some do it because their technique is poor, others to compensate for a low range of lateral rotation, and still others because of fatigue or simple carelessness. As a rule, if the patella points to the big or second toe in all positions of the limb, much damage is avoided. The dancer must learn and follow techniques adapted to individual physical abilities in order to avoid possible degenerative or traumatic conditions ascribed to overuse or misuse.

Degenerative Conditions

A force applied from above to the talar trochlea in the static foot is dissipated plantarward through the calcaneus posteriorly and through the metatarsal heads anteriorly. Dorsally, the force is dissipated through the midtarsal region.[5] Such a force would be expected to flatten the longitudinal arch, but it does not do so because the plantar soft tissue structures act as a tie-rod holding together the hind and fore parts of the foot against the resistance of the keystone construction of the midtarsus (figure 8-1). Movement of the dancer's feet changes the position of the talus in the mortise. When the foot is fully extended, the anterior tibial margin reaches a sulcus on the talar neck. When fully flexed, the posterior tibial margin reaches a sulcus on the posterior talar tubercle[6] (figures 8-2-A, 8-2-B, 8-2-C). This range uses the full arc of the talar trochlea, but dancers try to exceed it and cause the tibia to impinge on the talus anteriorly or posteriorly.[7]

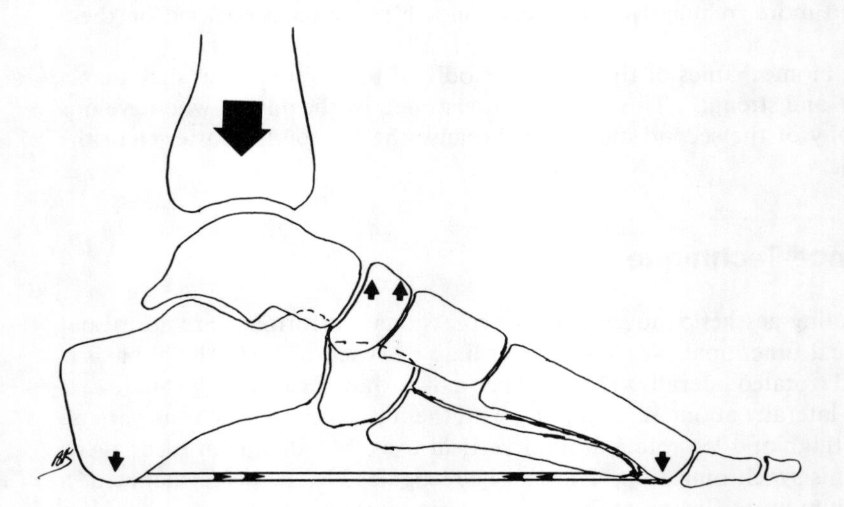

Figure 8-1. A downward force transmitted from the tibia (large arrow) through the talus is dissipated plantarward through the calcaneus and metatarsal heads (small single arrows) and dorsally through the midtarsus (double arrows). The longitudinal arch is not depressed because the keystone construction of the midtarsus and the tie-rod effect of the plantar soft tissues (arrowheads) prevent it.

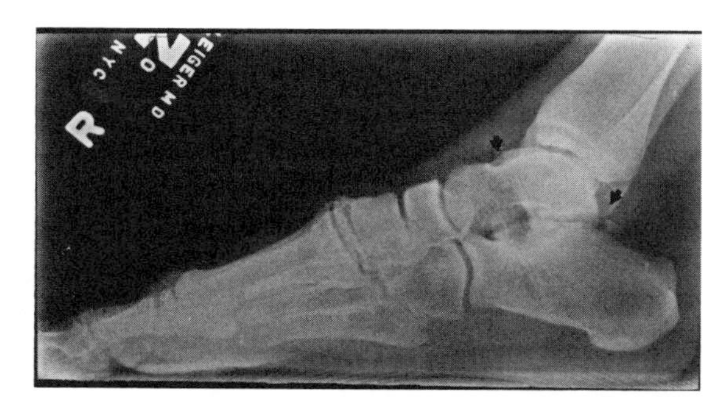

Figure 8-2-A. X-ray of a flexed foot showing a small os trigonum. The posterior tibial margin has not reached the sulcus on the posterior talar tubercle (arrow). The sulcus anteriorly on the talar neck is visible (arrow).

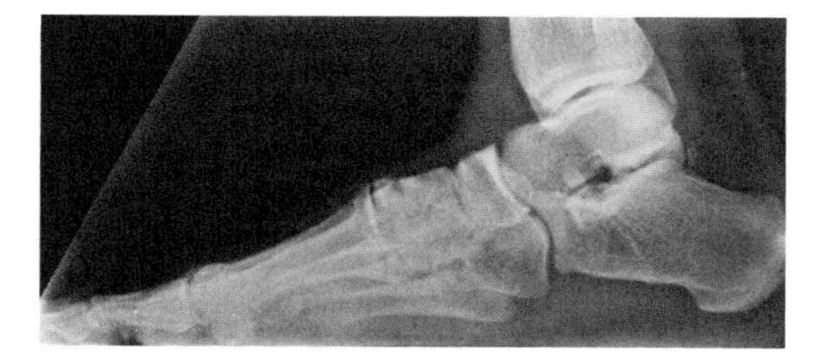

Figure 8-2-B. The same foot maximally extended impinges on the talar neck, and the posterior joint space widens. The longitudinal arch has maintained its height.

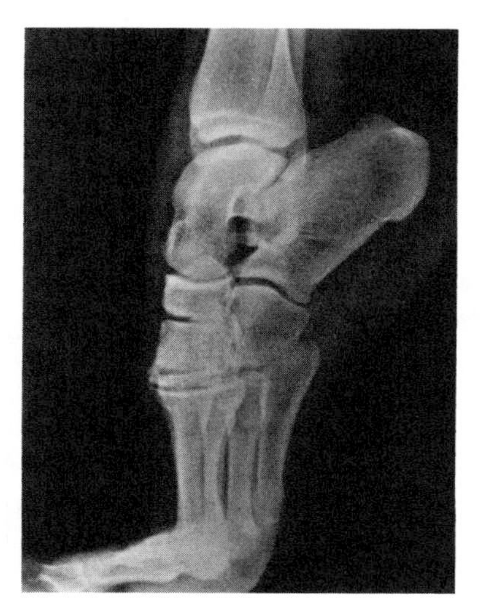

Figure 8-2-C. The same foot on *demi-pointe.* The talus is completely flexed and the posterior tibial margin impinges on the posterior talar tubercle. The metatarsals are aligned with the tibia, and the increased width of the anterior part of the subtalar joint indicates that this joint participates in this motion (compare with figure 8-2-B).

Anterior Impingement

The forcefully extended weight-bearing foot causes anterior tibiotalar impingement. Throughout their careers, dancers practice *pliés* "to stretch the heel cords" and increase their range of extension. This movement also stretches the posterior capsule and causes anterior tibiotalar impingement (figures 8-2-A, 8-2-B). With the passage of time and after many stretchings, exostoses form where tibia and talus meet (figure 8-3). Because the foot pronates as it extends, the talus and mortise rotate medially. This creates impingement between the anterior tibial margin and the talar neck and between the medial malleolus and the medial aspect of the talus. Exostoses form at both locations. The presence of impingement without exostoses or with small exostoses may cause no symptoms, but eventually the exostoses enlarge enough to cause pain, reduce the range of extension, and weaken the ability to push off.[7,8]

Anterior impingement is part of the technique of dance and cannot be eliminated, but when exostoses form, the dancer should be aware of it and should stop forcing the *plié*. Also, when the dancer is not dancing, shoes with mildly elevated heels should be worn. The exostoses are not reversible, but progression can be avoided or slowed by reducing impingement. The symptomatic ankle must be treated in the same fashion as the asymptomatic one; in addition, rest and nonsteroidal anti-inflammatory drugs may keep the patient dancing. Large exostoses induce inflammatory changes in the anterior capsule, the fat pad, and articular cartilage. The ankle then swells, and pain increases until the dancer can no longer perform. At this point, the dancer must decide

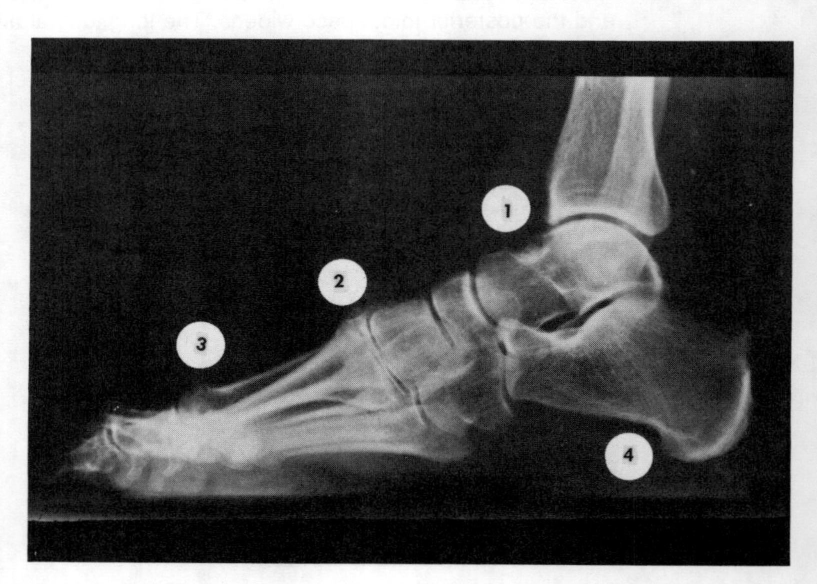

Figure 8-3. Lateral radiograph of a dancer's foot showing: (1) anterior tibio-talar impingement exostoses, (2) dorsal exostosis at the tarso-metatarsal joints, (3) dorsal exostosis on the first metatarsal head, and (4) calcaneal exostosis.

whether to stop dancing or to have surgery. If surgery is performed, the exostoses are excised through an anteromedial incision from the entire anterior aspect of the tibia, including the medial malleolus, and from the dorsal and medial aspects of the talar neck. The sulcus on the dorsum of the talar neck should be restored and the anterior fat pad excised. Surgery restores the ability to dance, but in 6-8 years, exostoses reform and symptoms may recur. If the dancer is still not ready to retire, the surgery can be repeated.

Young dancers with long, flexible feet have another problem related to anterior impingement. They have more than the normal range of motion in the midtarsal and talonavicular joints and the anterior facets of the subtalar joints (figures 8-4-A, 8-4-B, 8-4-C). Greater mobility increases the impact of these articular surfaces on one another and puts more strain on the supporting structures of these joints. Eventually, if extension is repeated often enough, the foot becomes weak, painful, and disabling.[7] The picture resembles a midfoot strain and is accompanied by pain in the plantar soft-tissue structures. Treatment of this condition is difficult in dancers because orthotics and shoe modification cannot be used while dancing. Such feet do not tolerate the strain of dancing, and students with them should not be encouraged to continue professional training. If a dancer with such feet survives the training, it is common for the dorsal exostoses of the midtarsal joints to develop.

Posterior Impingement

For the *pointe* or *demi-pointe* position, a dancer's foot flexes to align the metatarsals at 180° with the tibia.[4] In this position, the posterior talar tubercle is compressed between the posterior margin of the tibia and the posterior calcaneal facet (figure 8-2-C). If the posterior talar tubercle (or os trigonum) is enlarged, talar flexion is reduced, preventing complete alignment (figure 8-4-C). A dancer with this condition will repeatedly force flexion of the foot in the on *pointe* or *demi-pointe* positions, thereby causing posterior impingement. This, in turn, may cause any of the following conditions:

- Hypertrophied posterior talar tubercle or os trigonum
- Detached os trigonum
- Osteoarthritis of the posterior subtalar facets
- Heterotopic bone formation near the posterior talar tubercle
- Tendinitis of the flexor hallucis longus (In flexion, the tendon is compressed in its groove on the posterior talar tubercle. In extension, the tendon is stretched between the posterior talar tubercle and the sustentaculum tali. Repetition of these movements inflames the tendon and it swells. With continued repetition, the tendon degenerates and may rupture.)

Now that this syndrome is recognized,[9,10] its occurrence is frequently noted. It is serious enough that students who cannot align the foot and leg properly in the on *pointe* or *demi-pointe* position should be advised to study a dance form that does not require these positions. Professionals who are symp-

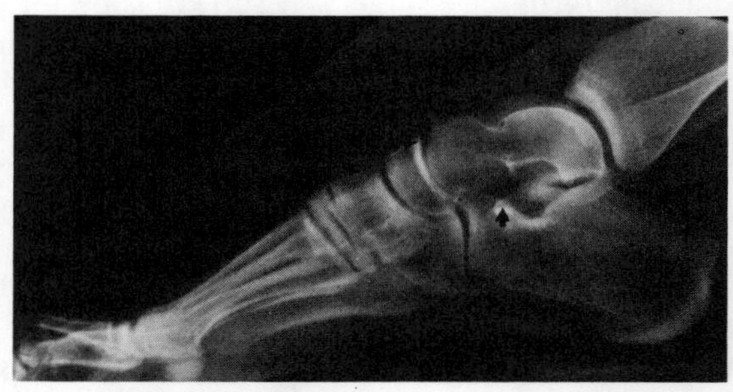

Figure 8-4-A. Radiograph of a foot in complete flexion showing posterior impingement and widening of the anterior part of the subtalar joint (arrow). The talar head projects beyond the dorsal cortex of the navicular (arrowhead). There is a well-formed longitudinal arch.

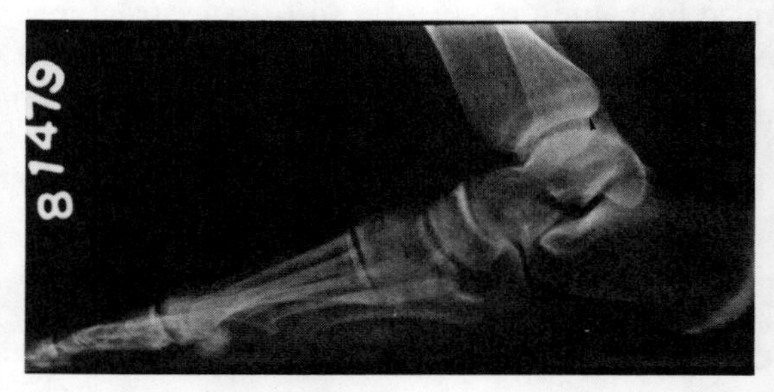

Figure 8-4-B. The same foot in complete extension showing anterior impingement and posterior widening of the ankle joint (small arrowhead) with closure of the anterior part of the subtalar joint. The dorsal cortex of the talar head is level with that of the navicular (large arrowhead). The longitudinal arch is depressed as compared with figure 8-4-A.

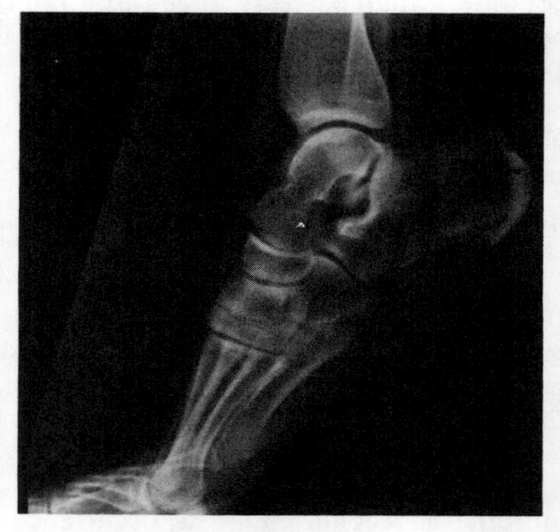

Figure 8-4-C. The same foot on *demi-pointe.* In spite of using all the talar flexion and achieving posterior impingement, the metatarsals are not in a straight line with the tibia (compare with figure 8-2-C).

tomatic should rest and take nonsteroidal anti-inflammatory medication until symptoms subside. They should then modify their technique and rechoreograph their work to reduce the frequency of movements causing impingement. Other local measures, such as soaks or massage (manual or ice), may be tried. If these measures fail and the dancer cannot perform, surgery must be considered.

Surgery is performed through either of two approaches: On the medial side, the incision is from behind the medial malleolus to the tubercle of the navicular. The posterior tibial tendon is released behind the malleolus and is retracted, avoiding the neurovascular bundle. The flexor hallucis longus tendon is located under the sustentaculum tali, on the posterior talar tubercle, or between the two. It is freed from the posterior talar tubercle and from under the sustentaculum tali. Retracting the tendon exposes the posterior talar tubercle or os trigonum. If an os trigonum is present, it is excised; if part of the posterior talar tubercle interferes with flexion, it is resected until there is no restriction to flexion. Severe degenerative changes in the posterior subtalar facets may warrant arthrodesis of that joint. A dancer would probably be unable to work with either severe arthritic changes or after arthrodesis.

A posterolateral incision can be used just lateral to the Achilles tendon to enter the plane between the flexor hallucis longus and the peroneals. The flexor hallucis tendon is followed to the posterior talar tubercle, from which it is released and retracted medially. If necessary, the tendon is released from under the sustentaculum tali, but it may be difficult to reach through this incision. The os trigonum and posterior talar tubercle are resected until there is no interference with flexion.

Either wound is closed by suturing skin; on the medial side, the posterior tibial tendon is replaced behind the medial malleolus, and its retinacular ligament is repaired before closure. If flexion is reduced because of a low talar trochlea, resecting the posterior tubercle will not increase the range.

Hallux rigidus may accompany posterior impingement. If the foot cannot align with the leg, the dancer compensates by pronating the big toe on *demi-pointe* or flexing the big toe interphalangeal joint (knuckle under) on *pointe.* In either case, abnormal stresses on the metatarsophalangeal joint of the big toe eventually cause osteoarthritis (figures 8-3, 8-5).

Early in the disease, a dancer can continue to work by changing techniques and choreography. The shoes worn for daily activities can be modified with a metatarsal bar or a metatarsal pad with a sesamoid extension. Dance slippers cannot be modified, nor can they hold an orthosis. Some dancers have used a rubber pad cut as a combination scaphoid and metatarsal pad with sesamoid extension. This pad is shaped by taping it to the foot for several days. When held in place by a snug dance slipper, it becomes a light, flexible orthosis. If the condition progresses, impingement can be relieved surgically.

A severe hallux rigidus prevents performance and may need surgical reconstruction. A Keller procedure produces a short, floppy toe that cannot be depended upon for dance. It may cause symptoms and recurrence of rigidity because weight bearing is abnormal. A capsular arthroplasty or a Silastic spacer implant[11] arthroplasty may relieve pain but cannot assure a return to

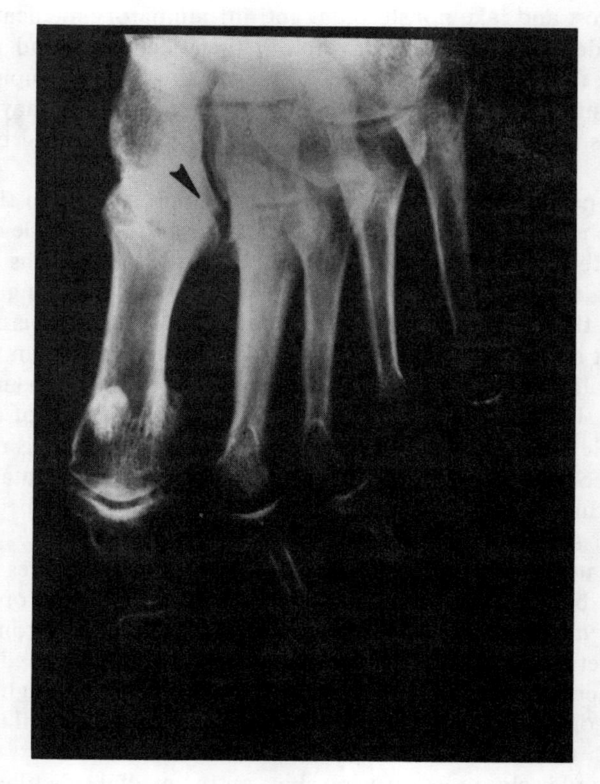

Figure 8-5. Dorsiplantar radiograph showing irregularity and cyst formation in the metatarsal head and proximal phalanx of the big toe, lateral deviation of the metatarsophalangeal joints of the lesser toes and subluxation of the middle toe. There are degenerative changes and heterotopic bone between the tarsometatarsal joints of the first and second metatarsals (arrowhead). This is another view of the same foot as in figure 8-3.

dance. The flexible Silastic joint prosthesis is not likely to withstand the functional demands of dance.

Degenerative Toe Disease

The trauma to toes during dance may lead to the development of many problems. The toes may deform and bursae and hyperkeratoses form over bony prominences (figure 8-5). Dancers pad their toes to protect these painful lesions, but the padding occupies space in a shoe and may crowd the toes. To fit, the shoes and dance slippers should be sized with the padding in place. Hyperkeratoses can be softened and bursae and fissures prevented by applying salicylic acid ointment twice daily for 5 days per week. Conservative measures usually keep the dancer working. Rarely needed, surgery to correct deformity should not be undertaken lightly. A reconstructed toe may not tolerate dance.

Heel Pain (Calcaneodynia)

The syndrome of pain on the plantar surface of the heel can have many causes, but in the dance population the most frequent are (figures 8-6-A and 8-6-B):[4]

- Calcaneal exostosis (figure 8-3)
- Plantar fasciitis
- Calcaneal fat pad atrophy
- Abductor hallucis myositis
- Subcalcaneal bursitis
- Calcaneal stress fracture
- Entrapment neuropathy of a posterior tibial nerve branch

Although heel pain may be caused by systemic disease of metabolic, inflammatory, or infectious origin, this is rare among dancers, in whom it is usually precipitated by either single or repeated trauma. The fat pad beneath the heel is organized into vertical, fibrous, fat-containing compartments.[12,13] This pad acts like a hydraulic shock absorber, but when the heel strikes a hard floor, compartments rupture and the fat disperses (figure 8-6-A). If enough compartments rupture, the pad flattens, atrophies, and no longer absorbs shock. The same injury causes trabecular microfracture and stress fracture, which heal with a residual area of sclerosis or an exostosis. Such an impact also injures the muscles and fascia attaching to the plantar and medial surfaces of the calcaneus. A loose shoe heel aggravates the situation because it does not contain the pad but allows it to spread and flatten. Thus, one or a combination of factors produces heel pain, and all may relate to a dance floor that is too hard for dancing.

Most patients are helped by symptomatic nonsurgical treatment, and this should be tried first. A 1/2-in. thick felt scaphoid pad taped to the foot with adhesive keeps the heel pad from spreading while relieving the tender area. Other methods providing effective pain relief consist of heel pads cut out under the tender area, flexible or firm plastic heel cups, orthotics, and shoe modifications. Mechanical support is helped by nonsteroidal anti-inflammatory drugs and occasionally by local infiltration of the tender area with lidocaine and steroid. If pain is unrelieved after three injections, this method is not likely to help.

If conservative measures fail and systemic disease is eliminated as the cause of heel pain, the clinical, neurological, and radiographic studies should be reviewed. If no definite diagnosis is established, a technetium bone scan will localize an active bony lesion, especially a stress fracture. A computerized axial tomography (CT) scan may show the pathology better than the radiograph, but the usefulness of nuclear magnetic resonance is still not known. Electromyography and conduction time studies are of help in establishing posterior tibial neuropathy. A negative test result, however, does not preclude a neuropathy. The studies should be done with the foot flexed and also extended maximally, because although conduction time is normal in flexion, it can be delayed in extension when the nerve is tensed. At surgery, the abductor hallucis and the

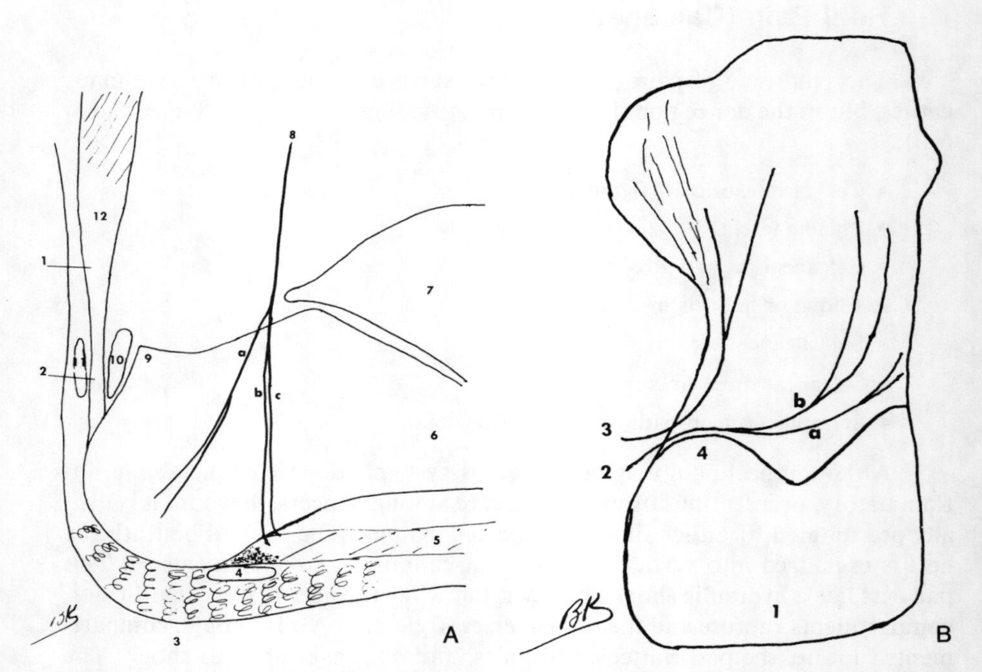

Figure 8-6-A. Sketch of heel from medial side: (1) Achilles tendon; (2) Achilles tendon-insertional area; (3) calcaneal fat pad; (4) subcalcaneal bursa with exostosis superior to it; (5) plantar fascia and abductor hallucis; (6) calcaneus; (7) talus; (8) posterior tibial nerve (a. medial calcaneal branch, b. lateral plantar branch, c. medial plantar branch); (9) posterior tubercle of calcaneus (Haglund's tubercle); (10) deep retrocalcaneal bursa; (11) superficial retrocalcaneal bursa; (12) myotendonous junction of Achilles tendon.

Figure 8-6-B. Sketch of plantar surface of calcaneus: (1) posterior end of calcaneus; (2) lateral plantar branch of posterior tibial nerve (a. motor branch to muscles of the fifth toe, b. remaining branches); (3) medial plantar nerve; (4) inferior tubercle of calcaneus.

plantar fascia are released from their origin. The posterior tibial nerve is explored, and its branches, including the motor branch to the little toe (figure 8-6-B), must be freed from fascial and bony entrapment. Exostoses are resected because they can cause pain and neural entrapment (figures 8-3, 8-6-A, 8-6-B).

Tendinitis

Tendinitis or tenosynovitis[14-16] is caused by overuse, misuse, anatomic anomaly, or a combination of these. The sheath of an inflamed tendon thickens, and the substance of the tendon degenerates and enlarges. This sequence causes snapping and locking of the tendon. In dancers, the Achilles and flexor hallucis longus are the tendons most often involved, but any tendon may be injured. Symptoms appear either suddenly or gradually, and the first manifestation is pain, followed by swelling, redness, and heat in the surrounding tissues. Pain is increased by active motion against resistance. Achilles tendinitis may be revealed in one of three ways: From 1 in. proximal to its insertion to the myotendonous junction, the tendon degenerates because of metabolic disease (especially gout) or overuse. At its insertion, Achilles tendinitis is caused by impingement of a prominent posterior calcaneal tubercle against the tendon when the foot is maximally extended (figure 8-6-A). Peritendinitis crepitans or paratendinitis causes the tissues around the tendon for all or most of its length to become swollen and crepitate.

The cause of flexor hallucis longus tendinitis has been discussed under the posterior impingement syndrome. Posterior tibial tendinitis is frequently associated with an accessory scaphoid, and peroneal tendinitis could be associated with a slipping tendon.

Dancers, impatient to work, may not rest long enough for the tendon to heal or may refuse to take nonsteroidal anti-inflammatory drugs. When symptoms subside enough to return to dancing, it is essential that the dancer learn to use the limb without overusing the involved tendons. Injection of steroids and local anesthesia relieves pain and encourages a dancer to resume dancing. But pain relief does not always mean that the tendon is healed, and continued misuse causes additional degeneration and even tendon rupture. After injection, the dancer should avoid using the tendon for 2 weeks, and afterward should be rehabilitated by progressively increasing the levels of activity until a normal level is reached without return of symptoms. Most tendons are symptomatic for a long time before rupturing. If symptoms persist or recur, tenography and CT scanning can help to clarify the pathology.[4]

If surgery is necessary, an adequate length of tendon and sheath is explored to determine the extent of tendon disease and the location of bone- or soft-tissue entrapment or impingement. If the Achilles tendon is involved, it should be determined whether the posterior calcaneal tubercle is impinging on the tendon and needs to be resected. With the foot both flexed and extended, the flexor hallucis longus tendon must be inspected in its groove on the posterior talar tubercle and under the sustentaculum tali. The retinacular ligaments at one or both locations can trap the tendon and may need to be released. The insertion of the posterior tibial tendon on the navicular should be examined, and if it is loose, the accessory navicular is removed and the tendon reattached. A slipping peroneal tendon is demonstrated when the foot is extended and is corrected if present. The tendon and sheath are debrided, and necessary repairs are made. At the end of the operation, the tendon must be intact and able to glide smoothly and freely in its bed. If the tendon required extensive debridement and repair, the ankle is immobilized long enough for healing to take place. Otherwise, a program of progressively increasing exercise and activity is followed until dancing can be resumed.

Bursitis

There are many synovial bursae about the foot and ankle located at points of friction[17,18] (figure 8-6-A). Adventitious bursae form in response to abnormal pressure or friction. Any bursa can become inflamed, but in dancers those about the heel are inflamed often enough to be significant. The onset, which may be sudden or gradual, is manifested by pain, swelling, and redness. The deep retrocalcaneal bursa lies between the posterior calcaneal tubercle and the Achilles tendon. Inflammation is caused by repeated extension of the foot, compressing the bursa between a prominent posterior calcaneal tubercle and the Achilles tendon. It may be difficult to distinguish between retrocalcaneal bursitis and insertional Achilles tendinitis, and the conditions may coexist. The subcalcaneal bursa is between the inferior calcaneal tubercle and the fat pad. It is injured by the heel's striking a hard floor. An adventitious bursa may form between skin and distal Achilles and calcaneus from shoe pressure. This swelling is called a "pump bump" because the pump is the kind of shoe most often responsible for the condition.

Relieving pressure, applying ice, and taking nonsteroidal anti-inflammatory medication is usually successful in treating this kind of bursitis. If this conservative treatment fails, surgery is the next step. The operation for excising the deep retrocalcaneal bursa is similar to that for insertional Achilles tendinitis, except that in the former the bursa is carefully excised. The surgery for the subcalcaneal bursa is the same as the surgery for heel pain. The adventitious bursa rarely needs surgery once shoe pressure is relieved; if pressure is not relieved, the condition will recur after surgery.

Shin Splints

Although shin splints are not a foot or ankle problem, the foot is secondarily involved. The condition is manifested mainly by painful leg cramps on activity. At first, the cramps subside with rest, but eventually they persist in spite of it. The disease has not been clearly defined, but its symptoms are caused by increased pressure within any of the leg compartments. The diagnosis is established by demonstrating increased pressure. If symptoms persist and are disabling, fasciotomy of the affected compartment may be necessary. The symptoms of tibial stress fracture resemble those of the anterior compartment syndrome, and in some patients with tibial stress fracture, an adjacent compartment may be swollen and under increased pressure. Rest and immobilization usually heal a stress fracture, and symptoms are relieved.

Trauma

Ankle Sprain

Ankle sprain is the most frequent injury in dancers and is often regarded as an inconvenient but benign injury.[16,19-21] However, the large number of patients with chronic symptoms after sprain indicates that this injury should be taken seriously and that factors causing chronicity should be sought.

A dancer sprains an ankle because of a misstep in which the foot is turned. This happens because the dancer is tired or careless, because the floor is defective, or because an object was on the floor that should not have been there. Pain is immediate, and walking becomes difficult or impossible. In a short time, the ankle swells over the injured ligaments, and a few hours later there is swelling and ecchymosis on the dorsal and lateral aspects of the foot. Movement is painful, and stress increases the pain. The injured ligament is tender to palpation, and this tenderness locates the affected joint.

Although the ankle is considered to be a single entity, it is actually a complex of three joints: talocrural (the main ankle), talocalcaneal (subtalar), and tibiofibular (syndesmosis). Any of these joints may be sprained, but the most frequent force tears the anterior talofibular ligament (figures 8-7-A, 8-7-B). The ankle is tender over the anterior surface of the lateral malleolus or in the

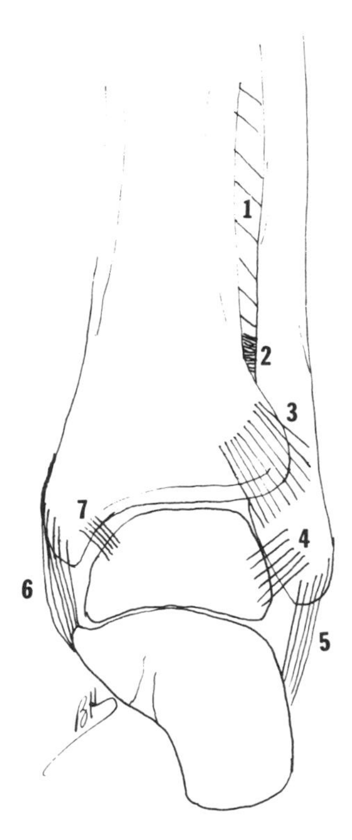

Figure 8-7-A. Sketch of ankle ligaments (frontal): (1) interosseous membrane; (2) interosseous ligament; (3) anterior tibiofibular ligament; (4) anterior talofibular ligament; (5) calcaneofibular ligament; (6) superficial fibers of deltoid ligament (anterior), tibionavicular and tibiocalcaneal ligaments; (7) dorsal tibiotalar ligament.

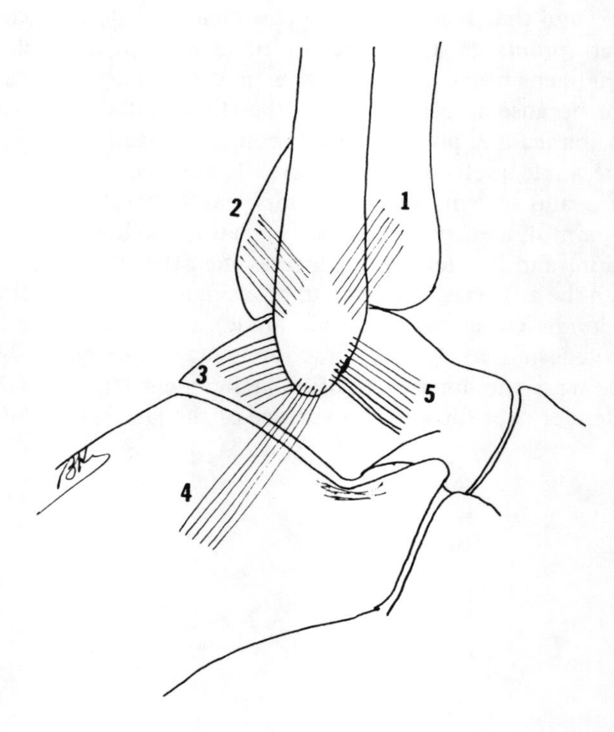

Figure 8-7-B. Sketch of ankle ligaments (lateral): (1) anterior tibiofibular ligament; (2) posterior tibiofibular ligament; (3) posterior talofibular ligament; (4) calcaneofibular ligament; (5) anterior talofibular ligament.

sinus tarsi. Less frequently, inversion tears the calcaneofibular ligament and the lateral subtalar capsule. This injury causes tenderness behind the lateral malleolus and on the lateral side of the subtalar joint. Because both are caused by inversion, a combined injury may result.[21] A third injury is caused by lateral rotation, or eversion, which tears the ligaments of the tibiofibular syndesmosis and the superficial fibers of the deltoid ligament (figure 8-7-C). It causes tenderness over the syndesmosis and the anterior aspect of the medial part of the mortise. To distinguish among them, the first injury might be called an ankle sprain, the second a subtalar sprain, and the third a syndesmotic sprain. The last is usually a more severe injury that has a longer course and poorer prognosis, and it often heals with heterotopic bone in the syndesmosis (figure 8-8). X-ray helps in diagnosis only if bony fragments can be seen at the site of ligament avulsion (figure 8-9).

The common sprain is a ligament injury that does not impair stability, but the absence of instability must be established before the condition is treated as a sprain. Physical examination may be all that is needed for diagnosis, but stress radiography[22] and arthrography[23] help to evaluate the extent of injury. If

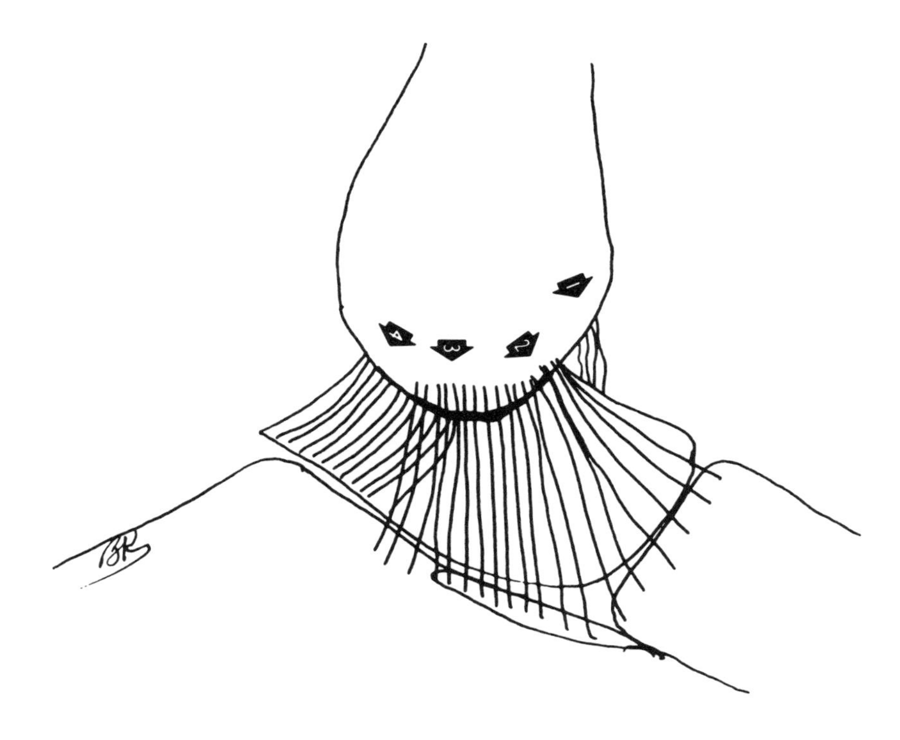

Figure 8-7-C. Sketch of ankle ligaments (medial): (1) dorsal tibiotalar ligament; (2) anterior tibionavicular ligament; (3) tibiocalcaneal ligament; (4) posterior tibiotalar ligament.

there is no instability, treatment is started by elevation, icing, and avoidance of weight bearing. Support helps to get patients on their feet. Ankle wraps, using compression pads and layers of elastic and nonelastic adhesive tape, are recommended. These are effective, but the dressing is bulky and will not fit a dance slipper when the patient is ready to wear one. At that time, a secure basketweave strapping of 1½-in. or 2-in. flesh-colored adhesive tape will fit the slipper, provide support, and be aesthetically acceptable. Walking is encouraged as tolerated, using a normal gait as nearly as possible. Unna's paste boot (soft cast) is popular, but it is bulky, and as swelling subsides, it becomes loose and ineffective. Splints can be effective, but these, too, are bulky and restrictive, and interfere with a dancer's return to work. Support is needed for 4-6 weeks, and strappings should be changed at least every 2 weeks and more frequently as activity increases.

Ankle Instability

When ligament injury is more extensive, joint stability is impaired.[20,21] On physical examination, inversion ankle instability is identified by an increased

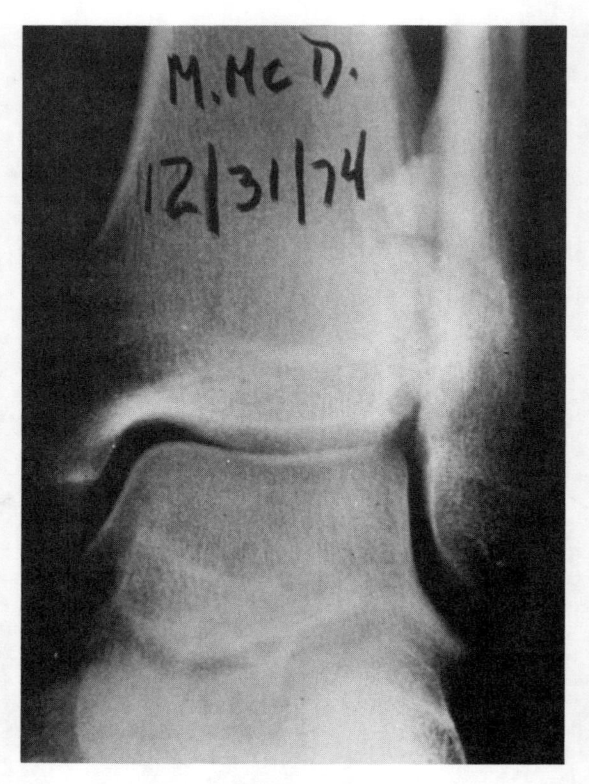

Figure 8-8. X-ray of tibifibular synostosis due to heterotopic bone formed after a syndesmotic sprain.

range of inversion and by feeling the talus tilt on inversion stress. Anterior instability is demonstrated by exerting forward pressure on the heel and backward pressure on the tibia. This displaces the talus anteriorly, and when the pressure is released, it replaces. Both kinds of instability result from lateral ligament tears. Subtalar instability, which has increased inversion but no talar tilt, is caused by tearing the calcaneofibular ligaments and the subtalar capsule.[21] Syndesmotic instability, present when the talus moves laterally and the space between the talus and the medial malleolus is wide enough to be felt, is caused by tearing of the syndesmotic and deltoid ligaments. Instability can be confirmed by anteroposterior radiographs under inversion and lateral rotation stress and by lateral radiographs with forward stress on the heel and backward stress on the tibia.[22] Contrast arthrography shows the size of ligament tear, but does not demonstrate instability.[23]

In most patients, fresh inversion ankle and subtalar instability can be successfully treated by plaster immobilization, but because of the special needs of dancers, surgical repair of the torn ligaments should be considered. After surgery, a plaster walking boot is worn for 4 weeks, followed by a program of progressive rehabilitation. The results of surgical repair are somewhat better than plaster immobilization, and the dancer should have the option to choose.

Syndesmotic instability may be accompanied by an eversion talar tilt. It

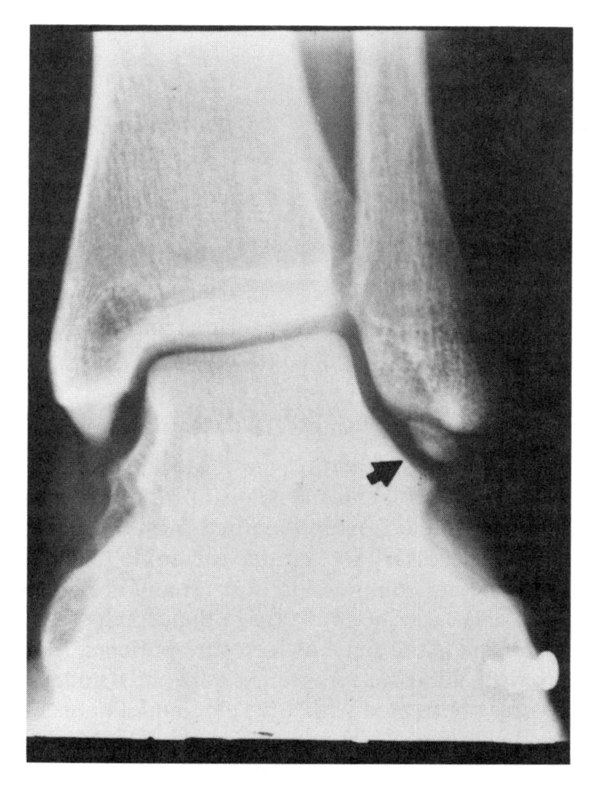

Figure 8-9. X-ray of ununited avulsed fragment from the distal end of the fibula (arrow).

can be successfully treated in an above-knee plaster with the knee flexed 30° and the foot plantigrade and rotated medially 15-20° to approximate the talus to the medial malleolus. The plaster is applied in sections, first below the knee. When it is dry, the foot is rotated medially and the plaster is extended above the knee.[24] After 4 weeks, the plaster is removed and the ankle reexamined for stability. If it is stable, a below-knee walking plaster is applied for 2 weeks. In the event of surgery, the syndesmotic and deltoid ligaments are repaired. Tibiofibular screw fixation should be avoided because it requires a second operation to remove the screw and because it results in increased heterotopic bone formation in the interosseous space.

Chronic Ankle Sprain

The chronic pain that often follows ankle sprain can be caused by many conditions, some of which are:

- Ligament malunion
- Chronic instability
- Talar articular contusions
- Posttraumatic talar cystification

- Heterotopic ossification
- Nonunion of avulsed bony fragments
- Tarsal tunnel syndrome
- Peroneal palsy
- Lateral compartment syndrome
- Reflex sympathetic dystrophy
- Chronic posttraumatic edema
- Pain of unknown origin

Chronic ankle pain following sprain is often serious and disabling and is best avoided by adequate treatment of the original injury.

Fracture Dislocation

Dancers often sustain minor fractures and dislocations of the toes, metatarsals (including stress fractures), calcaneus, distal fibula, and talar trochlea. Many of these are small-fragment fractures avulsed from bone at a ligament insertion, and this makes it necessary to examine the ankle for instability. Fractures of the sesamoid bone are compression injuries and are not accompanied by instability. Fracture of a large bone is rare in dancers.

Treatment for dancers is the same as for other patients. Most metatarsal fractures are treated with adhesive strappings and pads under the involved bone. Sesamoid fractures are treated with strapping and a dancer's pad, which is a combined scaphoid and metatarsal pad extended behind the sesamoids and under the first metatarsal. Walking is permitted if it can be tolerated. The strappings and pads are changed at 2-week intervals or less. Some fractures are treated with below-knee plasters, but an unstable oblique fibular fracture needs an above-knee, sectional, medial rotation plaster.[24] Small-fragment talar trochlear fractures rarely heal, and often become necrotic. These should be excised and the base drilled, but large talar osteochondral fragments can be replaced.[25]

The dance floor itself plays an important role in the production of disease or injury of the foot and ankle. A well-sprung floor improves performance and is less damaging. A hard floor increases the possibility of injury to the foot and predisposes to degenerative conditions of the foot and occasionally to osteonecrosis of the medial sesamoid. When an osteonecrotic sesamoid fragments, it may be confused with fracture, but the x-ray shows increased density, and in healing the sesamoid collapses and deforms.

Rehabilitation

Dancers should begin rehabilitation as early in the illness as possible. Deconditioning occurs rapidly in dancers, who need 2 days of rehabilitation for every day of inactivity. Rest and avoidance of weight bearing does not imply complete inactivity, and dancers should be encouraged to exercise while protecting the affected part. Floor exercises, which are a regular part of dance training, can be done without weight bearing. Exercises in a swimming pool are beneficial, although a pool is not always available, affordable, or acceptable to the dancer. Barre exercises are useful because support is provided while the injured limb is exercised with partial weight bearing. As the patient's condition improves, exercises are progressively increased within the limits of tolerance until a normal level is reached. During the rehabilitation process, a dancer may change choreography and technique to permit an earlier return to performance.

Drugs and Orthotics

Nonsteroidal anti-inflammatory drugs are useful in the treatment of painful degenerative and posttraumatic conditions. There are many such drugs, and all are useful. Naturally, if a particular drug is ineffective or if there are undesirable side effects, the drug should be changed. If the response is good, the drug should not be discontinued abruptly; rather, the dosage should be gradually reduced over several weeks before the drug is taken away.

Surface anesthesia with ethyl chloride spray is helpful in reducing pain and swelling. If this agent is overused or improperly used, the skin may be burned, but an intelligent, cooperative patient can use it effectively and properly. A fine spray is applied over the painful area until a light frost is noted. The spray is discontinued until a faint blush appears. The process is repeated several times and stopped when the skin stays red and does not return to a faint blush promptly. The application is repeated 2-3 times a day.

Local anesthesia by injection is also useful in the treatment of pain. Depending on circumstances, it may be used as a trigger zone rejection, regional block, or nerve block. Although pain has been relieved, the patient should return to activity gradually in order to be certain there is no mechanical weakness that will give way under the stress of dancing.

The use of steroids and local anesthesia by injection relieves pain and reduces inflammation, but provides a false sense of security. If the dancer returns to work too quickly, a diseased tendon or ligament may rupture completely. Other complications are granuloma formation at the site of injection and heterotopic calcification and ossification. Although the incidence is rare, intra-articular injections can lead to osteonecrosis or pyarthrosis. Because such complications end a career, steroids should be used in dancers with caution and only as a last resort.

As for supports and orthotics, any device worn on the foot creates an irregular surface on the sole of the foot. Adhesive strapping is the smoothest, but the edge of the tape can roll and stick to the floor if the foot is bare. When a device is worn on the foot, a slipper should cover it.

References

1. Stoller SM, Hekmat F, Kleiger B. A comparative study of the frequency of anterior impingement exostoses of the ankle in dancers. Foot Ankle 1984; 4:201.
2. Steindler A. Kinesiology of the human body. Springfield, IL: Chas. C. Thomas, 1955; 299, 376, 377.
3 Kleiger B. The anteversion syndrome. Bull Hosp Joint Dis 1968; 29:22.
4. Kleiger B. Foot and ankle injuries in dancers. In: Taveras JM, ed. Skeletal Radiol 1986; 5:131.

5. Manter JT. Compression forces in the foot. Anat Rec 1946; 96:313.
6. Wesley MS, Koval R, Kleiger B. Roentgen measurement of ankle flexion-extension motion. Clin Orthop & Rel Res 1965; 65:165.
7. Kleiger B. Anterior tibiotalar impingement syndromes in dancers. Foot Ankle 1982; 3:69.
8. O'Donoghue DH. Impingement exostoses of the talus & tibia. J Bone Joint Surg 1957; 39A:835.
9. Quirk R. Talar compression syndrome in dancers. Foot Ankle 1982; 3:65.
10. Howse AJG. Posterior block of the ankle joint in dancers. Foot Ankle 1982; 3:81.
11. Swanson AB. Implant arthroplasty for the great toe. Clin Orthop & Rel Res 1972; 85:75-81.
12. Tietze A. Ueber der architaktovischen aufbau des bindegewebes in der menschlichenfuszohle. Brun Beitrage zur Klinischen Chirurgie. 123:493-506. Trans & reprinted in Foot Ankle 1982; 2:252-59.
13. Blechschmidt E. Die architektur des ferstenpolsters. Gegenbaur's Morphologisches Jahrbuch 73:20-68. 1934. Trans. & reprinted in Foot Ankle 1982; 2:260-83.
14. Hamilton WG. Tendonitis about the ankle in classical ballet dancers. Am J Sports Med 1977; 5:84.
15. Sammarco JH. The foot and ankle in classical ballet and modern dance. In: Jahss MH, ed. Disorders of the foot. Philadelphia: WB Saunders, 1982; 626.
16. Thomasen E. Diseases and injuries of ballet dancers. Universitets-forlaget I Arhus, 1982; 26-27.
17. Sarrafian SK. Anatomy of the foot and ankle. Philadelphia: JB Lippincott, 1983; 256-59.
18. Sutro CJ. The oscalcis, the tendo-Achilles and the local bursae. Bull Hosp Joint Dis 1966; 27:76-89.
19. Hamilton WG. Sprained ankles in ballet dancers. Foot Ankle 1982; 3:99.
20. Kleiger B. Mechanisms of ankle injury. Proc Am Orthop Foot Soc 1974; 5:1.
21. Kleiger B, Ahmed M. Injuries of the talus and its joints. Clin Orthop & Rel Res 1976; 121:243.
22. Kleiger B, Greenspan A, Norman A. Roentgenographic examination of the normal foot and ankle. In: Jahss MH, ed. Disorders of the foot. Philadelphia: WB Saunders, 1982; 116.
23. Brostrom L et al. Sprained ankles II: arthrographic diagnosis of recent ligament ruptures. Acta Chir Scan 1965; 129:485.
24. Kleiger B. The treatment of oblique fractures of the fibula. J Bone Joint Surg 1961; 43A:969-979.
25. Kleiger B. Fractures of the talus. J Bone Joint Surg 1948; 30A:735.

9

THE LOOSE METATARSOPHALANGEAL JOINT IN DANCERS

Eivind Thomasen, M.D.

IN 1876, THOMAS G. MORTON published (in the *American Journal of Medical Science*) the classical paper, "A peculiar and painful affection of the fourth metatarsophalangeal articulation." In this paper, he cites a letter of Nov. 24, 1875, from his friend Dr. John H. Packard, who himself had had a foot neuralgia of the same form as Morton had described in his paper: "For several years a relaxed joint in the fourth toe of my right foot. They had always occurred in walking and the symptoms were perfectly distinct—deep pressure over the metatarsophalangeal joint is painful but does not bring on an attack unless long continued." He writes after the citation of this letter: "In this case it would appear that the neuralgia was in the first place caused by a sudden malposition of the metatarsophalangeal joint of the fourth toe, incident either to a relaxed state of the joint or to a partial rupture of the ligaments, which allowed the head of the bone to slip from its phalangeal articulation, thus subjecting the parts to unusual pressure."

Morton described 15 patients with pain in the fourth metatarsophalangeal (MP) joint, which was called neuralgia. In 8 of 15, it was possible to trace the neuralgia to an injury of the joint of the fourth toe. In several cases, where this neuralgia followed an injury, a rupture of the ligaments or parts about the joint of the fourth metatarsal was thought to have occurred. He imagined that the digital branches of the external plantar nerve might be bruised between the fourth and the mobile fifth metatarsals. In chronic cases, he believed that excision of the irritable MP joint with the surrounding soft parts would likely prove permanently successful. From this first paper concerning Morton syndrome, it is seen that the most effective treatment of this then obscure disease was resection of the fourth metatarsal joint.

In the literature, it has not been possible to find description of looseness in a solitary MP joint.

Anatomy

The MP joint (figure 9-1) has a metatarsal head with a convexity plantar-dorsal and side to side. The head is compressed side to side. The base of the first phalanx has an oval concave joint surface much smaller than the joint surface of the metatarsal head. The fibrous joint capsule on the dorsal side is rather thin, and is covered by the long and short extensor tendons continuing in an extensoral aponeurosis on the dorsum of the phalanges to the third phalanx.

The plantar fibrous capsule is thick. Known as the plantar ligament, it is attached firmly to the plantar side of the base of the first phalanx, but in the proximal end it is rather loosely connected to the metatarsal head behind the articular surface. The thick plantar ligament on the plantar side is connected to the fibrous tendon sheath for the two flexor tendons and proximally to the transverse metatarsal ligament. On the two sides of the joint are seen the collateral ligaments in the fibrous capsule. They arise from the sides of the metatarsal head and are directed distally and plantarward to the sides of the first phalanx. Vertical fibers from the anterior end of the plantar aponeurosis are connected to the sides of the plantar ligament and the fibrous tendon sheath.

The tendons of the interosseous muscles are situated dorsal to the transverse metatarsal ligaments; they are located on the sides of the fibrous capsule of the MP joint and fixed to the base of the first phalanx. These tendons, the fibrous tendon sheath, and the thick plantar ligament form a socket for the plantar side of the metatarsal head.

The movement in the MP joint is plantar-dorsal, but chiefly dorsal, with the base of the first phalanx moving up on the dorsal side of the metatarsal head.

Normally, the MP joint is stable for passive movement of the base of the phalanx on the metatarsal head, but in some cases there may be found a pathological subluxation by passive movement creating a loose joint, often causing metatarsalgia, with pain and tenderness of the joint. The joint is often swollen because of swelling of the synovial capsule. Such a loose joint is most common in the second MP joint, but may be found in other "small" MP joints.

The author has tried to find the cause of such a looseness of the MP joint and has, on a dissected foot, cut the collateral ligaments. After such an operation, the base of the first phalanx could be dislocated dorsally on the head, and the toe was loose.

Resection of the Metatarsal Head

Resection of the metatarsal head has been done in most of the operated cases. The joint is opened on the dorsal side, and the extensor tendons are pulled to the side. The front part of the head is resected with a rongeur, but not completely; the distal part of the neck with the fixation of the plantar ligament and the proximal part of the fibrous tendon sheath are not removed (figure 9-2). The toe is pulled distally, and the plantar ligament is cut from the plantar side of the first phalanx. An incision is made on both sides of the plantar ligament, and the ligament with the dorsal side of the fibrous tendon sheath is dissected free. The two flexor tendons are lying free in the bottom of the wound. The flap, consisting of the plantar ligament and the fibrous tendon sheath, is pulled up in front of the resection site of the metatarsal head as interposition in the joint and is sewn to the dorsal side of the first phalanx (figure 9-3).

This operation is similar to the Tupper interposition operation in the fingers after resection of the head of the rheumatic deformed metacarpal head, but in this operation the interposition of the volar capsule is turned the opposite way, with fixation distal on the phalanx. The intention with this interposition in the metatarsal joint is to prevent the toe from being subluxated on the dorsal side of the metatarsal head. The extensor tendons could have a tendency to do that. The opening of the fibrous flexor tendon sheath makes the flexor tendons free to pull the toe proximal phalanx against the interposed flap that holds the base of the first phalanx plantarward. The collateral ligaments are too thin to be sewn.

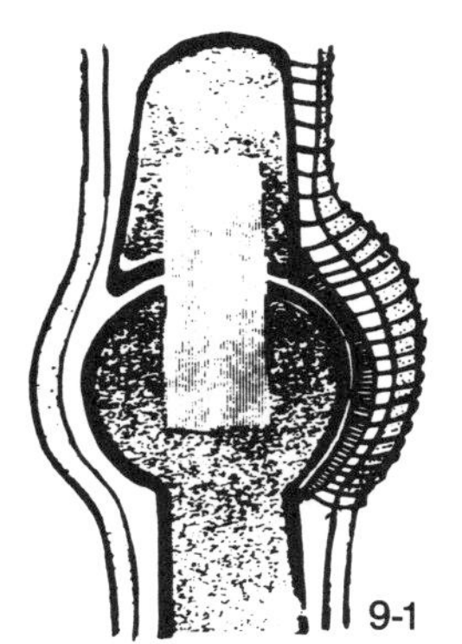

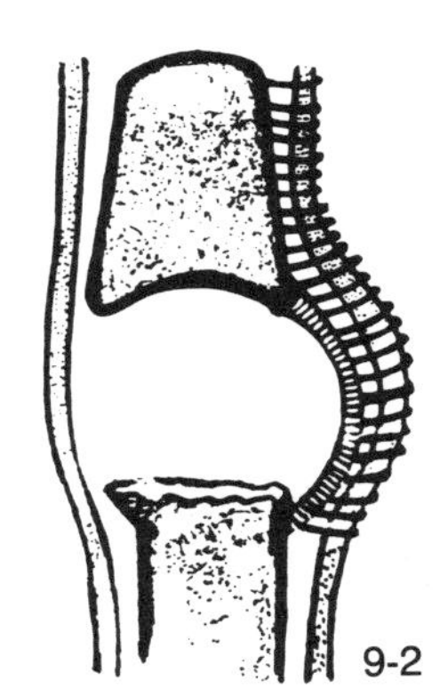

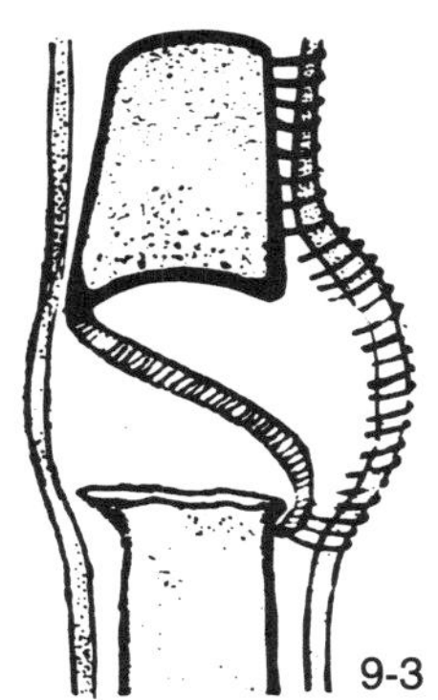

Figure 9-1. The metatarsophalangeal joint. On the upper side of the joint is seen the extensor tendon. On the plantar side is seen the thick capsule fixed to the metatarsal bone and the first phalanx and connected to the tendon sheath of the flexor digitorum.

Figure 9-2. The metatarsal head is resected to the fixation of the fibrous capsule on the neck of the metatarsal bone.

Figure 9-3. The fibrous capsule is cut free from the tendon sheath and is fixed to the dorsal edge of the first phalanx.

Case Examples of Loose MP Joints in Dancers

Case 1. A 27-year-old female dancer had an operation for a sprained ankle in 1971. Before this operation, she had metatarsalgia in both feet, mostly in the right. The author saw the patient in 1975. She had looseness in both second MP joints. The author resected the second metatarsal head on the right side, and after half a year, she was free of pain. Later, she had a resection of the left second metatarsal head, and 3 months later she was free of pain in both feet.

Case 2. A 56-year-old male choreographer and director in 1980 complained of pain from a hallux rigidus. The author performed a Keller Meary operation on the left hallux rigidus, with an excellent result. Four months later, the patient complained of metatarsalgia in the left second toe. The MP joint was painful and loose. In May 1981, the second metatarsal head was resected. The result was excellent.

Case 3. A 20-year-old female dancer had right metatarsalgia with pain when doing *relevé*. The author saw the patient in December 1980. The second MP joint was swollen and loose. X-ray showed a long and thick second metatarsal bone, and the joint space in the MP joint was wider than in the other MP joints. Resection of the second metatarsal head was done in January 1981. The joint capsule was distended. The result was excellent.

Case 4. In December 1979, the author performed a Keller Meary operation on the left foot of a 54-year-old male choreographer, with an excellent result. In September 1982, the patient complained of pain in the left second MP joint, which was loose. He underwent surgery in March 1983 for resection of the second metatarsal head. In March 1984 he was pain free and the second toe had a normal position.

Case 5. A 57-year-old female dance teacher had pain in the third MP joint in the right foot for 5 years. She was seen in May 1981. The third toe was loose and subluxated dorsally, and on the sole there was a callosity below the metatarsal head. The second toe was a hammer toe. She had a resection of the third metatarsal head and of the first interphalangeal joint of the second toe. After the operation, she had an inflammation in the wound on the second toe, but a year later she wrote that the foot was fine.

Case 6. A 27-year-old male dancer was seen by the author in November 1974. He had had right metatarsalgia, which had been treated with hydrocortisone injections, and had swelling and looseness in the right second MP joint. X-rays showed dislocation of the MP joint. The author resected the second metatarsal head. There was osteoarthrosis, with destruction of the cartilage. Five months later, he had swelling and pain, and a granuloma was removed from the space between the metatarsal bone and the toe. Pathology showed fibrous tissue with a foreign body granuloma. In June 1976, he underwent surgery for Morton's neurofibroma, and in 1980 he wrote that he had danced since 1976. The third toe had a tendency to overlap the distal part of the fourth toe, but he was still dancing.

Case 7. A 29-year-old male dancer had had surgery for an exostosis below the left heel bone, with good results. The author saw the patient in January 1984. He had pain at the first metatarsal head in the left foot. The first MP joint was normal, but he had a loose second MP joint and was experiencing pain and tenderness. The second metatarsal head was resected, with an excellent result.

10

DANCERS' SHOES AND FOOT CARE

Thomas M. Novella, D.P.M.

Introduction

The objective of this chapter is to help unravel the mysteries of bandages, tapings, paddings, and shoes and to explain what is involved in protecting the dancer's foot.

The essential question in nearly every dancer-physician encounter is, "How much time, if any, will I have to take off before I can safely return to dance?" The variety of salves, plasters, pads, and the like that dancers routinely and effectively employ indicates how much pain they withstand daily as well as how severe an injury must become before they seek professional help. The glib "Just stop dancing!" or "Take 3 months off!" are easy solutions for the doctor; but simple, well-planned measures such as paddings and tapings, dance shoe modifications, and street shoe orthoses may allow dancers to "selectively rest" an injury. This approach often allows them to continue some dancing without harming the injury site. Simultaneously, they may work on the underlying cause, such as a weak muscle group or incorrect technique.[1]

The greatest benefit a physician can provide in any microtraumatic injury is to determine the etiology. Once the underlying cause is corrected, the dancer can eliminate the pad or device as soon as reasonably indicated. Otherwise, a compensatory injury could evolve.[2] (It is safe to maintain the same attitude when prescribing anti-inflammatory medications for musculoskeletal overuse.)

These simple modifications will be more effective if the doctor is familiar enough with dance to predict all positions in which the dancer's foot must articulate with the floor. In paddings about a metatarsalgia, for example, the pad must border symptomatic areas from plantigrade foot position all the way up to three-quarters *pointe.* The scaphoid pad, which is commonly used for metatarsalgias, is by definition applied proximal to the metatarsal heads, but it is less effective than a long U-shaped pad for dancer's metatarsalgia.

Use of Padding

Plantar adhesive felt padding is used for:

- *Pontooning.* This modifies the weight-bearing surface of the foot to relieve injured areas from repetitive trauma by increasing the ground reaction at uninjured sites. It often permits continuance with dance.
- *Wedging.* Used to redirect or inhibit motion.
- *Proprioceptive Aid.* This may be attempted directly, as in a lateral forefoot wedge for ankle stability, or indirectly, by means of a gentle pad to remind the dancer of an alignment change.
- *Cushioning.* This is used in cases in which such a great percentage of the weight-bearing surface is affected that dispersion would be unrealistic. Foam works better here than felt.

The following sections discuss dance injuries that are amenable to this type of management and present details on techniques and materials involved.

Stone Bruises or Metatarsalgias

The dancer complains of pain, usually beneath a metatarsal head, while bearing weight strictly on the ball of the foot. Usually, no pain is present once full *pointe* is achieved (unless tight shoes are triggering a Morton's neuroma).[3] In severe cases, the pain will be present while wearing running or tennis shoes. The injury may be traceable to (1) stomping on *demi-pointe* without subsequent heel-contacting; (2) wearing "soft" *pointe* shoes after having been used to "hard" shoes (allowing more ready metatarsal-head contact); (3) doing more turns on *demi-pointe* than one is accustomed to (pirouettes and *chaînés* turns in particular); (4) dancing on particularly unyielding surfaces[4,5]; or (5) other mechanisms imparting increased ground reaction to the metatarsal head region.

The severity of the injury will in large part determine when the dancer may return to work. The following methodology may help to eliminate an individual's pain threshold in establishing the degree of severity in metatarsalgia.

Proceeding from least to most severe, degrees of pain metatarsalgia can be described as: (1) pain at the end of the dancing day; (2) pain landing in *temps levé;* (3) pain earlier in the day, abating; (4) pain earlier in class, abating; (5) pain landing in *sauté;* (6) pain descending stairs; (7) pain after class, persisting with every step; (8) pain at barre, persisting; (9) pain on getting up in the morning, persisting with every step; (10) pain not mitigated by weight bearing (neoplasia and Freiberg's infraction should be ruled out).

This synovitis, capsulitis, or other soft-tissue bruise should be differentiated from Freiberg's infraction, Morton's neuroma, metatarsal stress fracture, sesamoidopathies, fractured proximal phalanx, fractured supernumerary sesamoid, or torn metatarsophalangeal joint capsule.

Physical examination reveals tenderness to direct, relatively gentle palpation of the inferior aspect of the involved structures. Meticulous technique can usually delineate a vaguely circumscribed area and uncover indurated or focal masses representing scarring or "cysts."[6] It is painful to rise on *demi-pointe*. X-rays are often inconclusive for frank pathology. The involved metatarsals may be "dropped," or more often, fall long of the normal metatarsal length parabola.[7] Contiguous metatarsals may be too short or relatively hypermobile, thus causing an inordinate peaking of ground reactive forces at the chief complaint site.[8] A "splay foot," as is common in hallux valgus (which is almost universal in dancers[9,10]), may allow "spiking" of a single metatarsophalangeal joint to occur.[11]

Other associated findings often include a pes cavus with relative inflexibility at the ankle or midfoot (retaining impact trauma in the metatarsal head region[12]), short toes, or weak intrinsic digital muscles. If the examiner can easily resist plantarflexion of the distal *or proximal* phalanges, an occult weakness may be perpetuating the complaint, because digital weakness increases loading forces at the metatarsophalangeal joints.[13] Thus, *pointe* dancers who continue using rigid or "hard" shoes have less opportunity to develop intrinsic digital strength through articulating between *pointe* and *demi-pointe*. They are more susceptible to these or related injuries if the choreography calls for a bare foot or a ballet slipper. Similar loss of digital purchase no doubt causes chronic metatarsalgia in dancers who have undergone arthroplastic digital surgery, occasionally to such a degree as to prompt legal action.

Other muscles to be evaluated in assessment of metatarsalgias include the tibialis anticus, which decelerates foot slap after heel loading;[14] the triceps surae, which decelerates heel contact after forefoot loading; and the decelerators of pelvic tilt—the lower back, lower abdominal, and hip abductor groups—which stabilize pelvic tilt[15] and thus "ease the foot in for a landing." These occult factors should always be tested in overuse syndromes involving the foot or leg. Weakness of these muscles is likely to lead to overload in the distal extremity.

In establishing a primary diagnosis in such a compact area as the foot, it is important not to overlook other complaints or impending, subthreshold injuries. It should be remembered that dancers often wait for two or three injuries to accumulate before seeking help. This is especially true in metatarsalgias. A check should be made for radiographic or at least clinical signs of a stress fracture of the metatarsal shaft,[16] of an instability in the ankle, or of a bruise of the heel leading to forward weight shifting.

Finally, injuries to the foot are most often topographically accessible and lend themselves quite readily to palpation. Palpated findings are more reliable when the corresponding area of the uninvolved foot is simultaneously examined with equal pressure and direction of motion, to enable a subjective comparison.

Method

Less severe injuries can often be managed in such a way as to permit continued dance without significant rest if meticulously applied dispersive padding is used. The principles of dispersive padding are useful for dancers to know throughout their career. They will appreciate a doctor's sharing the information with them. The object of dispersive padding is to relieve injured areas from ground contact by overexploiting uninjured areas. Pads are applied to the portion of the foot bearing weight during maneuvers that typically cause pain. For example, in a second metetatarsophalangeal joint metatarsalgia, most contiguous uninvolved surface areas of the plantar forefoot can be considered candidates to help remove weight from the injured tissue.

Materials

Adhesive felt makes an excellent dispersive vehicle. It elevates uninvolved areas to perform a "pontooning" service for the injured tissue. Foam is usually inefficient because it packs. One can thin, skive, and stratify felt to a desired shape or thickness (figure 10-1). Adhesive felt will also more accurately stay in contact with the borders of the injury site than dispersive full-length insoles, which permit slippage and jamming of the injury into the dispersive cavity. Insoles have the added disadvantage of taking up more room in the shoe.

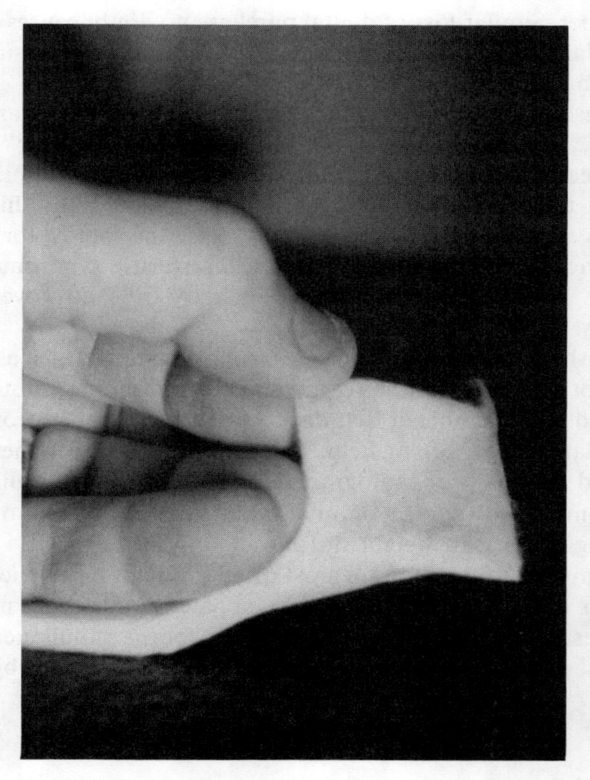

Figure 10-1. Adhesive felt can be thinned or stratified by snipping a corner (holding the scissors parallel to the plane of the adhesive) and then pulling the resultant ears apart.

Technique

1. By palpation, isolate the injured area *exactly* and if desired, delineate the injury geographically with a felt-tipped pen.

2. Visualize why the site received extraordinary stress. How far distally must the adjacent pontoons be placed to unweight a long metatarsophalangeal joint at high three-quarter *pointe*? Now outline the distal and proximal borders of the felt pontoons with the pen (figure 10-2).

3. Just after drawing the felt-tipped pen line, carefully press the paper backing of the adhesive felt into the line. This neat trick transfers the line to the backing. Then cut out and discard the apparent distribution of the injury and apply the remainder of the felt about the edges of the guidelines you drew on the skin. Angling the scissors at 45° to the surface while cutting will yield a beveled, more forgiving edge.

Selected Examples

Second Metatarsophalangeal Joint. The most common site for a stone bruise is the second metatarsophalangeal joint; it is usually the longest, thus

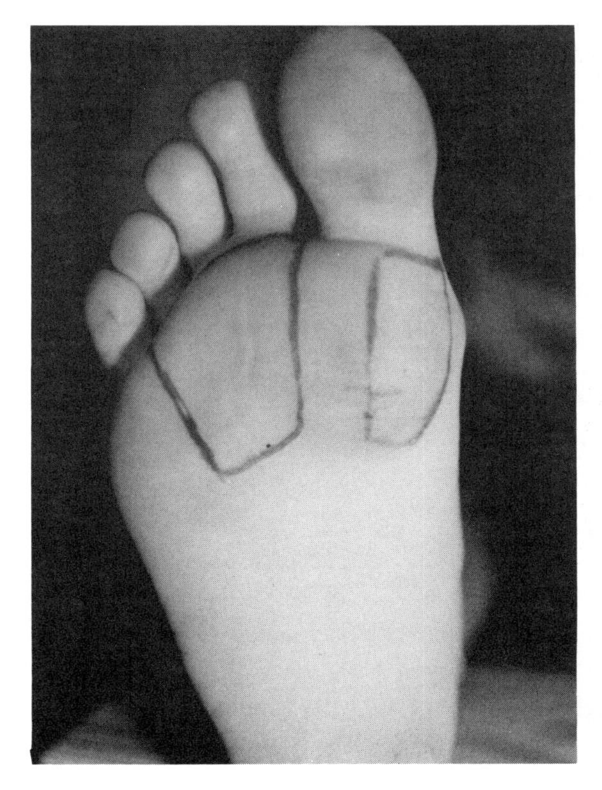

Figure 10-2. Felt-tipped pen line delineating asymptomatic areas about an involved fibular sesamoid.

the most vulnerable joint in *demi-* and full *pointe.* In addition, it is the most strongly anchored metatarsal at its base, leaving less shock-absorbing excursion in the joint. Evaluating the amount and quality of excursion available at the bases of the pontooning metatarsals, as well as the lengths of the symptomatic and pontooning metatarsals, helps determine the thickness of the pads as well as the surface area the pads must cover (figure 10-3).

Indiscriminate Bruise Pattern. Often, an area not simply limited to one metatarsophalangeal joint may be involved, but on the other hand, occasionally only a portion of a single metatarsophalangeal joint may be injured. In general, the larger the involved area, the less success one can expect with this padding technique. Often, after one area has been traumatized, other areas will bruise because of the dancer's guarding and compensatory weight shifting. Expect this if the problem is in the early postacute stage, making delineation, thus treatment, more difficult.

A traumatic etiology in cases involving such "spreading" metatarsalgias, especially if accompanied by swelling and/or larger-joint involvements, must be absolutely confirmed historically, lest an occult spondylopathy, Reiters syndrome, postinfection arthropathy, or other rheumatologic process be overlooked.[17] But if a violent misstep into a floor irregularity, for example,

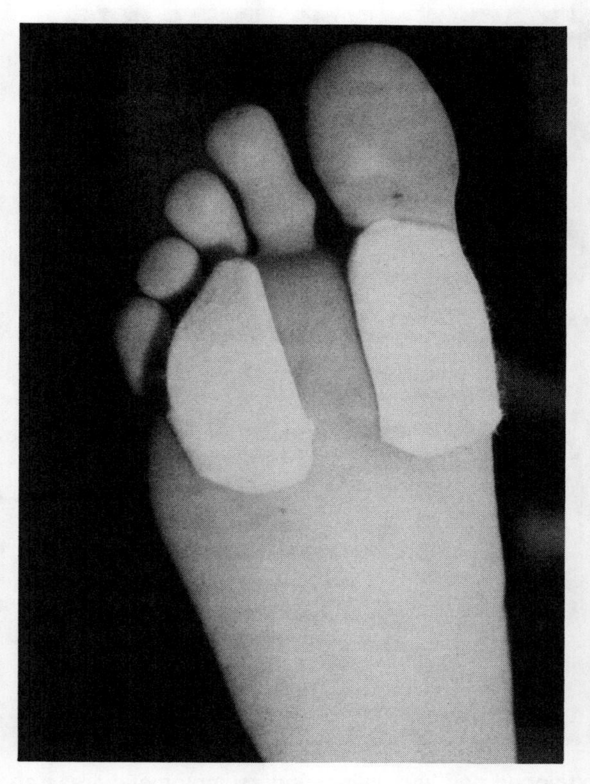

Figure 10-3. Padding for a second metatarsalgia.

confirms a traumatic etiology for an irregular-pattern metatarsalgia, attempts at felt padding can prove fruitful.

Adjunctive Measures

In addition to padding, postactivity localized ice massage (barring any neurovascular contraindications) is extremely useful, as also are intrinsic digital muscle-strengthening programs. Circumferential wraps about the metatarsus are helpful for a plantar soft tissue pad that is "spiked" by widely separated metatarsophalangeal joints. This often occurs in dancers who combine lax ligaments with hallux valgus.[18] These wraps are available commercially or may be fabricated with Elastoplast or adhesive tape (figure 10-4).

Fractured Supernumerary Sesamoid

The incidence of accessory ossicles beneath the fifth metatarsal head is 25-62%; the second, 4-18%; the third and fourth, 0%; and the first, 100%. Additionally, 50% of the population has an accessory bone beneath the interphalangeal joint of the hallux.[19] Swelling and ecchymosis may be a tip-off, but radiographic confirmation is required. Metatarsal head stress fractures, although uncommon, as well as transchondral or subchondral fractures should be ruled out. Fractured pedal sesamoids may persist symptomatically for 6-18 months.[20] Excision is not immediately advised, as subsequent metatarsophalangeal joint laxity could lead to chronic metatarsalgia and/or instability.

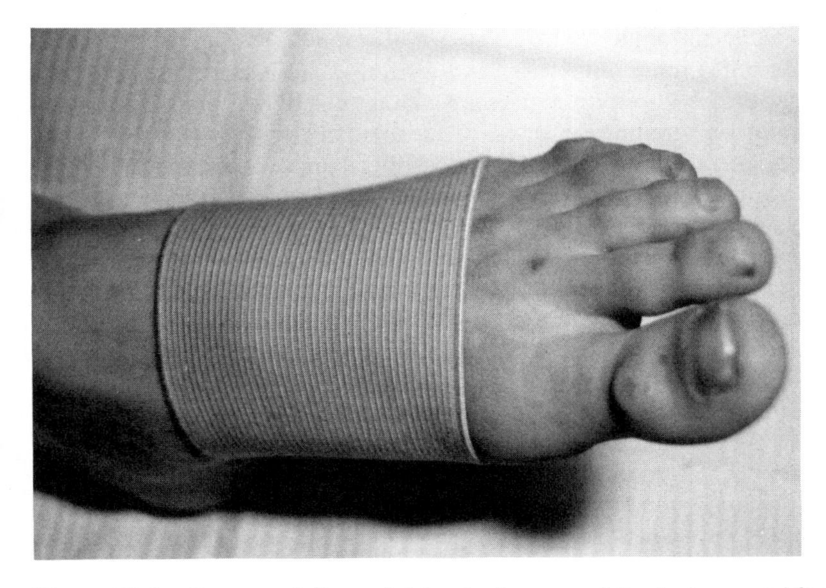

Figure 10-4. Commercially available elastic wrap of the instep, used for splay foot or metatarsal stress fractures.

Freiberg's Infraction

Freiberg's infraction, regarded as an avascular necrosis originating at the epiphysis of a lesser metatarsal head (usually the second), is a self-limiting disorder.[21] Continued dancing, however, can lead to growth plate avulsion and/or significant osteophytosis, both near-absolute impediments to a career. Erythema, swelling, tenderness dorsally as well as plantarly, and nonweight-bearing pain in a young adolescent, especially female, are the typical manifestations. These are subsequently confirmed by radiographic examination, which characteristically shows a flattening of the metatarsal head. Surgical intervention is usually not helpful. Rest and dispersive padding can help symptoms until the disorder runs its course. Certain authors recommend below-knee plaster immobilization. Others advise against immobilization because of ensuing atrophy and the extensive rehabilitation required to return to dance.[22]

Torn Metatarsophalangeal Joint Capsular Ligaments

In the acute stage of this injury,[23,24] the patient presents limping and reports having tripped, or having had some other mishap violent enough to have torn the proximal phalanx away from its metatarsal head. Patients presenting later in the course of this injury will complain of inability to *relevé* due to pain. Typical of a severe metatarsalgia, the dancer also admits to persistent pain while walking.

This injury should be differentiated from, among others, a dorsal bruise caused by a choreographic "fall to the knee" requiring weight bearing atop the metatarsophalangeal joints.

In addition to more tenderness and swelling than is normally seen in a simple plantar bruise, capsular injuries are characterized by apprehension signs as well as pain on attempts to displace the phalanx base dorsally or plantarward on the metatarsal head. Pure passive dorsal and plantarflexion is painful at end range, and crepitation, if present, is an ominous sign. X-ray evaluation usually shows joint space asymmetry or subtle signs of malalignment at the involved metatarsophalangeal joint. The greater the joint space asymmetry, the greater the likelihood that a transchondral and/or subchondral injury has taken place. Such an injury may require a Keller's operation at this lesser metatarsophalangeal joint to achieve walking comfort; unfortunately, this does not bode well for future dancing.

Noncartilaginous injuries should be locally immobilized (basket-weave taping to the adjacent toe and to the metatarsals, wearing a wooden-soled surgical shoe) and protected as effectively as possible with appropriate dispersive padding. An initial course of no weight bearing may be required. Dancing is suspended for 4-8 weeks, depending on the extent of the tear. Insufficient immobilization in the early course of this injury can leave the dancer with instability at the joint and recurrent metatarsalgia. As soon as the acute stage of the injury is over, active and/or galvanic strengthening exercises of the digital intrinsic muscles should be instituted.

For long-standing grade 3 injuries, which exhibit more pain when the examiner displaces the phalanx base dorsally or plantarward than when the joint is directly palpated plantarward, a different pad may prove useful. It would help to review the biomechanics of the lesser metatarsophalangeal joints at this time before describing the pad.

During closed kinetic chain dorsiflexion of the proximal phalanx in a *relevé (demi-pointe),* isolated pure dorsiflexion (spin about the axis) does not take place.[25] Because of the elliptical shape of the articular surface of the metatarsal head and its changing axis of rotation, a certain amount of dorsal displacement of the base of the proximal phalanx upon the metatarsal head must occur. It is this motion, as the examiner will note when he displaces the phalanx base during his clinical examination, that perpetuates this injury in *demi-pointe.*

Padding Technique

Use a square of 1/8-in. adhesive felt placed exactly beneath the involved metatarsal head. It should terminate distally right at the metatarsophalangeal joint line. It should not go beyond (that is, impinge upon the base of the proximal phalanx). In this way, dorsal gliding of the proximal phalanx can be limited to within an asymptomatic range, as the metatarsal head now has a starting point dorsal to its normal neutral position. Also, elevation of the metatarsal head reduces the dorsiflexion the proximal phalanx requires to achieve *relevé* (figure 10-5).

Another useful brace employs a strip of adhesive tape 2 in. wide and 4-5 in. long in which a hole is cut for each toe. The toes are inserted through the holes and the strip secured. (figures 10-6, 10-7).

Sesamoids

The term "sesamoiditis" is a catchall for pain in the region of the plantar first metatarsal head, but it is a misnomer just as "patella-itis" would be. Interpreted literally, the misnomer is a dangerous one for two reasons. First, it discourages further investigation as to the true tissue injured. Thus, accuracy of diagnosis is impeded. A wide variety of primary and secondary etiologies can cause trouble in this region. Second, the term defines itself as "inflammation of the sesamoid," which, like "patella-itis," does not actually occur and could lead one to give anti-inflammatory medications, systemic and/or locally injected, as primary therapy, perhaps later adding massage or ultrasound. If a fracture or stress fracture has not been ruled out and the diagnostic effort halted at the mere observation of swelling in the area, the above measures actually might do more harm than good.

A differential diagnosis of injuries in this area might include:

- Frank fractures of the sesamoids
- Stress fractures of the sesamoids[26]
- Sesamoid entrapment syndromes*[27,28]

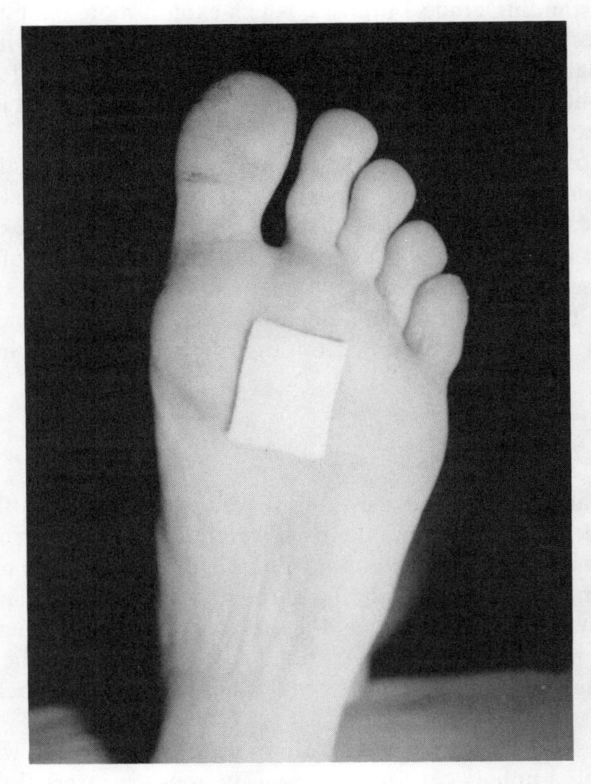

Figure 10-5. Pad affixed strictly beneath second metatarsal head to inhibit dorsal gliding of proximal phalanx.

- Chondromalacia of the sesamoid[29]
- Tendinitis of the flexor hallucis brevis
- Strained sesamoid suspensory ligament
- Neuritis
- Postsesamoid-excision incisional neuroma
- Ganglion cyst, intersesamoidal
- Osteochondritis of the sesamoids[30]
- Fractured base of proximal phalanx[31,32]
- Stress fracture of metatarsal head
- Arthritic (osteophytic proliferation, crista erosion, joint space narrowing) changes about the sesamoid–first-metatarsal-head articular surfaces.[33]

An acute sesamoid fracture should be treated primarily by complete avoidance of weight bearing for 4-6 weeks; stress fractures may require one week less off weight bearing. The dancer will be limited to getting around on crutches, which may already be in use at the time of the initial evaluation. The

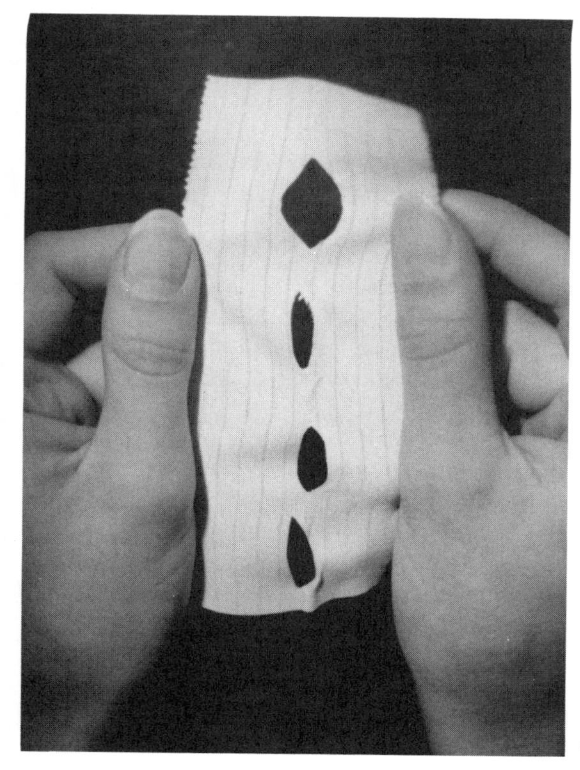

10-6

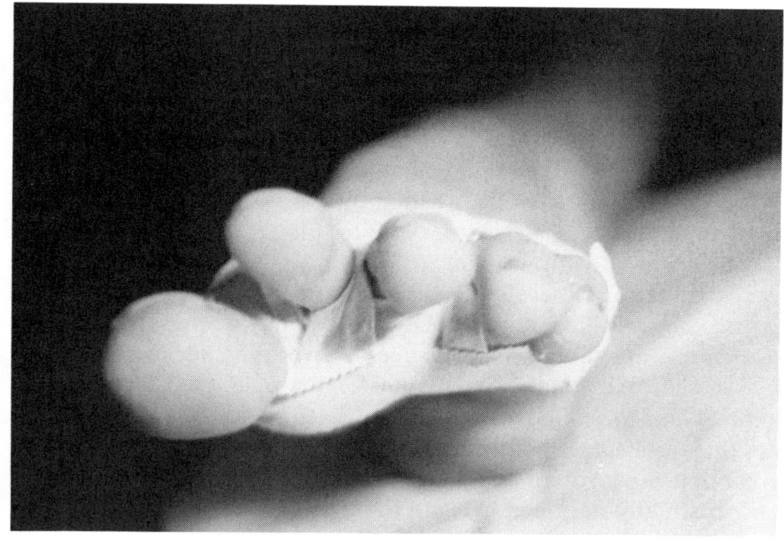

10-7

Figures 10-6, 10-7. Taping to arrest accessory motions in the toes.

area plantar first metatarsophalangeal joint region will be swollen, exquisitely tender to palpation, and almost always painful on any passive motion of the hallux. Resisted motion testing is discouraged at this time. Curiously, fractured sesamoids seldom become ecchymotic.

A fracture on x-ray will appear as one or more irregular semilinear radiolucencies in the body of the sesamoid. Displacement may not occur. Bi- or multipartite sesamoids should be ruled out. Axial or tangential views are suggested.

If the injury is neglected for a long enough period, the adjacent sesamoid often also becomes symptomatic. This circumstance greatly reduces the efficacy of sesamoid padding to afford weight-bearing comfort; also, it significantly impairs diagnostic efforts to determine the original lesion. Improper or insufficient treatment of an acutely fractured sesamoid could lead to 6-18 months or more of disability.

A stress fracture may not show up on plain x-rays, but may require both clinical judgment and a positive technetium 99 bone scan for confirmation.

Plaster immobilization is a standard treatment for acute sesamoid fracture, but it is not necessarily applicable to dancers because of the secondary muscular atrophy and loss of mobility that may result. Dancers understand this and will cooperate by avoiding weight bearing for the necessary period. Furthermore, attempts to immobilize the hallux could actually be contraindicated, as the distractile mischief of the flexor hallucis brevis upon the fracture fragments might be heightened.

While on the subject of differential diagnosis of sesamoid injury, the mechanism as alluded to by Root et al should be mentioned. Besides the obvious mechanism of direct impact, sesamoids may be injured by *entrapment*. The second metatarsal is normally longer that the first, so it can act as a prop in normal propulsive gait (and *demi-pointe*) to elevate the first metatarsal head. This allows the dorsiflexing hallux to easily pull the sesamoids beneath the metatarsal head. It becomes more difficult for the sesamoids to glide beneath the first metatarsal head if the first metatarsal exceeds or even approaches the second in length. This sets up the entrapment syndrome of the sesamoids between the ground and the first metatarsal head.

Classic cases present with complaints of weight-bearing pain in the sesamoid region, which is often relieved if the dancer walks "flat-footed" instead of propelling through the dorsiflexed toes at later phases of gait. Thus, *demi-pointe* cannot be achieved without pain.

Clinical examination is perplexing because tenderness to palpation often falls far short of the *relevé*-loaded pain. Discomfort may be present only during weight bearing. Depending on the degree of severity, tenderness to direct palpation may be elicited when active plantarflexion of the hallux is resisted from a maximally dorsiflexed position. Dorsoplantar x-rays are helpful (figure 10-8) because they immediately illustrate the overly long first metatarsal and may also reveal that the involved sesamoid (often the lateral or "fibular" one) appears more proximally stationed beneath the first metatarsal head than does its companion sesamoid. This presumably indicates that a tensile strain occurred upon the tendon attachment between the sesamoid and the base of the proximal phalanx.

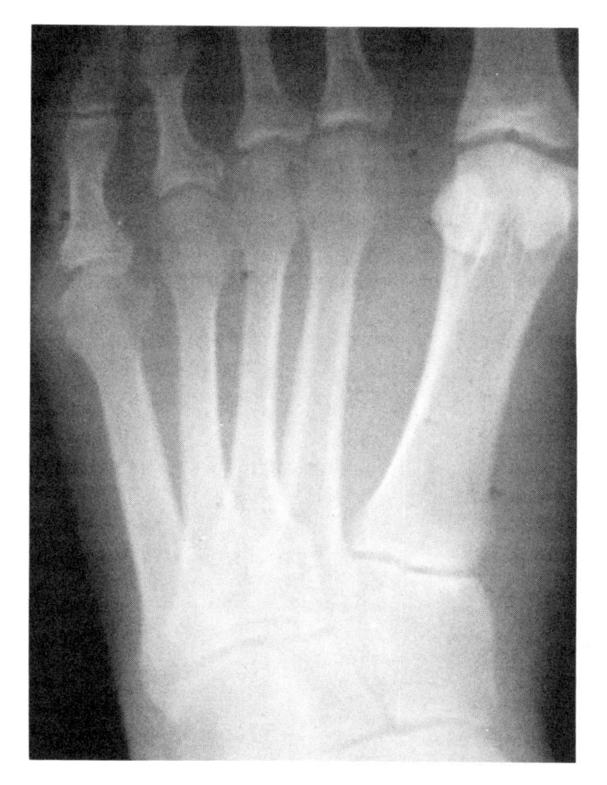

Figure 10-8. Radiographic illustration of the first metatarsal, which falls slightly long of the normal metatarsal length parabola, demonstrating proximally stationed fibular or lateral sesamoid.

If this foot type is present (long first metatarsal), then this syndrome will benefit from the classic "sesamoid pad" (figure 10-9). This pad elevates the first metatarsal in both plantigrade as well as in *demi-pointe* by functionally lengthening the lesser metatarsals. It must extend far enough distally to effectively lift the lesser metatarsals in full *demi-pointe*.

Nonentrapment injuries benefiting from this pad include stress or prestress fractures or old, inadequately treated fractures that are still painful upon weight bearing. These injuries are less successfully treated if they are old enough or serious enough to involve both of the sesamoids beneath a hallux. Therefore, if an appreciable tensile component to the injury also exists, wherein pain is elicited on clinical examination when hallux plantarflexion is resisted, then simple unweighting of the involved bone is not adequate for relief of symptoms. Healing is not easily promoted because the tensile strain upon the sesamoid mechanism is not eliminated, and the flexor hallucis brevis continues to fire to provide plantar stability to the first metatarsophalangeal joint in *demi-pointe.*

In these cases, one may only verify the efficacy of a dispersive pad by using it within a shoe with a rocker mechanism at the ball. This helps obviate hal-

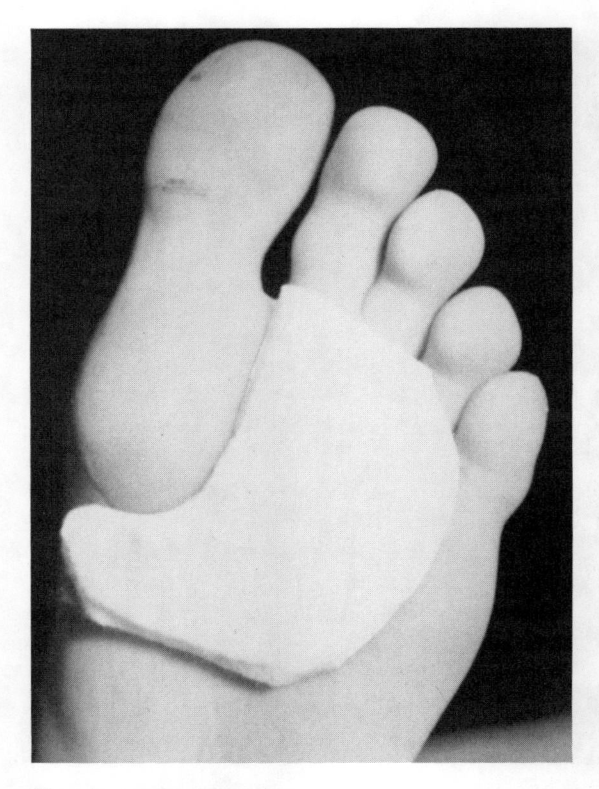

Figure 10-9. Classic sesamoid pad.

lux dorsiflexion. These shoes should have a wedge whose maximal thickness ($^3/_{16}$-$^3/_8$ in.) is beneath the average center of dorsiplantar rotation of the first metatarsophalangeal joint. The wedge should taper to zero thickness by the time it reaches the tips of the toes.[34] This allows the toes to rest on a flat footbed; the wedge essentially does the dorsiflexing for them. Wedges terminating proximal to the first metatarsal head, especially if they do not elevate it at all, will not work. Certain shoes available commercially have a small rocker effect. These include certain Famolare soles, Rockports, Tiger Epirus, and others. A custom rocker may be specified for fitting by a shoemaker. An additional benefit of a rocker mechanism is its ability to assist in heel-off. This can aid healing of Achilles tendinitis.

Sesamoid padding, as well as other dispersive padding at the ball of the foot, should take into account the parabolic silhouette of the metatarsal heads in a coronal section through the forefoot, the so-called "transverse metatarsal (head) arch." The apex of this arch is normally at the second metatarsal head. A pad must be thickest there to be fully efficient in lengthening the second metatarsal head. The pad tapers down gradually to least thickness by the time it reaches the fourth metatarsal head, following the silhouette of the transverse arch. The pad is usually not placed beneath the fifth metatarsal head, lest it rotate the body weight medially and increase ground-reactive force at the first metatarsal head. Affixing a little strip of felt beneath the asymptomatic companion sesamoid is also helpful (figures 10-10, 10-11).

Chondromalacia or malalignment syndromes may occur in the sesamoid-intersesamoid crista articulation. Tangential or axial roentgenographic projections may help to establish this diagnosis. It is often associated with early hallux valgus. The laterally drifting proximal phalanx carries the tibial sesamoid into the still-intact crista.[35] The injury may be appeased symptomatically with above-described modifications of the sesamoid pad, as well as by interdigital spacers to medially displace the hallux (figure 10-12).

Further efforts should be made to arrest the progress of the hallux valgus, such as strengthening of the intrinsic muscles investing the hallux, as long as the abductor hallucis does not laterally sublux the great toe on resisted plantarflexion. Otherwise, one might accelerate the formation of an established bunion deformity.[36] Benefit may be derived from street-shoe orthoses. Alignment modifications by a qualified dance or alignment teacher may help sort out technical errors potentiating the hallux valgus. Misfitted shoes are a simple consideration. If overlooked, they could foil exhaustive efforts to conservatively salvage a young foot from hallux valgus. Chondromalacia of the sesamoids or entrapment syndromes should have both clinical and the aforementioned radiographic criteria for differentiation from fractures. Extirpation of a sesamoid is a last resort, as it may potentiate a hallux abductovalgus or lead to instability of the hallux on *pointe.*

The flexor hallucis brevis, which envelops the sesamoid en route to its attachment at the base of the proximal phalanx, can be subject to tendinitis beneath the first metatarsal head. Typically, there is pain plantar to the first metatarsophalangeal joint upon resisting flexion of the great toe. Tenderness to palpation is usually absent. X-rays must be negative for fracture to confirm this diagnosis, although on the anteroposterior x-ray, the involved sesamoid may appear further from the base of the proximal phalanx than the one uninvolved.

Flexor Hallucis Longus Tendinitis

This injury, also known as functional hallux limitus, was initially described by Thomasen and is fairly common among ballet dancers.[37] Pain may be present in *relevé,* in *demi-* and *grand plié,* and even during walking. An atypical presentation can be pain at the posterior aspect of the talus. On examination, the pain may be produced by dorsiflexion of the foot with forced passive dorsiflexion of the hallux.

When the hallux dorsiflexes, the muscle fibers of the flexor hallucis longus become entrapped within the sheath that forms a tunnel for the tendon. The sheath is located at the posteromedial aspect of the talus. Active motion of the toes may cause palpable and even audible retromalleolar crepitation. Posterior tibial tendinitis may occur less frequently in dancers than in runners and must thus be carefully differentiated.[38] If hyperpronation is present, supinative in-shoe orthoses may relieve walking discomfort, as the flexor hallucis longus is a primary stabilizer of the subtalar joint against pronation. As indicated, ap-

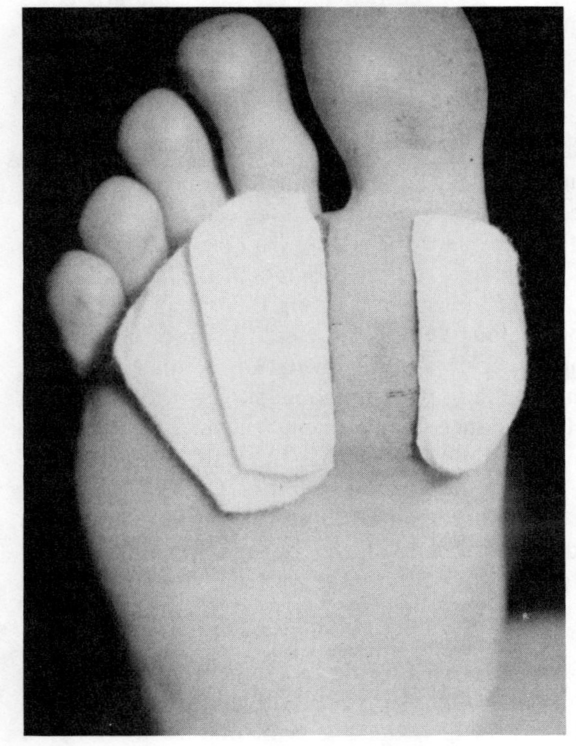

10-10

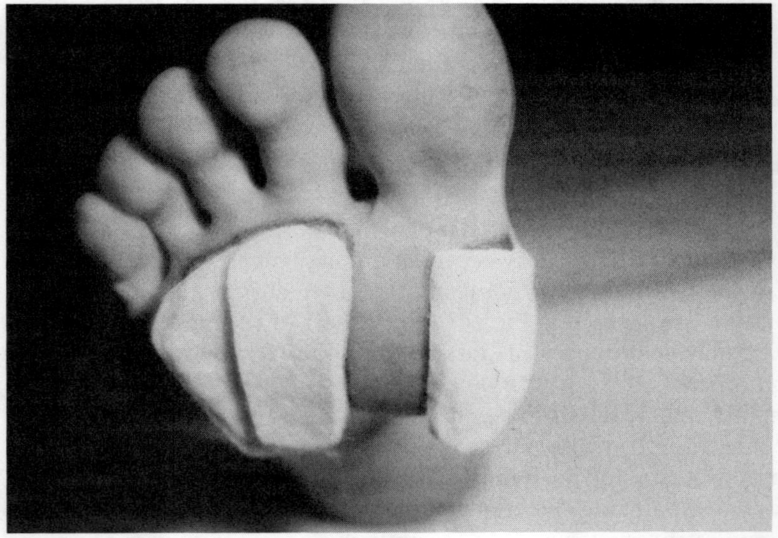

10-11

Figures 10-10, 10-11. Modified sesamoid pad exploiting tibial sesamoid to unweight fibular sesamoid.

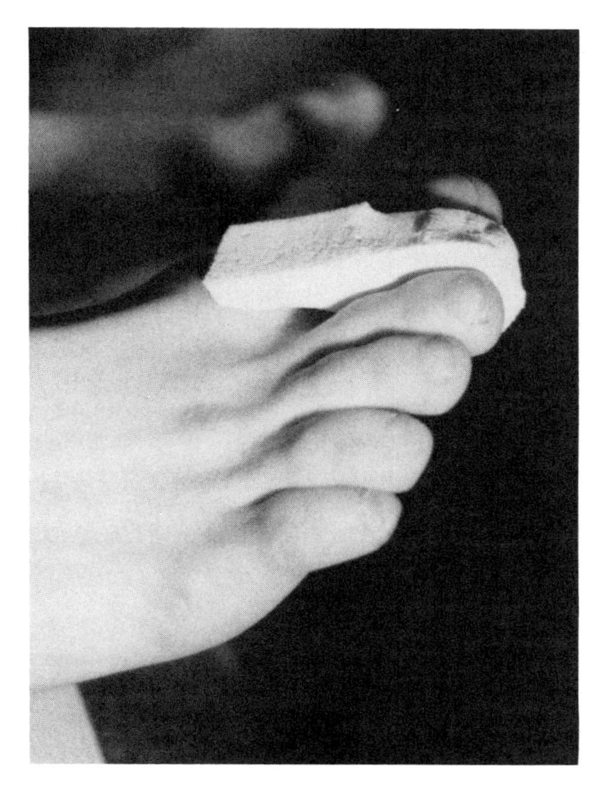

Figure 10-12. Interdigital spacer of 1/2-inch thick foam rubber to medially displace the hallux.

propriate stretching, strengthening, and proprioceptive therapy should be instituted for occasions when orthoses are not usable.

The flexor hallucis longus provides plantarflexory stability to the hallux in *demi-plié* and *grand plié* and medial stability to the ankle on *pointe.* This would explain its vulnerability. The tendon could be overtaxed while in *grand plié,* or even in *demi-plié,* forcing entrapment; while springing from a *demi-pointe* to a *pointe* position and vice versa, as in landing; while balancing on *pointe;* in dancers with lateral ankle weakness or instability (as a hyperabducted compensatory mechanism to achieve stability); and in dancers whose limited hip turn-out forces abduction at the foot on *pointe.*

This injury typically waxes and wanes, especially in those who have tenosynovial crepitation, or "trigger toe." These dancers take time off to let the injury calm down, and some go on to surgery. A pad that may help in the less acute case is a square of 1/8- to 1/4-in. felt beneath the medial forefoot. This decreases the total range of motion through which the flexor hallucis longus must support the body's center of mass at the ankle. It also decreases the tensile strain upon the tendon at its maximally taut position. Caution should be exercised in using this pad to avoid potentiating laterally unstable feet or ankles. Additionally, the pad may exacerbate preexisting sesamoid pathology.

Physical therapy is valuable in managing this condition. Full-blown cases can go on to stenosing tenosynovitis or trigger toe, requiring surgery.

Morton's Neuroma

Clinical assessment by examination of the foot with fingertip pressure from the plantar surface may elicit a palpable, even audible, clicking sensation that is strongly suggestive of Morton's neuroma. The typical presentation involves shooting pain emanating from the metatarsal head region into the toes. Some patients complain of numbness instead of, or in addition to, pain. A neurologic examination may demonstrate diminished touch sensitivity of the adjacent toes reduced not only in suspected neuromas but also with interdigital keratomas, particularly if the objective findings outweigh the complaint. A few dancers with this neuroma present with abscessed soft corns and underplayed symptoms.

This condition, usually the result of excessively tight shoes, may cause loss of sensation in the interdigital space. It occasionally responds to padding. The current theory states that Morton's neuroma involves pinching of nerve tissue between the metatarsal heads, usually the third and fourth, causing thickening of the neurilemma and leading to a chronic state. Because the condition is aggravated by tight shoes (and thus is more common in ballerinas than in modern dancers) and cumulative slamming of the foot, it may be relieved by tennis shoes or dispersion. Conservative therapy includes not only padding but sometimes taping, the use of orthoses for street shoes, physical therapy, and perhaps injections of hydrocortisone. If these measures are not successful, surgical excision of the nerve tissue may be necessary.

In the nondance mode, the condition may be addressed conservatively by various pads. In the dancer, the choices are limited, both from a functional and practical perspective. The most frequently used pad for a Morton's neuroma consists of a cuneiformlike felt wedge affixed plantar and proximal to the metatarsal heads to spread them apart. The purpose of the pad is to relieve the nerve of transverse metatarsal head compression without subjecting it to the direct pressure of the pad. Unfortunately, this pad relies on a plantigrade (heel and ball in simultaneous contact) stance to be effective. Dancers spend a great percentage of their time in forefoot or toe contact only, considerably diminishing more caudal ground-reactive forces required by the pad to separate the metatarsal heads. Still, tapings and dispersive pads following the guidelines set forth under metatarsalgia, as well as the cuneiform wedge, occasionally work. A simple half-size increase in shoe length or width sometimes is a more successful answer, because feet have a tendency to "grow" as time goes on. An adult ballerina may have finally exceeded a shoe tightness threshold because she is still wearing the same size she wore when she was 17.

Drawbacks in Use of Pads and Tapes

The drawbacks involved in using pads, tapes, orthoses, and the like include:

1. Encouraging dance without seeking to eliminate the cause of the injury. A warning sign of a more serious impending injury may be ignored, or other compensatory injuries might develop.

2. Constricting the artistic fluidity of a dancer's movement. This applies especially to tapings required for ankle stability, which can thus be self-defeating.

3. Upsetting a dancer's proprioceptive "feel for the floor,"[39] particularly in the case of forefoot or toe paddings. A patient must be warned to break in a pad gradually before using it for allégro or performance.

4. A pad may *directly* cause another injury. A dispersive pad to relieve one bruised metatarsal head may cause a contiguous one to bruise or even fracture. This could happen if a once-injured sesamoid is used as part of a pontoon.

Some ankles lack dorsiflexion after heel contact. This may impart too much ground-reactive force to the padded metatarsal heads.[40] Osteophytes at the anterior talotibial joint sufficient to produce this side effect are not rare in dancers.[41] The depth of the *demi-plié* should first be checked before padding is used beneath the forefoot.

A wedge beneath the medial forefoot may cause a sprained ankle in patients with lateral instability.

A too-stiff *pointe* shoe orthosis may cause a ballerina to force *tendu* or *pointe,* leading to Achilles tendinitis.

5. The appliqué may *indirectly* cause injury. A dancer may have to devise a subconscious technique change, like foot hyperpronation, to relieve dysfunction in the lower back.[42] This may cause discomfort in the ankle. A too-aggressive taping of the ankle could reignite the back injury.

6. Sometimes, a device is useful during only a portion of the day's activities. For example, street-shoe orthoses may contribute carryover relief, so that a problem is less acute during dance. An effort should be made to achieve a pain-free state during nondancing time.[43]

7. Some appliqués may be acceptable for class, but their bulk or appearance may make them inappropriate for performance. Only as much material as is necessary to gain the desired result should be used.

8. Physical therapy and alignment modification should be instituted as soon as reasonable. Unfortunately, these adjuncts are not always within the dancer's means. If this is the case, it is paramount that the physician provide the patient with appropriate exercises, along with advice on local care, street shoes, daily activities, and follow-up. Materials not readily purchased over the counter, such as adhesive felts and elastic tapes, should be made available at minimal cost, with explicit instructions and warnings as to their use.

9. Adhesive felt is less effective in individuals who sweat heavily. Pretape sprays or adhesive tape binders sometimes help, as may tincture of benzoin.

10. Adhesive dressings changed too infrequently to allow hygienic routine can lead to contact dermatitis or can promote growth of surface organisms. They should not, of course, be applied over broken or infected skin. Upon removal, they can worsen epidermal fissures or so-called skin splits.

Limited Ankle Dorsiflexion

As discussed earlier, ground-reactive forces are increased at the forefoot if the ankle lacks adequate dorsiflexion. In some cases, this is due to a lack of mobility in the joint itself. Cumulative forces or a traumatic injury may have lessened normal mortise diastasis.[44] Sometimes forefoot-loading forces are increased by tightness in the gastrocnemius or, less often, in the soleus. Not infrequently, osteophytosis at the anterior talotibial joint margin limits dorsiflexion.

Regardless of the cause, if a limitation to ankle dorsiflexion exists, forces upon the forefoot will be increased as the tibia proceeds forward over the foot (*demi-plié,* landing, *fondu,* fifth position, etc.) Unaddressed, this underlying deficiency can greatly lessen the effectiveness of conservative treatment.

The situation can be helped with stretching exercises of the gastroc-soleus and therapeutic mobilization to facilitate normal distal tibiofibular joint mobility and/or talocrural mobility in ankle dorsiflexion.

Additionally, strengthening exercises of the decelerators of heel-loading (lower back, lower abdominals, and hip abductors, which soften pelvic tilt,[45] and in dancers who are forefoot-first contactors, calf muscles) diminish compressive forces at the ankle. Strength in this group also slows down the forward momentum of the tibia upon the talus.[46] Rest, therapy, alignment or technique modifications, and other conservative measures may provide an alternative to a surgical cleanup of the anterior ankle joint.

Heel Lifts

In anterior ankle impingement syndrome, the structures at the front of the ankle are "pinched" in dorsiflexion *(plié).* In other cases, limited dorsiflexion may be the cause of a separate complaint. During acute stages, one may "cheat" around this defect by suggesting that the dancer use a heel lift, in effect to exploit some of the posterior curvature of the talar dome upon which new dorsiflexion can be achieved.

To work, a heel lift must be thick enough (at least 3/16 in.) and noncompressive. Jazz shoes, which have a thin heel rise, may help. A felt heel lift inside a slipper or affixed by Elastoplast to the foot inside the slipper may also work. But felt heel lifts tamp down quickly, requiring frequent replacement.

Another method involves using the rear two-thirds of a ballet slipper. One cuts a ballet slipper in two at the juncture just proximal to the metatarsal heads. (A heel lift should not be extended beneath the metatarsal heads because its slope will be nullified. Doing this is not desirable in anterior impingement syndromes.) The rear portion, elastics affixed, is worn; the front portion is discarded. The dancer then puts on a normal pair of ballet slippers and is thus wearing a nonslip heel lift within the shoe. Some manufacturers such as Repetto make ballet slippers with a heel lift.

Some ballerinas order "three-quarter-shank" *pointe* shoes, a feature that both enhances the arched appearance of the foot on *pointe* and increases the flexibility of the shoe. But this also places the ankle in a "negative heel" situation; so that counterproductive forces caused by any lack of dorsiflexion in *plié* are increased. It is often difficult for a dancer to change to a full-shank shoe just for the benefit of a heel lift. A full-shank shoe may induce an Achilles tendinitis, as the dancer now has to plantarflex with more force against the shank in order to achieve *tendu* or *pointe.*

A word of caution about heel lifts. If one foot requires a heel lift, there must be a good reason for not giving the uninvolved foot a lift, lest an iatrogenic leg length difference be created.[47] This could result in symptoms in the lower back, sacroiliac joint, hips, or knees. Usually, lifts should be considered short-term solutions.

Incompletely compressible heel lifts made by Viscolas, Sorbothane, Spenco, or PPT may be used for injuries characterized by excessive heel impact.[48] These injuries include calcaneal impact syndromes (heel bruises, stress fractures, etc.); Achilles tendinitis caused by guarding against heel contact after heel bruises,[49] thus increasing tensile load on the calf; cuboid subluxation syndromes; tibial stress fractures; and hip, sacroiliac, and lower back shock syndromes. Calf strength also should be examined.

Tapings

The possible side effects of every taping should be weighed against the desired effect. For example, ankle tapings, which would seem so useful, often are too cumbersome to be effective if they are in the least bit too robust. Of all athletic pursuits, dance and gymnastics require the greatest fluidity and range at the ankle. This requires a taping to be both unobtrusive to deep *plié,* yet substantive in high *relevé,* or vice versa. This is what defeats most tapings (and dance-shoe orthoses). The absolutely confining tapings of the football player must be modified to allow the dancer to get on with technique. Strengthening and proprioceptive therapy should be stressed during periods requiring tapings.

The type of tape used is also a major consideration. A lot of motion must be allowed for ballet, so the tape must have elasticity. A too-rigid tape could cause an overuse tendinitis. Elastikon is a good choice. If great range is not desired, as in a splay foot or an instability at a metatarsophalangeal joint, then a less elastic but contouring tape, such as Kendall Curity, provides stability. It is good practice, whenever possible, to use a foam underwrap to diminish the likelihood of adhesive-induced dermatitis, abrasions, or blistering.

In conditions such as plantarfasciitis, posterior tibial tendinitis, or strains of plantar ligaments or at the metatarso-cuneiform joints, stresses upon the arch are increased as *demi-plié* deepens. In addition to or instead of a heel lift, one may wish to instruct a dancer in the use of tape that can absorb some of the forces of a deepening *demi-plié.* This requires elastic tape, applied moderately stretched to a foot in a partially plantarflexed position. The tape is applied circumferentially about the instep and arch in such a direction as to supinate (clockwise, right foot; counterclockwise, left foot). The circumferential wrapping continues proximally to firmly envelop the heel and then terminates 1 in. above malleolar level. As the *plié* deepens, the tape stretches between anterior ankle and posterior heel and thus absorbs force.

Another useful taping is a simple circumferential wrap of either elastic or adhesive tape strictly about the metatarsus. As mentioned earlier, this can help a metatarsalgia caused by a splay foot. It also helps uninjured metatarsals splint a healing second, third, or fourth metatarsal stress fracture, and it can help arrest symptomatology of a hallux valgus. If metatarsal splay is occurring, the transverse head of the adductor hallucis muscle exerts a harmful rotational force on the base of the first (and fifth) proximal phalanges. An elastic metatarsal binder with a removable metatarsal pad is available commercially and can save the dancer time and tape money.

The number and variety of tapings that could be applied to the foot is nearly infinite. Many apparently identical injuries are mitigated by structural or choreographic circumstances that dictate individualization. The simplest way to devise a taping is to try to understand the initiating and precipitating mechanisms of injury, then constructing the tapes to inhibit the mechanisms.

It helps when the practitioner asks the dancer the try the appliqué in typically painful positions. What is comfortable during an in-office trial is not going to be as effective after 4-6 hr. of dancing, but if symptoms are not reduced at the in-office trial stage, it is unlikely that the taping will be very helpful during dance.

In-Shoe Orthoses

Although street-shoe orthoses may be helpful in keeping symptomatology at a minimum during nondance activities, dance-shoe orthoses are often unsuccessful because:

1. The underlying reason for the complaint, such as pronation or flattening of the arch during *plié*, often is caused by very strong forces, such as anterior tibiotalar impingement in *plié*. Any orthosis robust enough to countermand those forces would be intolerably inflexible and would inhibit artistic movement.

2. A foot in *plié* is longer than a foot in *relevé*. Thus, an orthosis used to help an injury brought on in plantigrade stance is often too long in *relevé*, and cuts into the toes.

3. In-shoe orthoses that add bulk to the arch region of a slipper affect the cosmetic appearance of the foot by making the arch appear flat.

Surprisingly, dance-shoe orthoses, in both ballet slippers and *pointe* shoes, are occasionally successful. In some cases, a "cookie" built up of successive layers of 1/4-in. adhesive felt and placed into the arch region of the slipper can give good results. In other cases, particularly where cosmetic appearance is a factor, a shell of heat-molded polyurethane/polyvinyl about 1/8 in. thick is useful until it flattens (2-6 months). Because it is flexible, this device can also incorporate forefoot wedging or dispersion. Orthoses work best for dancers whose arch does not flatten in *demi-plié;* in those who do lose their arch in *demi-plié,* a heel lift incorporated in the orthosis may allow it to work.

Dance Shoes

The question is often asked, "What is the main difference between foot injuries sustained by modern dancers and those sustained by ballet dancers?" Aside from stress fractures, ankle sprains, and tendinitis, which are common to both, the answer is, "Most modern dance injuries are caused by the lack of protection of a shoe, whereas most ballet injuries are caused by the constriction or technique contingent upon the shoes."

Aerobic Dance Shoes

The forces applied to the foot during aerobic dance include repetitive loading at the ball and, to a lesser extent, the heel, and dorsiflexion at the metatarsophalangeal joints, particularly the more medial ones. Abduction-eversion or adduction-inversion forces load the forefoot on tiptoe or plantigrade, normally while the other foot is in contact with the floor. Ankle extension and flexion are also required.

A primary service of the shoe is to cushion impact for the ball of the foot during repetitive jumping in place. Should the participant have a history of impact-related mishaps, such as metatarsalgias, sesamoidopathies, metatarsal stress fractures, neuromas, Achilles tendinitis, or "shin splints" (tibial stress fractures), a softer shoe should be chosen. The shock-absorbing capability can be augmented by installing Spenco, Viscolas, Sorbothane, or other shock-absorbing insoles, particularly if the dance surface is concrete, or metal, or an otherwise unsprung floor. The shoe should be checked periodically by the wearer. A midsole that has been "compacted' or an outer sole that has worn away will have lost much of its ability to protect. This is why using aerobic dancing shoes for street wear should be discouraged. Resoling, in which only the outer sole is replaced, can still leave the wearer with a compacted and non-protective midsole.

It is also important that the tread of the aerobic shoe be as uniform as possible. Bizarre patterns and large waffle plugs can impinge upon or abut susceptible metatarsophalangeal joints, particularly if the participant has a plantarflexed first ray or a particularly long first, second, or third metatarsal.

Aerobic shoes should be light in weight to allay anterior leg fatigue. They also must provide lateral stability at the heel while in heel contact (supportive counter, sole not narrower than counter) and at the ball while in ball contact. If the upper easily cascades over the sole at the ball, the sesamoids or the fifth metatarsal can be spiked. The instability could also lead to an ankle sprain.

The shoe should also have some shank stability to discourage adduction of the midtarsal joint, an occult cause of inversion sprains in feet having hyperadduction available to the oblique axis of the midtarsal joint. This is more often seen in a pes cavus.

Jazz Shoes

These are soft, close-fitting slipper shoes that lace up, have a thin sole, and have a heel rise of 1/4 in. They have no counter reinforcement. Besides their intended use, they are helpful for allowing some dance or barre exercises during low-grade Achilles tendinitis or other injuries helped by heel lift.

Ballet Slippers

Ballet slippers (figures 10-13 and 10-14) are flexible, thin, and close fitting. They are made of canvas or leather. They are usually purchased a little tight because they stretch. An overly tight slipper is not recommended for constant use, as it can lead to symptoms characterized by digital malalignment. Dancers sometimes interchange their slippers right to left to vary pressure on single toes and to prolong shoe life. Dancers with long great toes often do not interchange. Dancers also stitch elastic bands to their slippers to help hold them on and provide a bit of support.

Ballet slippers are worn by male ballet dancers. Male ballet dancers do not wear *pointe* shoes to perform, but do occasionally work out in them, presumably to facilitate speed and strength.

All slippers and shoes are useful if tapings or pads must be applied, as they help prevent the appliqué from knurling. They also hide the plasters.

Character Shoes

Character shoes are designed differently for men and women. Men's character shoes can be fairly robust, sometime over-the-ankle boots, with supportive counters and shanks. They have a 5/8- to 3/4-in. heel. They are ideal vehicles, when indicated, for orthoses. Character shoes for women have a stocky Cuban heel 1 1/4 to 1 3/4 in. high. Built on a wide ball/narrow heel last typical of a dancer's foot, they employ a strap about the front of the ankle. They also have stable counters and fairly rigid shanks occasionally reinforced with metal.

Tap Shoes

Tap shoes are similar to character shoes. Their essential features are, of course, their acoustically tuned taps of a specific thickness and shape at toe and heel. The tap at the ball ends in an arcuate shape beneath the proximal phalanges. The remainder of the ball is cushioned with scored soling rubber. An occult cause of sesamoid injuries, either bruising or tensile, lurks in tap shoes whose rubber has thinned sufficiently beneath the first metatarsal head to exert both a hyperdorsiflexory and impact-type stress at the first metatarsophalangeal joint.

Flamenco or Spanish Shoes

These are like tap shoes. Some, by tradition, substitute scores of tiny brads hammered beneath the toe and heel for taps.

Pointe Shoes

Pointe shoes* enable the ballerina to *relevé sur les pointes.* They are rigid in the toe and relatively inflexible in the shank. They are covered with satin, which both absorbs sweat and provides traction. They are worn with ribbons which, correctly affixed, can provide beneficial support. They come in various

*Some valuable information on *pointe* shoes was supplied by Brenda Anderson.

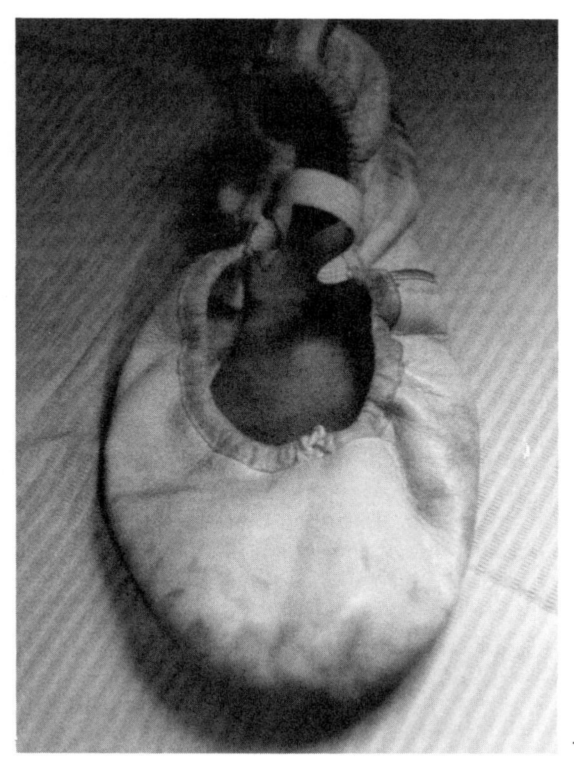

10-13

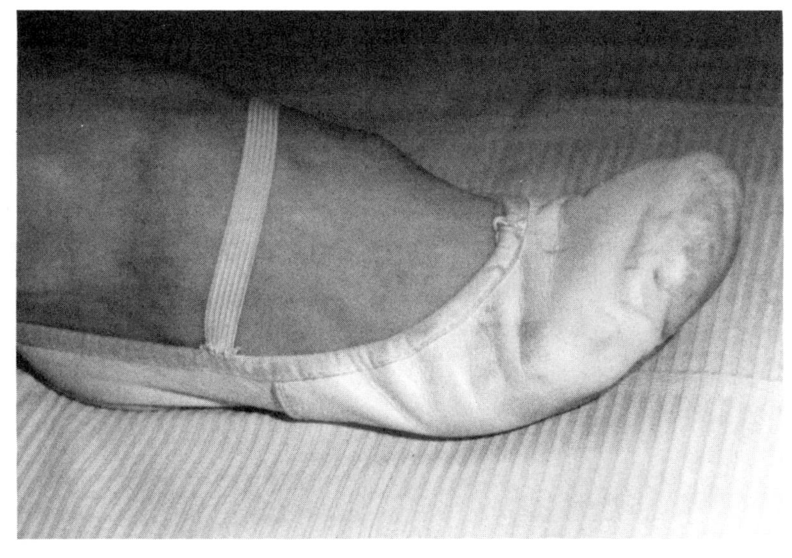

10-14

Figures 10-13, 10-14. Ballet slippers. Note flexibility.

lengths and standard or "combination" (different ball and heel width) lasts. They are often custom-ordered by a ballerina, who orders many pairs, months in advance, from her favorite supplier. When a ballerina receives her shoes, she first bangs the toe box against something to get the right "feel." These shoes can cost upwards of $30 to $35 per pair and are usually good for only one performance. Needless to say, the cost of *pointe* shoes is a major factor in the wardrobe budget of a dance company.

The shoe should be long enough so the heel doesn't pop out due to inadequate depth at the "counter." The wear pattern beneath a ballerina's heel therefore should extend only 1/2 in. or so caudad to the shank (figure 10-15). A farther-back wear pattern would indicate that the shoe is too short, and could cause excessive gripping with the toes to keep it on. Curling and digital pressure points or cramping or metarsalgias can ensue.

The vamp, or reinforcement of the toe box, is available in various shapes and lengths. The vamp should be chosen so that it does not cut dorsally into any bony prominence such as a metatarsal head. The length of the vamp should be determined by the angle of inclination that the metatarsals make with the floor. In other words, a pes cavus with a high metatarsal inclination angle requires a longer vamp to act as a brace while on *pointe.* This helps prevent falling or "knuckling" forward.

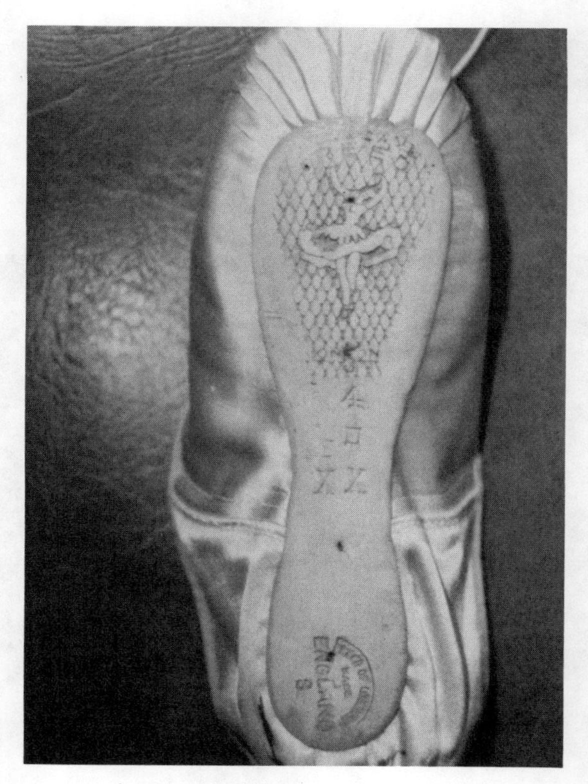

Figure 10-15. Bottom of a *pointe* shoe. Note line in heel area denoting caudal terminus of weight pattern for proper sizing.

Another consideration is the placement of a dancer's ribbons. If the ribbons are placed too far forward of the heel, thus affixed in mid-arch to give a more elegant, "high-arched" appearance to the foot, the heel of the shoe may tend to flip off the foot. The ballerina might then have to supplement the heel grip with elastics across the ankle tied to the rear part of the shoe. This could irritate synovial structures in the front of the ankle. Additionally, much of the supportive function of the ribbons is lost if they are forward-affixed. The dancer must then tie her ribbons so tight that she may cause pressure-induced problems about the prominence of the ankle where the ribbons cross. One patchwork solution that evolves is to splice 1¼-in. strips of elastic into the ribbons at the points of prominence.

To avoid many of the above problems, the ribbons should be affixed to the shoe at a point just distal to where the counter meets the upper when it is folded forward.

Unfortunately, the appearance of the foot in the *pointe* shoe is often a dancer's or a choreographer's chief concern. A few dancers have presented asking for surgery on asymptomatic feet to actually give them a higher arch or to give them a "bunion" (neither request was granted). Some patients refuse to increase their *pointe* shoe size by even one-half size because they are afraid their feet will look "too clunky." Consequently, they suffer recurrent soft corns and digital abscesses requiring expensive, time-consuming treatment.

Another consideration is the shape of the toe box. Dancers with medial or lateral unsteadiness while on *pointe* should choose a square, broad box rather than one that is very narrow or rounded. Dancers with recurrent fibular stress fractures or posterior impingement syndromes should avoid *pointe* shoes with excessively "winged-out" toe boxes.[50] Posterior impingement syndrome involves limitation of motion and pain in the posterior ankle on *relevé*. It is often associated with an accessory bone in the posterior joint space (os trigonum or Stieda's process) or with anterior ankle laxity after repeated sprains.[51] The latter allows the talus to displace excessively forward while in maximal plantarflexion, imparting an abutment force between the trigonal plateau of the calcaneus and the tibial plafond.

These dancers should inspect the toe box in the sagittal section. If the plantar aspect of the box is longer than the dorsal aspect, the dancers must hyper-*pointe* at the ankle to bring the full surface of the toe box in contact with the floor. Thus, they should order or modify their shoes so that the plantar part is shorter than the dorsal part (figures 10-16, 10-17). Excessive hyperextension at the knee should also be controlled by hamstring strengthening and alignment modification. Otherwise, a dancer may have to hyper-*pointe* the ankle to compensate and maintain balance.

Pointe shoes must also be evaluated for their rigidity. Dancers who wear very rigid or "hard" shoes don't develop as much strength in their toe muscles. This weakness can be an occult cause of such injuries as Achilles tendinitis and metatarsal stress fractures in dancers called on to dance barefoot or in ballet slippers when they must land in *demi-pointe* without the protection of *pointe* shoes.

Returning to *pointe* too soon after a long layoff can cause new injuries, such as Achilles tendinitis. During a 10- to 14-day return period, the dancer

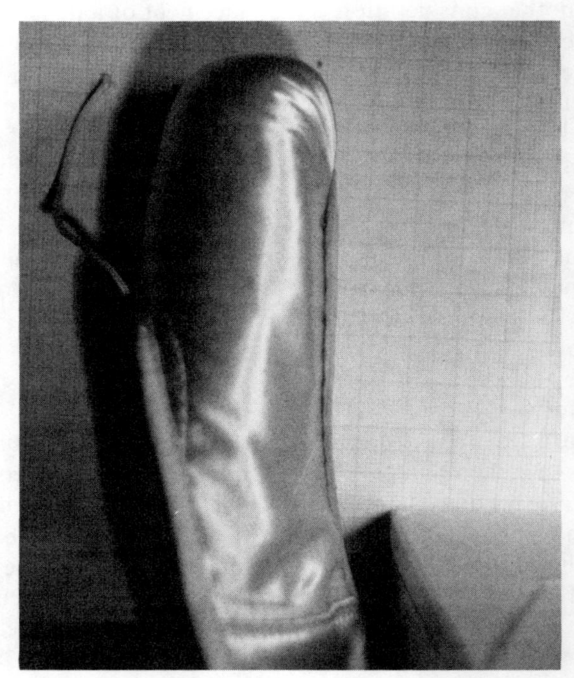

10-16

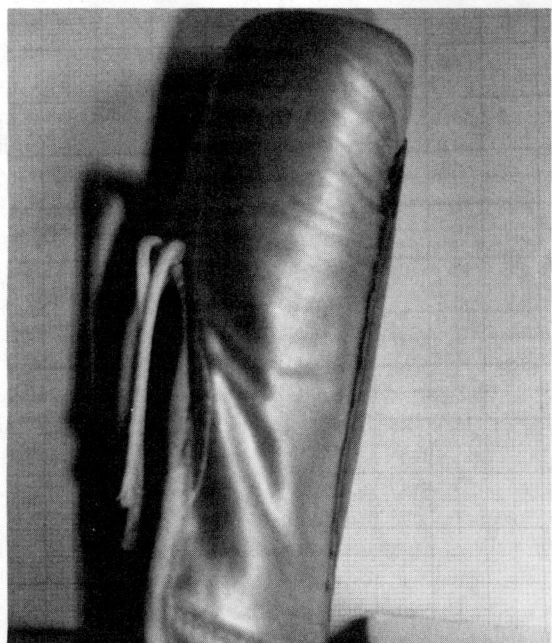

10-17

Figures 10-16, 10-17. This *pointe* shoe as examined from the side (figure 10-16) is not longer plantarly than dorsally. This requires more pointing from the ankle to bring the toe of the shoe into contact with the ground than does the shoe in figure 10-17, which has a shorter plantar length.

should take non-*pointe* class in "soft" or old *pointe* shoes rather than ballet slippers, as the former will provide more support on returning to class.

It is important that the dancer monitor her shoe size, especially in late adolescence. Although she may have "stopped growing," her feet may continue to expand, leading to pressure problems, especially at the proximal interphalangeal joints, atop the hallux, between the toes, or at the toenails.[52] One's feet may be mismated in size, especially length, not only at the first toe, but at any digital antimere. If a half size or greater difference is present, a dancer should buy one pair of shoes that exactly fit the smaller foot and another pair that fit the larger one. Because *pointe* shoes do not come in left/right, there are no economic ramifications.

Commonly, ballerinas apply adhesive plasters to blister-prone toes. They position wads of lambs wool or paper towels to even out toe lengths that would otherwise be uncomfortably staggered on *pointe*. Some place a small square of paper toweling over all their toes before they put their points shoes on. This helps absorb sweat, thus adding to the life of the shoe, and provides a little cushioning.

Skin and Nail Problems

Onychomycosis

Onychomycosis, or fungal infection of the toenails, is a near universal condition among dancers. It appears at a much earlier age and in a more full-blown form than it does in the general population, particularly in those who subject their toes to intensive trauma, namely ballerinas. Onychomycosis is difficult to treat, but with the exception of ballerinas who happen to put particular stress on their great toenails, treatment is seldom necessary. Even in the nondance population, the condition is difficult to cure. Since trauma will recur, cure should not be sought. The nail may be kept thin by filing the plate occasionally, but it should not be removed, lest the fleshy tip of the toe become painfully bulbous or the thin skin atop the proximal phalanx press uncomfortably into the toe box.

Chronic fungus infection of the toenails may be controlled or completely eliminated in some persons by the oral administration of griseofulvin. This may have to be continued for as long as 6 months as the new nail grows out, but it may prevent the deformity of the terminal phalanx that often results from chronic onychomycosis. A suitable preparation is Fulvicin P/G 330. These tablets contain ultramicrosize crystals of griseofulvin. The adult dose is one tablet every 12 hours. Patients taking this medication should be warned that photosensitivity may occur, and that they should avoid unnecessary exposure to strong sunlight or ultraviolet light. If skin rash occurs (rarely), the medication should be discontinued. With prolonged usage, blood count and renal and hepatic function should be monitored periodically.

Traumatic Nail Deformity

Chronic trauma to the nail as the result of the toes being jammed into the tight toe box may result in hematomas under the nail, improper treatment of which results in deformity of the nail plate and bed. It may not be possible to correct this result, but it can be prevented by encouraging the dancers to have the acute injury treated promptly and properly.

Onychocryptosis (Ingrown Toenail)

The most frequent cause of onychocryptosis is incorrect trimming technique, wherein the distal edge of the nail is trimmed too short of the distal skin corner (hyponychial-ungua labial juncture).[53] Hallux valgus, tight *pointe* shoes, and hypertrophied nail folds can bring on the condition.

The dancer should be advised about the causes and correction of ingrown toenail, including the rationale of the time-honored "cutting the nails straight across." This allows the nail edge to always remain distal to the skin corner, lest the forward tuft of skin be impinged by a nail deep within the nail fold. If this happens, self-care often amounts to trimming farther and farther back, with successive increases in pathology and symptoms.

Barring any evidence of infection, nail-edge hooks, or pyogenic granulomas, which must first be eliminated, the nail may be salvaged from operation by teasing a wisp of cotton beneath its edge and affixing the cotton to the site with flexible collodion.[54] The cotton must be hooked beneath the proximal edge and extend to the distal edge. The procedure may cause discomfort. Then the dancer is encouraged to leave the cotton in or have it monitored to assure it is in place. It must remain there long enough (usually several months) to enable the distal corner of the nail to advance above and beyond the tuft of skin.

In deeply ingrown nails, a local anesthetic may be necessary to excise any hooks of nail. After suitable measures are taken and any infection eliminated (soaks, appropriate antibiotics, topicals), the above cotton technique should be employed.

In cases in which a hallux abducto valgus is forcing the second toe to press on the lateral aspect of the great toenail, an H-shaped pad of 1/2-in. nonadhesive foam rubber can be employed to diminish pressure at the hallux nail groove (figure 10-18). Any hyperkeratosis that may have accumulated in the groove should also be meticulously debrided.

Traumatic Onycholysis

Onycholysis, or partial to complete avulsion of a nail from its bed, is not an infrequent occurrence in dancers. This occurs particularly in the great toenail of male modern dancers, or in ballerinas with onycholysis secondary to onychomycosis. The dancer's practices in cutting the nails should be learned; the nails should not be left too long in the center or they will be prone to catch inside the toe box and be torn.

Barring any evidence of infection subungually, which requires removal of all plate above the infection, or of onychocryptosis at the intact edge proximal to the tear, the portion of the nail plate partially attached may be saved by taping it down with the nonadhesive part of a Band-Aid; this allows the plate to

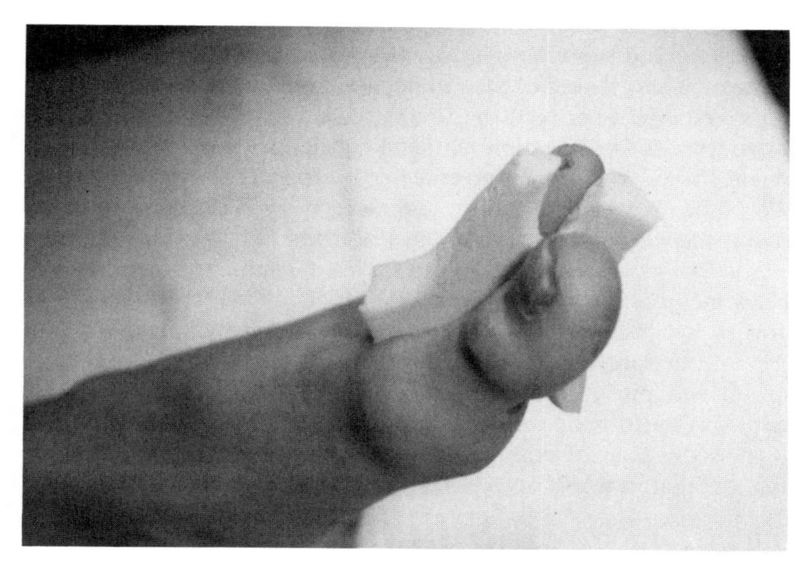

Figure 10-18. "H"-shaped pad to relieve lateral hallux ingrown toenail in hallux valgus.

protect the distal phalanx from pressure. Usually, a new nail plate grows forth inconsequentially. Occasionally, as it advances, it catches the distal toe flesh, which may then become a bulbous tuft. If possible, cotton packing should be placed beneath the leading edge of the nail if symptoms arise.

Corns

Corns are focal hyperkeratoses at the pressure-liable points of the toes. They are most often seen atop the second or fifth proximal interphalangeal joint in ballerinas, but these sites are usually self-managed. They can occur at any bony prominence in the forefoot, particularly between the toes, atop the first interphalangeal joint, atop a metatarsophalangeal joint, at the tip of a distal phalanx (occasionally overlying an exostosis), or atop any interphalangeal joint. Occasionally, the fifth toenail is replaced by keratinoid tissue resembling a corn, and can hurt.

The unwillingness of a ballerina to change to the next larger shoe size aggravates such a pressure-induced problem. Trauma to the hallux, leading to medial instability on *pointe,* may cause a lateral cascade of ground-reactive forces terminating at the fourth interdigital space, causing a soft corn there. Toe length, if not staggered but uniform, can also lead to recurrent and especially problematic soft corns, particularly between the second and third and fourth toes (figure 10-19).

If corns continue to recur on one foot only, it should be determined whether the feet are the same size. Fifth metatarsal fractures, common in dancers, may cause a shortening or an adducted angulation of the fifth metatarsal, leading to recurrent corns in the fourth toe web.

In any dancer with corns symptomatic enough to bring them to the doctor, debridement should be meticulous enough to assure that no pressure abscess underlies the keratoma. These lesions are usually infected with *Staphylococcus epidermitis,* although *S. aureus, β-hemolytic Streptococcus, Escherichia coli,* or *Proteus mirabilis* occasionally will be cultured. Familial history of diabetes mellitus should be ruled out. Interdigital sensoria should be assessed. After all hyperkeratotic and necrotic tissue is debrided, local and (if indicated) systemic measures are taken to control infection. No pressure should be exerted on the site until healing occurs.

Elimination of pressure on the site to allow reorganization of the underlying fat cushion is the goal of conservative treatment. If shoes are properly sized, padding and lamb's wool can be tried. Through ingenuity and necessity,

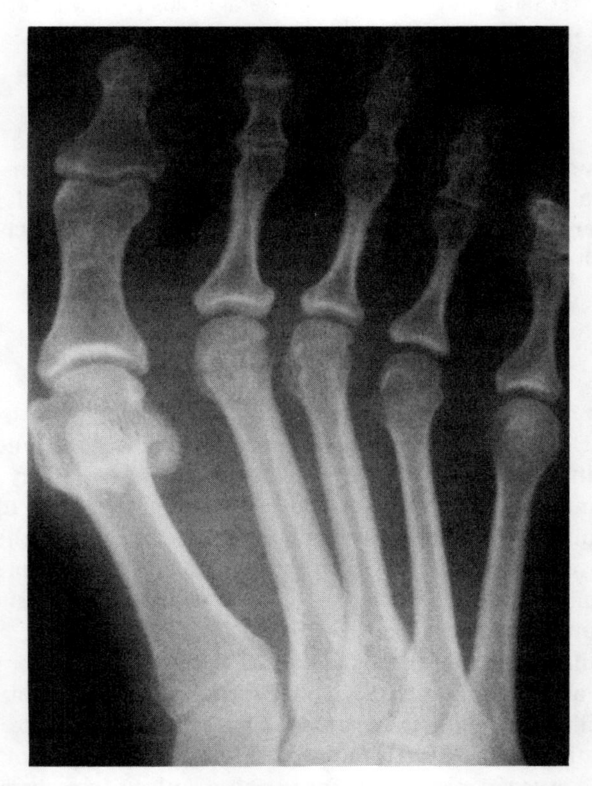

Figure 10-19. A soft corn exists between the second and third proximal interphalangeal joints of this dancer's foot due to even toe length as demonstrated by the radiograph of her foot.

a seasoned ballerina will have developed quite successful padding techniques as she has become more and more familiar with the peculiarities of her feet combined with the requirements of her technique. Rarely can a practitioner improve upon what years of trial and error generate. The occasional dancer whose attempts at self-care are not fruitful may be helped with various types of dispersive padding such as felt doughnuts or horseshoes surrounding the prominence. Quick-curing silicone rubber devices can also be most helpful for shielding and windowing pressure-induced lesions (figures 10-20, 10-21).

Indiscriminate use of keratolytic plasters can exacerbate these conditions if dancers are overzealous in repeated applications. They should be advised that a "cure" cannot be effected unless the focus of pressure is relieved. The cause of hyperkeratosis should thus be explained to the dancer (and all patients suffering from this condition).

Many ballerinas undergo surgery to eliminate soft corns. Although many patients are pleased, if too much tissue is removed, leaving a toe flail or weak, a chronic metatarsalgia of the corresponding or contiguous metatarsal head could result. A weakened lateral toe could lead to recurrent ankle instability. If a jagged bony edge is left at the surgical site, then symptoms may subsequently be exacerbated rather than eliminated. In cases of soft corns, syndactylization or simple exostosectomy seem to yield the most successful results.

'Toughening-Up'

The knots, corns, bony eminences, thickened toenails, and muscular bulk that characterize a dancer's foot are the result of long hours of stress. Young females who are just beginning to do a lot of *pointe* work or even seasoned ballerinas returning from a 10-month layoff from back injury[55] often report pain at toenail or digital pressure points now conspicuously devoid of adaptive hypertrophy. At this point, one realizes the value of these knots and corns and the potential danger involved in indiscriminate debridement of every asymptomatic hyperkeratosis on a dancer's foot. But this pressure point pain may be a blessing in disguise, a signal lest the dancer undertake choreography too rigorous for her lessened strength, endurance, and proprioception. Returning to *pointe* work too soon almost guarantees another injury.

Verrucae

Warts, which are viral and contagious, are frequently seen on dancers' feet. Slippers or clogs should be worn in showers and changing rooms. Warts often appear at pressure points and hurt during positions or movements that create the pressure. An inauspicious and not infrequent site of presentation is beneath a hallux sesamoid.

The lesions are characterized by their papillomatous, hyperkeratotic, and dry surface well demarcated from the surrounding skin lines. They are often more tender to transverse compression (pinching) than to direct palpation. In dancers, verrucae plantares occur much more frequently than do focal solitary

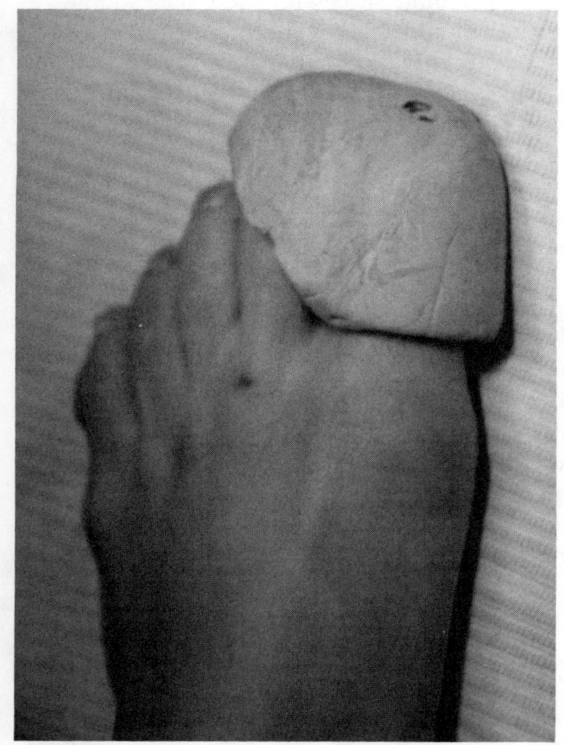

10-20

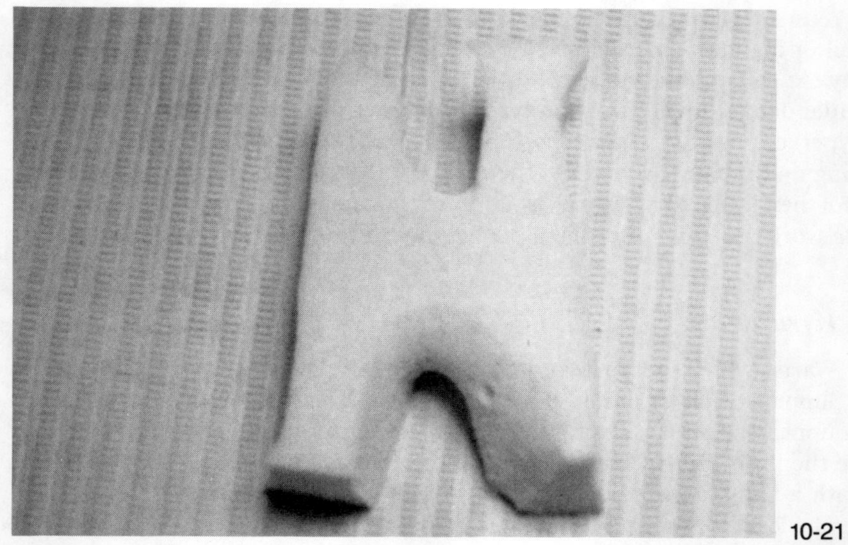

10-21

Figures 10-20, 10-21. Typical symptomatic keratoma dorsal to the medial interphalangeal joint in a *pointe* dancer, and a fast-curing silicone putty device whose inner contour matches the toes and outer contour matches the toe box (Moldable Podiatric Compound; Multi-sil; Silisoft; Otoform-K).

pressure-induced plantar hyperkeratoses. Dancers usually develop flatter, more diffuse plantar hyperkeratoses, although verrucae may be peppered within diffuse hyperkeratoses.

Recent research indicates that most untreated verrucae will spontaneously resolve in about 5 years. I have seen a number of cases where plantar verrucae had been too aggressively treated, leaving the patient with painful weight-bearing scars producing hyperkeratosis and requiring continuing attention thereafter.

Ordinarily, verrucae are difficult to eradicate. The great variety of treatment procedures attests to that. They often recur after treatment, presumably because the entire viral inoculum had not been removed about the lesion's periphery. No wart is easy or simple to treat; all treatments have their drawbacks. Therefore, only the symptomatic or the rapidly spreading lesions should be treated.[56] A treatment that is least likely to cause a painful weight-bearing scar should be chosen.

A relatively benign technique involves daily applications of salicylic acid in a collodionlike base (Viranol, Duofilm, Salactic Liquifilm) combined with frequent home abrasion with a coarse pumice stone (which should not be used elsewhere on the body). A no. 15 scalpel might be used at home or on tour if the dancer is manually dexterous enough and has been instructed in safe technique, but this approach does involve considerable risk. Periodic visits to the practitioner to monitor progress ensure that nonverrucous tissue is not being damaged. Dispersive pads can help to relieve pain. The technique has the advantages that work time is not lost, pain is usually quickly relieved, and the dancer does not need to keep the site dry. The disadvantage of this method is that effecting a cure usually takes from 6 weeks to 6 months.

Pulsed ultrasound has also been used with success in certain cases.[57,58] Care should be taken when applying ultrasound at the sesamoids, the heel, or any possible stress fractures or open growth plate.

In rare cases in which more immediate treatment is necessary and surgery is required, care must be taken to assure that the fatty layer beneath the epidermis is not invaded, producing a painful scar.

Skin Splits (Epidermal Fissures)

Fissures, or rips in the skin, are more common in modern than in ballet dancers. They are most often seen under the metatarsal heads, between the toes, or at the heel. The skin is callused, dry, and nonresilient. It is prone to tearing when the dancer turns on the heel or ball, imparting a shearing stress to the skin. Dry skin exacerbates fissures. Dryness may be caused by such factors as diet, oil gland inactivity, hyperkeratosis formation, or barefoot dancing on floors that have been left with deposits of rosin following a *pointe* class. Occasionally, a localized cellulitis warranting cleansing and other appropriate measures is found at the depth of the fissure.

Fissures are difficult to eliminate if dancing must continue. Steps to eliminate them include cleansing, topicals, and debridement of peripheral hyperkeratosis. Tapings, applied butterflylike across the rift and covered by a circumferential foot wrap of Elastoplast help to prevent dehiscence. Combining the above with nightly occlusive dressings of emollients also proves helpful.

Conclusion

Working with dancers is both challenging and rewarding. It is challenging because the practitioner must work within the gray zone of neither overtreating to the point where a delicate career-ending balance might be broken nor doing so little as to be ineffective. The work is rewarding in that to achieve an occasional success in a most demanding population, one must always remain open to the "could be's" and "what if's" while waiting for the "Aha's". What one learns in working successfully with a dancer will benefit all phases of a physician's practice.

The practitioner should not approach any dance injury with a "face-value" attitude, but rather try to place the individual's injury and treatment history in proper time sequence. Changes occurring in frequency, choreography, floors, teachers, shoes, or sideline jobs are factors that govern the element of accuracy in a diagnosis. Searching for the underlying cause, while carefully and deliberately treating the symptomatic manifestations, offers the best guarantee for success.

References

1. Doxey GE. Management of metatarsalgia with foot orthotics. Orthop Sports Phys Ther 1985; 6:325.
2. Root M, Orien W, Weed J. Normal and abnormal function of the foot. In: Clinical biomechanics, vol 2. Los Angeles; Clinical Biomechanics Corp, 1977; 115-16.
3. Cailliet R. Foot and ankle pain. Philadelphia: FA Davis, 1970; 140-41.
4. Werter R. Dance floors. J Am Podiat Med Assoc 1985; 75:355.
5. Seals J. A study of dance surfaces. Clin Sports Med 1983; 2:557-61.
6. Mann RA, Reynolds JC. Interdigital neuroma: a critical clinical analysis. Foot Ankle 1983; 238-43.
7. Ibid.
8. Kravits S et al. Osseous changes in the second ray in ballet dancers. J Am Podiat Med Assoc 1985; 75: 346-48.
9. Sparger C. Anatomy and ballet. New York: Theatre Arts Books, 1976; 89.
10. Sammarco GJ. The foot and ankle in classical ballet and modern dance. In: Jahss MH, ed. Disorders of the foot. Philadelphia: WB Saunders, 1982; 1630.
11. Cailliet R. op. cit. 140-41.
12. Glancy J. Orthotic control of ground-reactive forces during running (a preliminary report). Orthot Prosthet (autumn) 1984; 38:15.
13. Root M, Orien W, Weed J, op. cit., 224.
14. Sheffield FJ et al. Electromyographic study of the muscles of the foot in normal walking. Am J Phys Med 1956; 35:223-25.
15. Porterfield JA. Dynamic stabilization of the trunk. J Orth and Sports Phys Ther 1985; 6:272.
16. Sammarco GJ, op. cit. 1637.
17. Ball J. Enthesopathy of rheumatoid and ankylosing spondylitis. Ann Rheum Dis 1971; 30:213.
18. Root M, Orien W, Weed J. op. cit., 406-08, 435.
19. Serrafian. Anatomy of the foot and ankle, Philadelphia: JB Lippincott, 1983; 85.

20. Sammarco GJ, op. cit., 1655.

21. Gregg J, Das M. Foot and ankle problems in the preadolescent and adolescent athlete. Clinic Sports Med 1982; 1:143-44.

22. Tachdjian M. The child's foot. Philadelphia: WB Saunders, 1985; 312-15.

23. Sammarco GJ, op. cit. 1656.

24. Ashley M. Dancing for Balanchine. New York: EP Dutton, 1984; 131-137.

25. Kaltenborn FM. Manual therapy for the extremity joints. 2nd ed. Oslo: Olaf Norlis Bokhandel, 1976; p.88.

26. Van Hal ME et al. Stress fractures of the great toe sesamoids, Amer J Sports Med 1982; 10:122-28.

27. Sammarco, GJ. Forefoot conditions in dancers, pt 2. Foot Ankle 1982; 3:95.

28. Root M, Orien W, Weed J, op. cit., 56-60.

29. Apley AG. Open sesamoid. Proc R Soc Med 1966; 59:120.

30. Kliman M et al: Osteochondritis of the hallux sesamoid bones. Foot Ankle 1983; 3:220-23.

31. Yakoe K, Mannoji T. Stress fracture of the proximal phalanx of the great toe: a report of three cases. Amer J Sports Med 1986; 14:240.

32. Sammarco GJ, op. cit. 1655.

33. Root M, Orien W, Weed J, op. cit., 278-83.

34. Fishman S et al. Lower limb orthoses. Atlas of orthotics (Am Acad Orth Surgeons). St.Louis: CV Mosby, 1985; 209.

35. Cailliet R, op. cit., 13-14.

36. Sparger C, op. cit.

37. Hamilton WG. Stenosing tenosynovitis of the flexor hallucis longus tendon and posterior impingement upon the os trigonum in ballet dancers. Foot Ankle 1982; 3:74-80.

38. Fond D. Flexor hallucis longus tendinitis: a case of mistaken identity, and posterior impingement syndrome in dancers, evaluation and management. J Orth and Sports Phys Ther 1984; 5:204.

39. Hamilton WG. Sprained ankles in ballet dancers. Foot Ankle 1982; 3:99.

40. Schreiber LF. The law of locomotor stability. J Natl Assoc Chirop 1951; 41:19-27.

41. Kleiger B. Anterior tibiotalar impingement syndrome in dancers. Foot Ankle 1982; 3:69-73.

42. Beekman S et al. A preliminary study on asymmetrical forces at the foot-ground interphase. J Am Podiat Med Assoc 1985; 75:351.

43. Sammarco GJ, op. cit., 1655.

44. Kapandji IA. The physiology of the joints, vol 2. The lower limb. New York: Churchill-Livingstone, 1970; 151-53.

45. Inman V, Ralston H, Todd F. Human walking. Baltimore: Williams & Wilkins, 1981; 103-05.

46. Root M, Orien W, Weed J, op. cit., 195-203.

47. Woerman A, Binder-Macleod S. Leg length discrepancy assessment: accuracy and precision in five clinical methods of evaluation. J Orth and Sports Phys Ther, 1984; 5:230.

48. Jahn WT: Viscoelastic orthotics: Sorbothane 2. J Orth and Sports Phys Ther (winter) 1983; 4:174-75.

49. Jorgensen U. Achillodynia and the loss of heel pad shock absorbency. Am J Sports Med 1985; 13: 128-32.

50. Howse AJG. Posterior block of the ankle joint in dancers. Foot Ankle 1982; 3:81-84.

51. Kapandji IA. The physiology of the joints. vol 2. The lower limb. New York: Churchill-Livingstone, 1970; 146.

52. Teitz C et al. Pressure on the foot in pointe shoes. Foot Ankle 1985; 5:216-21.

53. Howse AJG. Disorders of the great toe in dancers. Clin sports Med 1983; 2:503.

54. Dixon GL. Treatment of ingrown toenail. Foot Ankle 1983; 3:254-55.

55. Micheli LJ. Back injuries in dancers. Clin Sports Med 1983; 2:482.

56. Sammarco GJ, op. cit., 1634.

57. Bartolomei FJ, Biggs EW. Ultrasonic energy in the treatment of verruca plantaris. Curr Podiat 1982; 31:(2):16.

58. Tropp BE. Ultrasound in verruca plantaris: report of a study. J Am Podiat Med Assoc 1967; 57:326.

59. Vaughn D. Direct method versus underwater method in treatment of plantar warts by ultrasound. Phy Ther 1973; 53:26.

11

THE DANCER'S KNEE

Ronald Quirk, F.R.C.S., F.R.A.C.S.

Introduction

INJURIES OF THE KNEE in dancers are relatively common. Several years ago, the writer analyzed 2,113 ballet injuries he had personally treated over a period of 20 years and found that 17.3% of these involved the knee.[9] Because the whole scope of knee surgery changed dramatically during this time, detailed analysis of cases over such a period becomes meaningless. Some of the operations that were standard practice 20 years ago are now outmoded, and some conditions that are now well recognized were unknown then.

Among the changes that have affected the management of knee injuries in dancers, arthroscopy and the development of arthroscopic surgery stand out.[2] Many of the conditions that could only be guessed at 20 years ago can now be studied in great detail through the arthroscope. Probably knee injuries represent a greater percentage of the ballet injuries that present to doctors nowadays because dancers know about new methods of diagnosis and treatment and are more likely to come forward rather than just put up with their discomfort.

The Adolescent Knee

It is generally agreed that the adolescent knee presents a special problem in diagnosis and treatment. The term "adolescent" was defined by Kennedy[7] as the age group between 12 and 18 years, and this period corresponds with the period of great development in young dancers. By the age of 12, a girl may have begun to show promise and will already be thinking of a career in ballet. Probably she will soon be taking part in daily classes. By the age of 15, she very likely will have started full-time ballet studies, with 6 hours or more of dancing each day. By the age of 18 she should have graduated and will be ready to take her place in a professional company.

The increasing load of dancing thus occurs during the exact period when diagnosis is most difficult and treatment hardest to evaluate. In addition, most ballet students are females, and the female adolescent knee provides more diagnostic pitfalls than its male counterpart. Often an adolescent girl will present with a very convincing clinical picture of a meniscus tear, and yet in most cases no tear will be detected. Some conditions, such as Osgood Schlatter disease, are confined to the adolescent period.

The Dancer's Knee

The average dancer's knee is little different from the average in the population. It is true that top dancers, especially females, tend to show persistent deviations from the average, but these individuals have passed through a process of selection on their way to the top, and it is these deviations that have allowed them to leave their opposition behind.

The ballet world is like a pyramid. The broad base includes all the young hopefuls, mostly girls, who start at the age of about 5 years and continue until their own limitations or conflicting interests make them give up. The ballet physique is seen in its most developed form in those expert dancers who are at the tip of the pyramid.

It is obvious to any member of a ballet audience that the knees are used a lot in dance, but the artistry of the dancers conceals the full magnitude of the strain. Dancers work close to their limit much of the time, and knee injuries may be caused by one or more of the following factors: (1)unsuitable physique, (2) faulty technique, (3) overuse, or (4) traumatic incidents.

The pattern of knee injuries in ballet is quite different from that seen in football and similar sports. Whereas a football player is often thrown off balance when his foot is fixed to the ground, a dancer is usually in complete control, with the foot free to turn at all times. Thus, meniscus lesions are relatively uncommon, and severe ligamentous injuries extremely rare; however, disorders of the extensor apparatus and problems with the patellofemoral joint are very common.

Anatomy

The normal anatomy of the knee is dealt with comprehensively in other texts; the purpose of this section is to review briefly some of the terms that will be used later in the chapter.

Bones

The knee is really three joints in one. The lower end of the femur is expanded into the medial and lateral femoral condyles, and these articulate with the medial and lateral tibial condyles to form the main part of the knee joint.

Soft tissue attachments separate the medial and lateral compartments of the joint. The third part of the joint, between the patella and the anterior surface of the lower femur, is often referred to as the patellofemoral joint.

The patella is a sesamoid bone, and its posterior surface is a reflection of how it articulates with the lower femur in various degrees of flexion of the knee. The largest part of the patellar articular surface is taken up by the medial and lateral facets. Smaller superior and inferior facets are seen above and below, and the "odd" facet is a thin strip on the medial side of the medial facet.

Capsule and Synovial Membrane

The fibrous capsule is very complex, being deficient in some areas, and in others being thickened by expansions from the tendons of muscles that surround the joint. The synovial membrane is the most extensive and complex in the body. It extends upward beneath the quadriceps tendon to form the suprapatellar pouch. Below the patella, the synovial membrane is separated from the patellar tendon by the infrapatellar pad of fat, and this is projected to either side as the medial and lateral alar folds.

Ligaments

The main ligaments are four in number: the two collateral ligaments and the two cruciate ligaments. The tibial collateral (medial) ligament is a broad, flat band that joins the lower femur to the upper tibia. It is closely applied to and blended with the fibrous capsule, and because of its attachments it tends to limit the mobility of the medial meniscus. The fibular collateral (lateral) ligament is, by contrast, a rounded band that passes from the lower femur to the head of the fibula without being attached to the capsule or to the lateral meniscus. The anterior and posterior cruciate ligaments are attached above to the condyles of the femur within the intercondylar notch and below to the intercondylar area of the tibia.

Menisci

The menisci are crescentic structures that pass around the periphery of the joint and fill the gap between the rounded femoral condyles and the almost flat tibial condyles. The medial meniscus is tethered to the medial ligament, whereas the lateral meniscus is more freely mobile. This is thought to partly explain the fact that medial meniscus tears outnumber lateral meniscus tears by about 10 to 1. The exact function of the menisci is arguable, but experience has shown that complete excision tends to cause degenerative changes in the same compartment of the knee. Because of this, considerable efforts are made now to remove as little meniscal tissue as possible.

The Extensor Apparatus

The quadriceps muscle consists of four parts: the rectus femoris, vastus lateralis, vastus medialis, and vastus intermedius. These four heads converge to be inserted into the upper pole of the patella and by fibrous expansion into the capsule of the knee joint. The patella is a sesamoid bone within the quadriceps tendon, but it is so large that it effectively separates the muscle from the patellar tendon, which is its tendon of insertion. This tendon is inserted into the tibial tubercle, which is at the upper anterior part of the tibia. Abnormalities in the extensor apparatus cause many of the problems seen in dancers. These will be discussed in detail later.

The Hamstrings

The muscles at the back of the thigh divide into two groups whose tendons can easily be felt behind the flexed knee. On the medial side are the semimembranosus and semitendinosus and on the lateral side are the biceps femoris. The tendons of sartorius, gracilis, and semitendinosus insert into the upper part of the medial surface of the tibia, forming the pes anserinus.

Bursae

Bursae around the knee joint are quite numerous, and four of them are prone to cause problems. The prepatellar bursa is large and lies between the lower part of the patella and the skin. Two infrapatellar bursae, one superficial and one deep, lie in front of and behind the patellar tendon. The anserine bursa lies between the tendons of the sartorius, gracilis, and semitendinosus where they insert into the upper tibia. The semimembranosus bursa lies between the tendon of semimembranosus and the medial head of gastrocnemius.

Anatomical Variations

Genu Varum and Genu Valgum

A survey of successful dancers will show many examples of both of these variations, together with a small number whose legs are perfectly straight. It has long been recognized in ballet circles that the extremes of these two types have quite different characteristics as dancers, and they are distinguished by having different names.

The *arqué* dancer (figure 11-1) is bowlegged and has powerful, tightly knit muscles with short muscle bellies and long tendons. Arqué dancers are remarkable for their quickness and their ability to leap high. Most leading tennis players have this type of leg, often to a very marked degree.

The *jarreté* dancer (figure 11-2) is knock-kneed, with longer and weaker muscle bellies and relatively shorter tendons. The jarreté dancer is often looser and more supple, and is remarkable for elegant clarity of movements and beauty of position.

These two types of dancer are as different from each other as tenors are from basses in singing, and it can be a serious mistake, possibly leading to injury, to ask one type to undertake the roles of the other.

Genu Recurvatum

Hyperextension of the knees ("swayback knees") is a common trait in dancers. In many cases, it is an expression of the dancer's natural hypermobil-

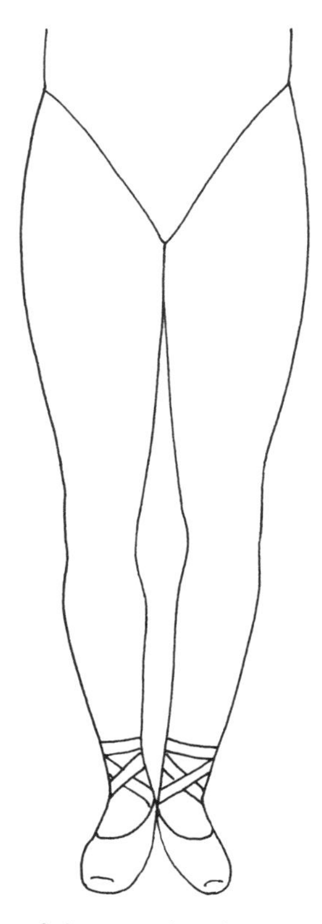

Figure 11-1. An arqué type of dancer, showing genu varum.

ity[1] (figure 11-3) and is paralleled by hyperextension of the elbows (which are not affected by ballet training). Hyperextension is, however, presumably aggravated when young dancers are asked to "pull up" their thigh muscles for long periods in class. In the course of pulling up, they forcibly extend the knee during periods of growth and development, and older dancers sometimes show a degree of recurvatum that is quite outside the normal range (figure 11-4).

Hyperextended knees can cause problems in technique. For example, they prevent a proper first position unless certain adjustments are made. These problems can be overcome, however, and some of the finest dancers have marked recurvatum. This has come to be regarded in the ballet world as aesthetically pleasing, so it is unfortunate that it is also associated with an increased incidence of anterior knee pain. In some cases, the resulting laxity of the anterior capsule contributes to malalignment problems, and in others the hyperextended knee causes compression of the infrapatellar fat pad.

Tibial Variations

The main tibial variation causing problems in dancers is external tibial torsion, in which there is a twist in the tibial shaft so that the medial malleolus lies anterior to the lateral malleolus, and the foot is rotated somewhat outward.

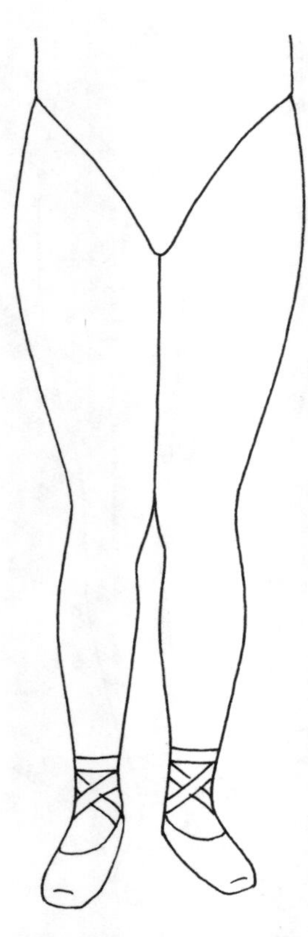

Figure 11-2. A jarreté type of dancer, showing genu valgum.

This deformity is said to be seen more often in knock-kneed children and is known to be associated with inset hips (although a child whose hips remain inset is unlikely to go far in ballet). With the feet in parallel, the dancer will have "cross-eyed" patellae that turn in toward each other. Fortunately, this position is not assumed frequently in ballet. Of more significance is that external tibial torsion is associated with a laterally placed tibial turbercle, and this may lead to patellar malalignment problems.

Patellar Hypoplasia

In general, the patella conforms in shape to the trochlear notch on the front of the lower femur, but some patellae are hypoplastic (figure 11-5), and this can predispose to subluxation. Wieberg has devised a widely accepted method of classification of hypoplasia based on axial radiology,[12] but the details are beyond the scope of this chapter.

Femoral Hypoplasia

The lower femur has a shallow groove in its anterior surface called the trochlear notch. In general, this corresponds to the shape of the patellar articular surface, and the groove is deep enough to give a good measure of lateral sta-

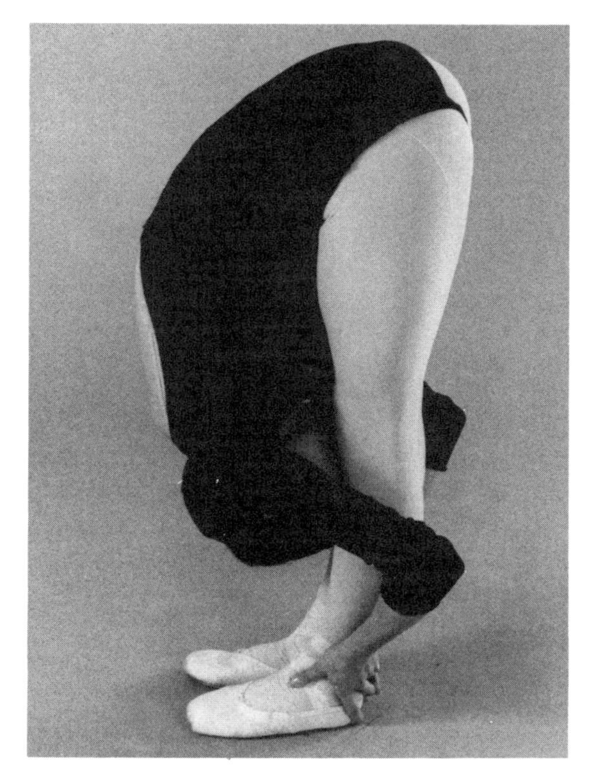

Figure 11-3. There is a process of natural selection in the ballet world, and those who reach the top usually have a natural hypermobility of all their joints, including the knee.

bility to the patella. The lateral femoral condyle usually extends forward a little farther than the medial femoral condyle, and this confers some added stability. Hypoplasia of the lower femur involves shallowness of the trochlear notch (figure 11-5), often with a deficient lateral condylar ridge. Hypoplasia of the patella and the femur often exist in the same knee.

Patella Alta

The height of the patella (and thus the length of the patellar tendon) varies widely. The term for a high patella is *patella alta*, and for a low patella, *patella baja*. The diagnosis can be made in many cases by simple clinical examination and can be confirmed radiologically by the method of Insall and Salvati (figure 11-6). A lateral radiograph is taken with the knee in 30° of flexion, and the greatest diagonal length of the patella is compared with the length of the patellar tendon. If the length of the patella divided by the length of the tendon equals $1.0 \pm 20\%$, the patella is considered normal. Figures of less than 0.8 indicate patella alta, and figures of greater than 1.2 indicate patella baja.

Patella alta is common in female dancers and is often associated with patellar hypoplasia. The high position of the patella puts it above the deepest part

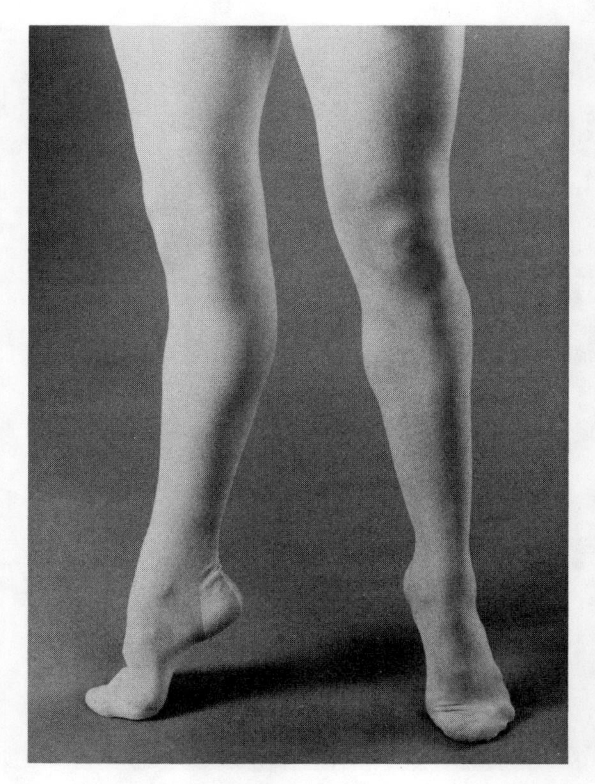

Figure 11-4. A typical genu recurvatum in a leading dancer.

of the trochlear notch, which further adds to the lateral instability. Patella alta is thought to reduce the efficiency of the quadriceps mechanism, resulting in an increase in quadriceps contraction and hence a greater incidence of overuse syndromes such as patellar tendinitis and Osgood Schlatter disease. Sometimes the patella may be so high that the infrapatellar fat pad is uncovered, and the knee has two swellings instead of one (figure 11-7). This double hump, or "camel sign," is a frequent finding in female dancers. Patella baja is extremely uncommon in dancers.

Increased Q Angle

The Q (quadriceps) angle is a useful measurement in cases in which patellar instability is suspected. To make the measurement, the patient is asked to straighten the knee and contract the quadriceps. The center of a goniometer is placed over the center of the patella. One arm of the goniometer is pointed at the anterior superior iliac spine and the other at the tibial tubercle. The angle between them is the Q angle (figure 11-8). Most authorities consider that a Q angle of less than 15° is normal, though Hughston[6] considers anything over 10° abnormal. A high Q angle is not in itself diagnostic of patellar subluxation, but it is important when found in conjunction with other signs of instability.

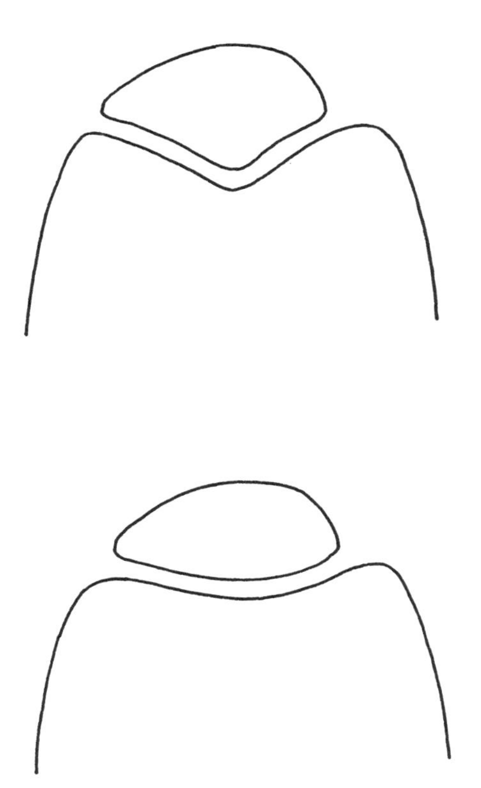

Figure 11-5. A normal-shaped patella lying in a deep trochlear notch (top) has inherent bony stability. However, when there is hypoplasia of both patella and femur (bottom), patellar subluxation is much more likely.

Clinical Approach

History Taking

Taking a history from a dancer follows the usual pattern, but is greatly facilitated if the doctor is familiar with elementary ballet terminology. Dancers are not always good at expressing themselves outside their own familiar language; moreover, the doctor's familiarity with ballet terms adds greatly to the patient's confidence.

It is useful first to know at what age dancing began. In girls, this is usually about the age of 5, but in boys, it is in the mid- to late teens. Girls should be asked at what age they began dancing on *pointe*. It is also necessary to know how many hours of ballet training are currently being done, because so many ballet injuries are due to relative overuse. For the same reason, it is useful to know whether there is an examination, audition, or important performance in the near future, as this will nearly always mean an extra work load, which may precipitate an injury.

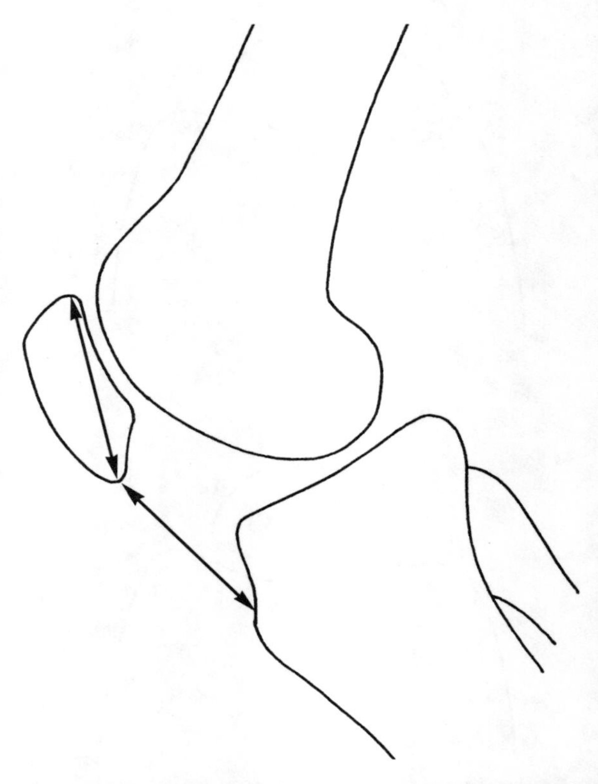

Figure 11-6. Method of Insall and Salvati for confirming the presence of patella alta (see text).

It helps to know whether the dancer is engaged mainly in classical or in modern dance, because injuries from these differ considerably. Modern choreographers often show scant respect for their dancers' normal anatomy, and I have seen as many as three identical injuries come from one class due to the teacher's ignorance. If one is associated with a particular company or school, it soon becomes apparent if a particular teacher is producing an abnormally high number of injuries.

In assessing a knee injury, I have found that the five most useful lines of inquiry are:

1. *Pain.* Where is it situated? How often is it felt? What aggravates it? What relieves it?

2. *Noises.* Is there a sharp click or a grating sound? From what part of the knee does the sound come? Is the sound associated with pain?

3. *Swelling.* Is it constant or intermittent? What makes it worse? Is it local or general? Does it feel like fluid?

4. *Giving way.* How often does this occur? Is it associated with pain, or with any abnormal "going out" feeling in the knee?

5. *Locking.* Is this true locking, with a mechanical block to full exten-

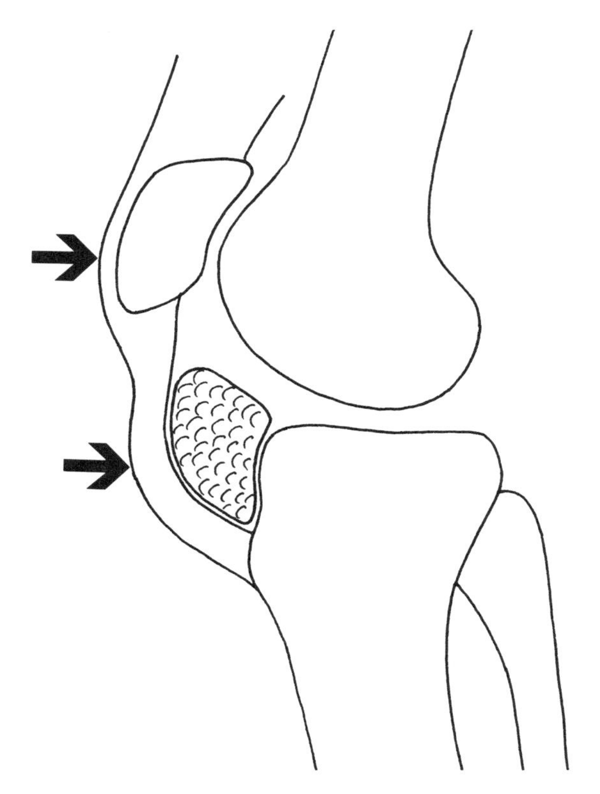

Figure 11-7. "Camel" sign. The high patella uncovers the infrapatellar fat pad, so that there are two swellings on the front of the knee (shown by arrows).

sion, or is it a momentary unwillingness to move the knee due to pain? How long does the knee remain locked? How often does it lock?

Examination

Dancers often come wearing tights, and are used to having their body position observed while wearing them, but they must be persuaded to remove them so that the whole of both lower limbs can be seen. To begin, observe the patient's gait, and note the presence of varus, valgus, or recurvatum. Tibial torsion can be seen while the patient is standing, and the "camel sign" is often best seen in the standing position. Next, have the patient sit with the knees bent at 90° over the edge of the examining table. Tibial torsion is now more obvious, and enlargement or tenderness of the tibial tuberosity can be checked. Note the position of the patellae to see whether they are high or low, and whether they incline medially or laterally. Have the patient flex and extend the knee from 0–90° while you observe the tracking of the patella, and feel for any crepitus.

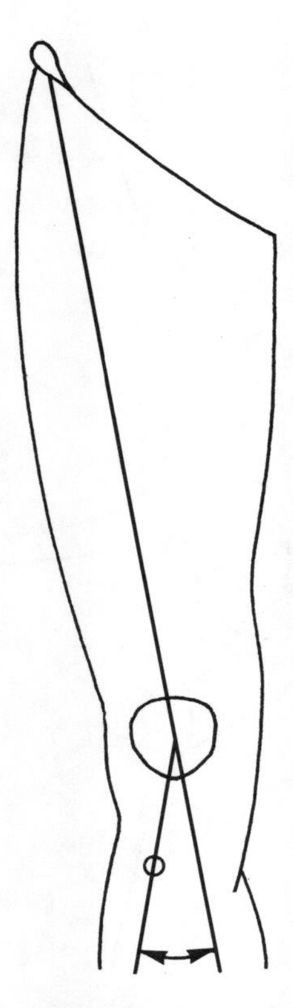

Figure 11-8. The Q angle is the angle between a line joining the anterior-superior iliac spine to the center of the patella and another joining the center of the patella to the tibial tubercle.

Check for vastus medialis dysplasia (loss of muscle bulk on the medial side of the knee, just above the patella).

Now have the patient lie on the table with the knees straight. Measure the Q angle. Note the presence of an effusion and any wasting of the quadriceps. Move the patella in all directions, with and without a compressing hand on it, and note any crepitus or pain. By pushing one side of the patella down, the other will be forced up, and it is then easy to check for tenderness under the patellar margin by pressing the finger toward the patellar articular surface. A plica will be felt as a tender band on the medial aspect of the joint close to the patella. Passive flexion and extension of the knee may reproduce the popping sound characteristic of this condition.

Finally, support the knee across your own thigh, flexed to about 30°. Firmly displace the patella laterally and check for an apprehension sign, indicating patellar instability. The knee may now be examined in the usual way for meniscal tears or ligamentous instability if either of these is suspected.

Radiography

X-rays should always be taken of injured dancers' knees to rule out such conditions as Osgood Schlatter disease, osteochondritis dissecans, or loose bodies. Always have an axial view taken in 30°, 60°, and 90° of flexion. Most patellar subluxation is seen best at 30-45° of flexion and usually disappears by 90°, so routine axial views with the knee at 90° will seldom show anything useful. If patella alta is suspected, a lateral view in 30° of flexion is needed in order to measure the relative lengths of the patella and the patellar tendon.

Arthrography

Although the advent of the arthroscope has somewhat reduced the need for double-contrast arthrography, it still has a place. Minor degrees of patellar subluxation are sometimes better seen when contrast medium in the joint accurately delineates the joint surfaces. Meniscus lesions and loose bodies are often well shown.

Nuclear Bone Scan

This is of limited use in the knee, although it is very helpful when a stress fracture of the patella is suspected. Stress fractures are hard to diagnose with confidence by any other means, but the diagnosis is important because a stress fracture may progress to a complete fracture if jumping is allowed to continue.

Arthroscopy

This relatively new technique is of enormous importance in the assessment and treatment of common knee conditions in dancers.[2] In trained hands, it is a minor procedure, and it gives far more information about the state of the joint than any other investigation. Our understanding of patellofemoral problems, especially chondromalacia, has been greatly enhanced by arthroscopy.

Conditions that can be easily diagnosed arthroscopically include:

- Meniscus tears
- Tears of the cruciate ligaments
- Suprapatellar plica
- Chondromalacia patellae
- Patellar subluxation
- Chondral softening and erosions
- Osteochondritis dissecans
- Loose bodies

Treatment

Reassurance

Dancers are used to the idea of living with pain and are quite content to "work through" an injury provided that they are reassured that they are not doing any serious damage. Many ballet injuries are very minor, only becoming important because of the extraordinary demands made on the dancer's body. Treatment is often difficult for a dancer to fit into a busy schedule, and if the doctor feels that an injury can heal with no treatment, then none should be given.

Advice on Technique

It is unlikely that a doctor can give useful advice on the aesthetic side of ballet unless he has himself been a dancer, and this is an area where we should not trespass. However, a doctor can often, on a purely medical basis, give technical advice that would help the injury to heal.

It would pay any doctor who proposes to treat dancers to read an elementary book on ballet technique and to sit in on a few ballet classes. In addition, if each ballet injury can be discussed with the appropriate teacher, a pattern will soon begin to emerge.

Many knee injuries are due to overuse, in which the dancer, the teacher, and the parents often enthusiastically collaborate. If there are also errors of technique, then the problem is compounded, because correct classical technique has evolved partly as a protection against injury. Injuries are "choreographed into" many modern ballets, in which dancers are asked to kneel on a hard stage, perform impossible lifts, and otherwise put themselves at risk. The correction of technical mistakes is often a crucial part of treatment, and in some cases it is the only treatment required.

Rest

Rest is probably the most unpleasant word in the English language to a dancer, yet it is an essential part of medical treatment. This seeming impasse can often be resolved by redefining what is meant by rest. If, when first presenting an injured knee, a dancer is told that he or she must "take three months off" or "give up ballet," another doctor will be consulted straightaway. On the other hand, if the dancer is told to avoid jumping for a week but that everything else is permissible, this will probably be accepted, and for many knee injuries this is enough.

Dancers have many ingenious ways of doing their daily routine on the floor instead of standing up (a "floor barre"), and this can spare an injured knee while at the same time preserving general fitness. It is possible to do most ballet movements standing in a pool, with the water supporting most of the body weight. With a little thought and ingenuity, it is usually possible to keep dancers going in some way and thus speed their eventual recovery.

Physical Therapy

A good physical therapist with an understanding of ballet is a great asset in the treatment of knee injuries. Methods of treatment will vary from one therapist to another, but the aim in all cases is to preserve the maximum of quadriceps strength coupled with full mobility. Fortunately, a number of dancers are now turning to physical therapy as a second career, and they should be ideally placed to give informed treatment to other dancers.

Medication

Medication has little place in the treatment of common knee injuries in ballet. Analgesics are sometimes required, and nonsteroid anti-inflammatory preparations are sometimes of some help, although in most cases they are not. Aspirin seems to help with some cases of chondromalacia. Steroid injections are widely used in sports medicine, but they too have little place in the treatment of knee injuries. On no account should injections be given into the substance of the patellar tendon, as this may predispose to rupture of the tendon.

Strapping and Bracing

Strapping is popular in some circles, but I have found it of little help in the treatment of knee injuries. Some cases of chondromalacia are now being treated by a method of strapping that tends to pull the patella into a central position and thus minimize subluxation. Some success has been claimed, but the method must still be regarded as experimental. Knee braces of the sort worn by football players are seldom if ever required by dancers.

Open Surgery

Since the advent of arthroscopic surgery, the indications for open operation have diminished. However, open surgery may still be required in such conditions as:

- Bipartite patella
- Bursitis
- Jumper's knee
- Patellar tendinitis
- Osgood Schlatter disease with a loose bone fragment
- Loose bodies
- Patellar realignment
- Ligamentous injuries (rarely)

Arthroscopic Surgery

Arthroscopic surgery has advantages for both the surgeon and the patient. The arthroscope gives a far better view of the knee joint than is obtained through an average arthrotomy. With practice, the operating time is not greatly increased. Very precise removal of tissue ensures that as much tissue as possible is spared. Postoperative recovery is remarkably swift compared with open surgery.

Following are examples of operations that are very suitably performed through the arthroscope:

- Meniscectomy
- Lateral capsular release
- Chondrolysis of the patella for chondromalacia
- Excision of a medial suprapatellar plica

- Removal of loose bodies
- Synovial biopsy

Capsular and Ligamentous Injuries

Turn-Out

The turned-out position of the feet in classical ballet is not just an affectation, but has a sound anatomical basis. If a dancer stands with the feet parallel and abducts the leg at the hip, the range of movement is quite limited because the greater trochanter soon comes into contact with the wall of the pelvis. When the leg is externally rotated at the hip, however, the trochanter moves out of the way, and the leg can then be raised as high as the dancer's ligamentous laxity will permit. Most dancers have no idea why they turn out, but it is a part of ballet technique, and they tend to be quite competitive about it. In trying to show that they have a better turn-out than the next student, they tend to rotate the foot out farther than the hips, thus putting a torsional strain on the whole leg (figure 11-9). The result can be pain in the hip, knee, ankle, or foot.

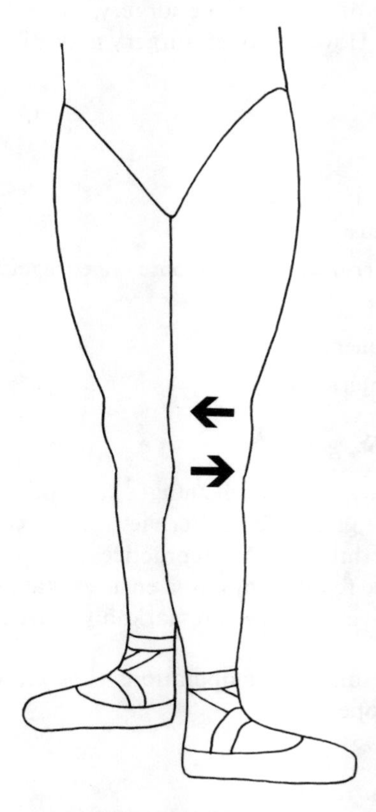

Figure 11-9. Excessive turning out of the foot creates a torsional force up the leg, and this may cause injury to the medial side of the knee.

In the knee, the dancer usually complains of a diffuse, poorly localized pain on the medial side of the knee, presumably due to a chronic ligamentous injury. Examination often reveals nothing more than some vague tenderness. The pain can be quite troublesome, and if the doctor is unaware of the problem, it is likely to remain undiagnosed. This is a good example of an injury resulting entirely from faulty technique. If the foot is not turned out any more than the hip, the pain will soon vanish.

Sprained Ligaments

Minor sprains of the knee ligaments are quite common, especially in male dancers. Often the cause is landing awkwardly from a jump, although sometimes the pain seems to result from repeated minor trauma. Usually, the only treatment needed is to avoid activities that produce the pain for a few days. In more severe cases, physical therapy and anti-inflammatory medication may help.

Partial Ligament Tears

These tears, which are relatively uncommon, are usually due to a fall or mishap. The knee may be swollen or bruised, and there will be localized tenderness in the region of the tear. Stressing the knee in the appropriate direction will reproduce the pain. Most cases I have treated have involved the upper attachment of the tibial collateral (medial) ligament. Treatment is the same as for a ligament sprain, except that the rest will need to be more prolonged and more complete.

Major Ligament Injuries

These injuries are extremely rare in ballet. I have seen only one major injury, in a male dancer who lost control in the rehearsal studio, collided with the piano, and fell with his leg twisted under him. He was left with a degree of anteromedial rotary instability that prevented his return to dancing major roles, but he did not suffer serious inconvenience otherwise.[8] He elected not to have surgery because at the age of 35 he was almost ready to retire from dancing.

Other authors have reported a greater incidence of ligament injury. Thomasen reports 17 cases of ligament rupture, including one acute rupture of the medial ligament, which was successfully repaired.[10] The other 16 cases were seen too late for primary repair and were not treated surgically. I agree with Thomasen's view that it would be almost impossible to get a dancer back to full activity after a knee reconstruction.

The Extensor Apparatus

Anterior Knee Pain

Pain around the front of the knee is a very common complaint in dancers. Many of the conditions to be discussed below present with anterior knee pain, and it is convenient to list them here for reference.

1. Pain above the patella
    - Tear of the lower quadriceps
2. Pain level with the patella
    - Prepatellar bursitis
    - Bipartite patella
    - Stress fracture of patella
    - Subluxation or dislocation of patella
    - Excessive lateral pressure syndrome
    - Chondromalacia
    - Plica syndrome
    - Meniscus lesion
    - Ligament sprain
    - Pain due to forced turn-out
    - Osteochondritis dissecans
3. Pain below the patella
    - Jumper's knee
    - Patellar tendinitis
    - Infrapatellar bursitis
    - Fat pad syndrome
    - Osgood Schlatter disease
    - Contusion of tibial tubercle
    - Pes anserinus bursitis

Muscle Strain

Muscle strains in the region of the knee are confined almost entirely to the lower fibers of the quadriceps close to the upper pole of the patella. Minor strains in this region are not uncommon because of the explosive contraction of the quadriceps during the more vigorous movements of ballet. Usually, avoidance of jumping for a few days is the only treatment required.

Bipartite Patella

This is a congenital condition in which the patella is divided into two very unequal parts, joined by fibrous tissue. It is seen in less than 1% of patellae. Occasionally, the patella may be in three or more parts. This condition is usually painless, although with the overuse that occurs in ballet, pain localized to the region between the two fragments is sometimes felt. Examination reveals localized tenderness in the same area. The condition is often diagnosed when x-rays are taken because of anterior knee pain. It is often hard to see the lesion on anteroposterior views, but it often shows up well on axial views (figure 11-10).

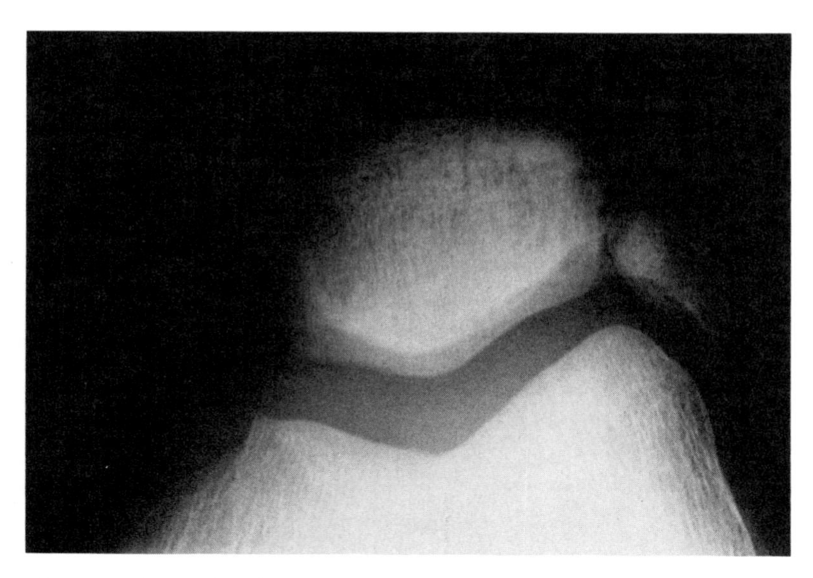

Figure 11-10. Bipartite patella. The separation between the two fragments is usually best seen radiographically in an axial view.

It is a common error to suppose that the most obvious abnormality seen must be the cause of the patient's symptoms, and many knees have been wrongly operated on because the bipartite patella was blamed for the pain. Only when the patient failed to respond following surgery was the knee thoroughly evaluated and the correct diagnosis made. Before excising the small fragment, the knee must be fully assessed, preferably including arthroscopy to exclude patellofemoral pain. In cases in which the pain really does come from the bipartite patella, excision of the small fragment is curative.

Fractured Patella

This is an uncommon injury in dancers. The few examples I have seen have resulted from powerful contractions of the quadriceps rather than from direct trauma. Usually, the lower pole of the patella is avulsed during an awkward or heavy landing from a jump. One leading male dancer from the Australian Ballet had been suffering from recurrent pain in the region of the patella for some weeks. In retrospect, this was probably a stress fracture. As he pushed off at the start of a big leap, he felt his knee being "torn apart"; at surgery, it was found that he not only had fractured the lower pole of the patella but also had severely torn the quadriceps expansions (figure 11-11). The small bone fragment was excised and the expansions carefully repaired. After prolonged rehabilitation, he returned to the same highly athletic style of dancing as before.

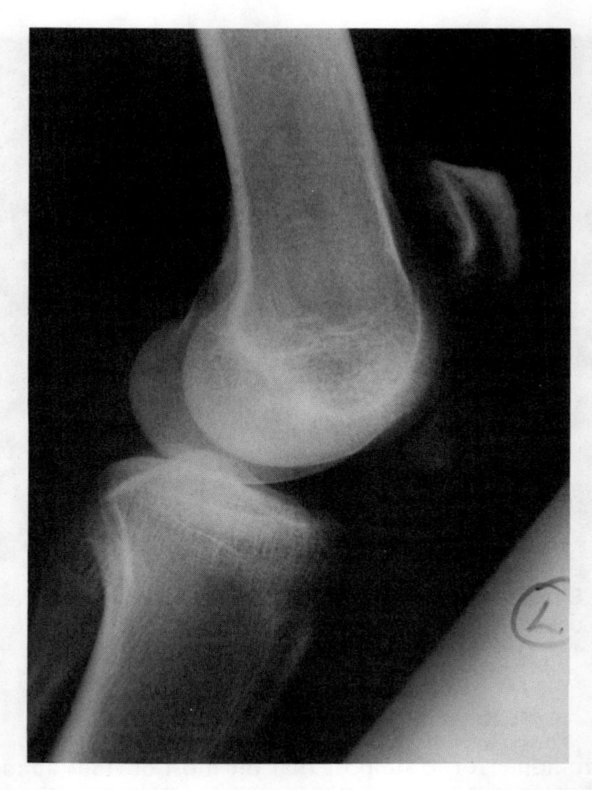

Figure 11-11. This patella fractured as the dancer was taking off for a big leap, and was probably weakened by a pre-existing stress fracture.

Stress Fractures

These are found from time to time in the patella, and Devas describes the problem well.[3] Any pain that seems localized to the patella and that does not have another explanation suggests a stress fracture. Plain x-rays are usually of no help; the diagnosis can be made with certainty only by performing a nuclear bone scan. If a stress fracture is found, the treatment is rest, which should be as complete as possible, even to the extent of using crutches for some weeks. If there is even the suspicion of a stress fracture, all jumping should be avoided, because there is danger that the fracture may become complete, and the problem is then much more serious.

Bursitis

There are many bursae around the knee (figure 11-12), but the four which I have seen causing trouble in dancers are:

1. *The prepatellar bursa.* This may become inflamed by kneeling on a hard stage or by repeated bending of the knee. It presents as a fluid-filled swell-

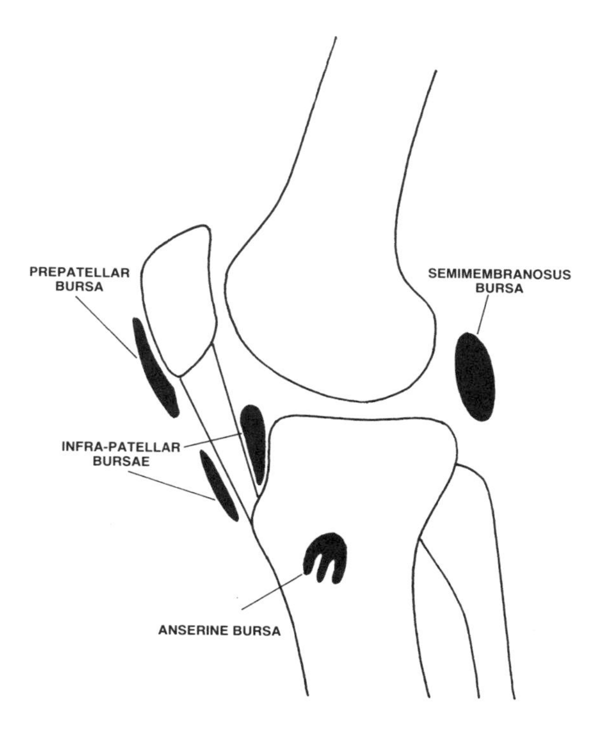

Figure 11-12. Bursae around the knee joint, which tend to become symptomatic in dancers.

ing that is clearly in front of the patella, distinguishing it from an intra-articular effusion.

2. *The superficial and deep infrapatellar bursae.* These cause a similar swelling, but lower down, in the region of the patellar tendon and tibial tubercle.

3. *The anserine bursa.* This bursa, which lies on the upper part of the medial surface of the tibia, sends prolongations between the attachments of the tendons of sartorius, gracilis, and semitendinosus. This is a relatively uncommon site for bursitis in dancers, but deserves to be mentioned because it is sometimes overlooked.

4. *The semimembranosus bursa.* This lies on the medial side of the back of the knee, and when distended is often referred to as a Baker's cyst. The presence of a Baker's cyst is often associated with an effusion within the main joint cavity, and arthrography often shows that there is a communication between the cyst and the knee joint. This can be verified at operation.

Although I have seen inflammation of all the bursae mentioned above in dancers, most cases have been mild and have healed with rest and conservative treatment. The Baker's cyst is the only one of the four that has required surgical excision.

Jumper's Knee

Jumper's knee, as we use the term, refers to a partial tear of the patellar tendon just inferior to the lower pole of the patella.[10] It is quite a common complaint, especially in male dancers who dance very athletic roles. Presumably, the original injury is an acute tearing of some of the upper fibers of the patellar tendon due to the explosive pull of the quadriceps during a leap. Before the injury has time to heal, it is aggravated by further jumping, and a chronic injury develops, with a small area of granulation tissue at the site of the original tear.

The dancer will complain of pain just below the patella, felt very sharply when taking off or landing in a jump. Examination of the knee reveals an extremely localized area of tenderness that can be palpated more easily if the upper pole of the patella is pushed down toward the femur, thus making the lower pole more prominent. If the pain can be reproduced by extending the knee against resistance, the diagnosis is strengthened. It is sometimes difficult to distinguish this condition from pain arising in the patellofemoral joint or from patellar tendinitis, and a useful confirmatory test is to inject the tender area with a small volume of local anesthetic. If the dancer can then jump without pain, the diagnosis is almost certain.

Treatment initially is by the avoidance of jumping, helped by electrical treatment from a physical therapist. If the pain eases, then jumping can be resumed, but only after a careful scrutiny of the dancer's technique is made to ensure that there is no technical fault that may cause a recurrence.

The correct way to land from a jump is with a gentle but definite bend of the knees, which allows progressive deceleration and takes the shock out of landing. This movement is known as a *demi-plié*. Some dancers having a poor *demi-plié* injure themselves in landing rather than taking off.

When conservative treatment fails, surgery is necessary. The aim of surgery is to excise the area of granulation tissue. Unfortunately, this is usually closer to the deep surface of the tendon and is difficult to find without doing considerable damage to other structures. A method used by Eivind Thomasen of Denmark is as follows (figure 11-13): Under local anesthesia, a small transverse incision is made at the lower pole of the patella. The upper part of the patellar tendon is exposed and probed with a fine needle until the tender spot is found. Further local anesthetic is injected down the needle, which is left in situ as a guide to help in finding the lesion. The fibers of the patellar tendon are separated on either side of the needle close to the patella. The characteristic lesion is an area of grey, glistening granulation tissue slightly larger than a grain of wheat. Occasionally, there is also a small flake of bone avulsed from the lower pole of the patella. Excision of the abnormal tissue provides satisfactory relief of pain in most cases. It is worthwhile repeating here that under no circumstances should steroid injections be used to treat this condition, because they weaken the tendon and may cause it to rupture.

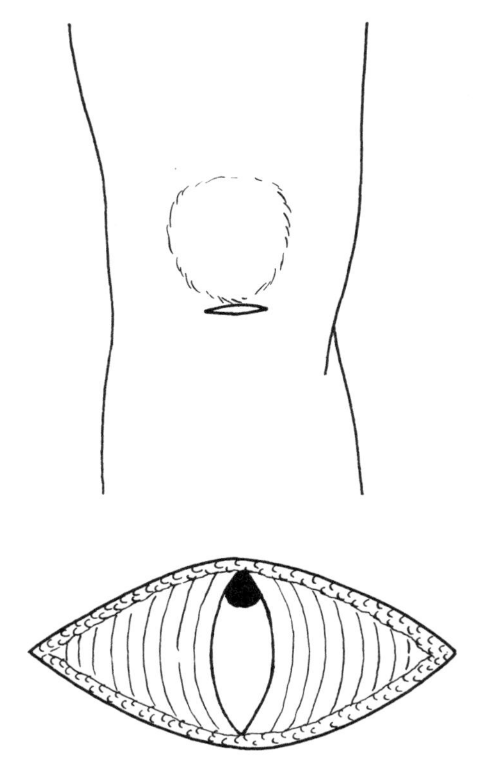

Figure 11-13. Operation for jumper's knee. The skin incision is shown (top). When the fibers of the patellar tendon are separated (bottom), an area of granulation tissue is revealed (black area).

Patellar Tendinitis

Patellar tendinitis is less common than jumper's knee, but is still quite common in dancers. It is seen more often in male dancers, although females develop it as well. The precipitating factor is an increase in the total volume of work, such as occurs during rehearsals for an important performance, especially if there are a lot of steps requiring load bearing on a bent knee.

The pathological changes are the same as in tendinitis elsewhere, with inflammation, thickening, and contracture of the sheath, and the formation of adhesions between sheath and tendon. The dancer feels pain related directly to activity and extending from the lower pole of the patella to the tibial tubercle. Crepitus is sometimes felt, but is far less prominent in the knee than it is in the tendons around the ankle. Examination may reveal slight swelling, tenderness, or crepitus on movement. It is often hard to be certain whether crepitus is coming from the tendon itself or is being transmitted from the patellofemoral joint.

In most cases, rest, physical therapy, and anti-inflammatory medication will relieve the problem; if activity is then moderated, a recurrence can be avoided. In resistant cases, surgery offers good prospects for relief. A transverse incision is made at the midpoint of the tendon, and the tendon sheath is split from end to end. Adhesions between the sheath and the tendon are divided. If there is swelling of the tendon itself, it is worth separating the fibers in a couple of places to ensure that there are no areas of focal degeneration within the tendon.

Contusion of the Tibial Tubercle

In modern ballet, dancers are often required to kneel on a hard stage, "walk" on their knees, or even do "knee spins." Because the tibial tubercle is prominent in the kneeling position, the tissues over it may become contused and the skin callused or abraded. Occasionally, the superficial infrapatellar bursa also becomes inflamed.

The solution is simply to remove the cause. If choreographers cannot be persuaded to revise their ballets, then at least dancers can wear knee guards in rehearsal and subject their knees to trauma only during the performance.

Osgood Schlatter Disease

This condition is sometimes incorrectly referred to as Osgood-Schlatter's disease. Osgood and Schlatter were two men who independently described the radiographic appearance of this condition. The term "disease" is also incorrect, inasmuch as this is a traction injury to the epiphysis of the tibial tubercle. Osgood Schlatter disease is quite common in athletic adolescent males, and is particularly common in young dancers. There is enlargement and sometimes deformity and fragmentation of the epiphysis of the tibial tubercle. A similar condition is described in the lower pole of the patella under the name Sinding Larsen Johanson syndrome.

The patient presents with a history of increasing pain from activities involving forceful extension of the knee, such as cycling or climbing stairs. Ballet movements that aggravate the pain include *pliés, fondues,* and jumps. Usually, the swelling is sufficiently marked to have been noticed by the patient. Examination reveals a tender swelling of one tibial tubercle, and forced extension of the leg against resistance produces pain in the same area.

A lateral x-ray will show the epiphysis as enlarged, elongated, and fragmented (figure 11-14). There may be a loose fragment visible. It is important also to form some estimate of how close the epiphysis is to uniting with the main shaft of the bone, as this has a bearing on prognosis.

The first and most important part of treatment in a youngster is to reassure the child and his parents that this is a benign and self-limiting condition. Anything the patient wishes to do is permitted, and he is told that when the tubercle unites with the main part of the tibia, the pain will usually go away. Any treatment beyond this is a waste of time.

If pain persists into adult life, further x-rays should be taken to rule out the presence of a loose fragment. This is always found above the tubercle deep to the lowest fibers of the patellar tendon (figure 11-15). If pain is sufficient to warrant removal of the fragment, a small transverse skin incision is made just above the tibial tubercle. The fibers of the patellar tendon are separated without cutting them, and the bone fragment will easily be identified. Although the

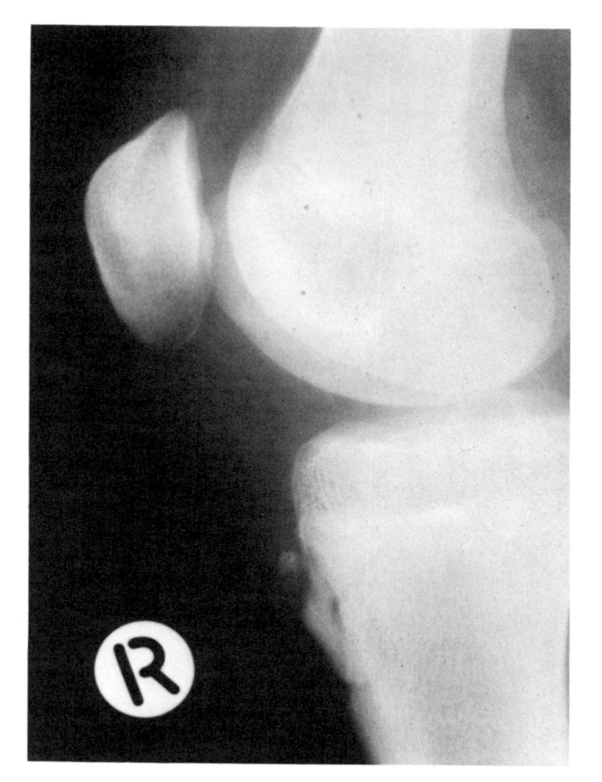

Figure 11-14. Typical appearance of the tibial tubercle in Osgood Schlatter disease.

fragment is fairly mobile, it is always attached by fibrous tissue to the tubercle, and sharp dissection is needed to remove it.

Exostoses Around the Knee

A problem occasionally encountered in young dancers is an isolated exostosis, usually of the lower femur but occasionally of the upper tibia. The most common site is on the medial side of the lower femur about 2 in. above the knee joint. Exostoses of this sort are thought to be caused by failure of resorption of bone as the lower femoral epiphysis migrates distally during growth. The dancer sometimes presents because of a small, hard lump on the inner side of the knee. In many cases, the lump was noted because of pain in the region. During the forceful and repetitive movements of ballet the exostosis interferes with the action of vastus medialis, and increasing discomfort results.

Clinically, the exostosis is felt as a small, hard, nonmobile swelling on the medial side of the lower femur. X-rays show the exostosis clearly (figure 11-16). It should be remembered, however, that there is usually a cap of cartilage on the exostosis, and, because this is radiolucent, the x-rays give a misleading impression of the size of the exostosis. It is always larger when seen with the naked eye than it is radiographically.

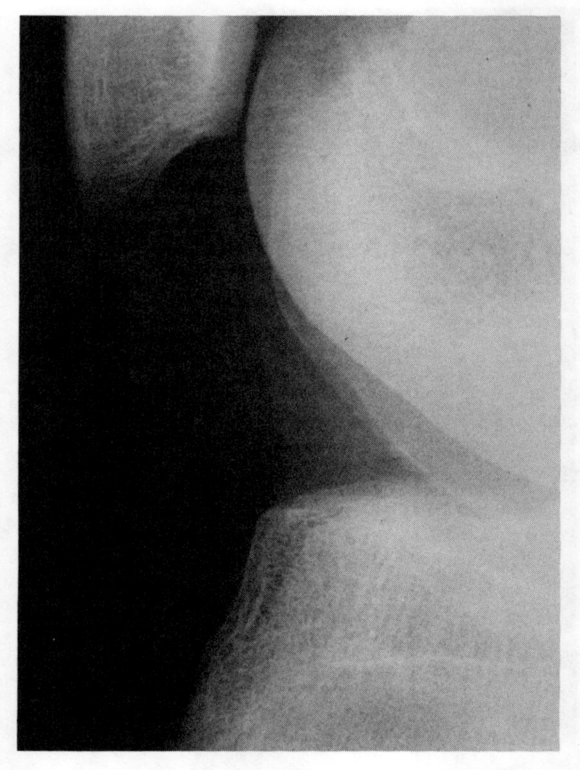

Figure 11-15. Old Osgood Schlatter disease with a loose bone fragment deep to the patellar tendon.

If the dancer has come only because of the finding of a painless lump, then explanation and reassurance are the only treatment required. When the swelling is interfering with the movements of ballet, excision is advisable. A short, vertical incision is made and the fibers of the vastus medialis carefully separated to expose the exostosis. The bony swelling is then carefully removed flush with the surface of the femur, using either an osteotome or bone nibblers. Excision of the exostosis should give complete relief of symptoms.

Patellofemoral Problems

The articulation between the patella and the lower femur is a potent source of problems for the dancer. The body type that is best suited to ballet tends to have the sort of knee that predisposes to patellofemoral conditions that include subluxation, dislocation, excessive lateral pressure syndrome, and chondromalacia.

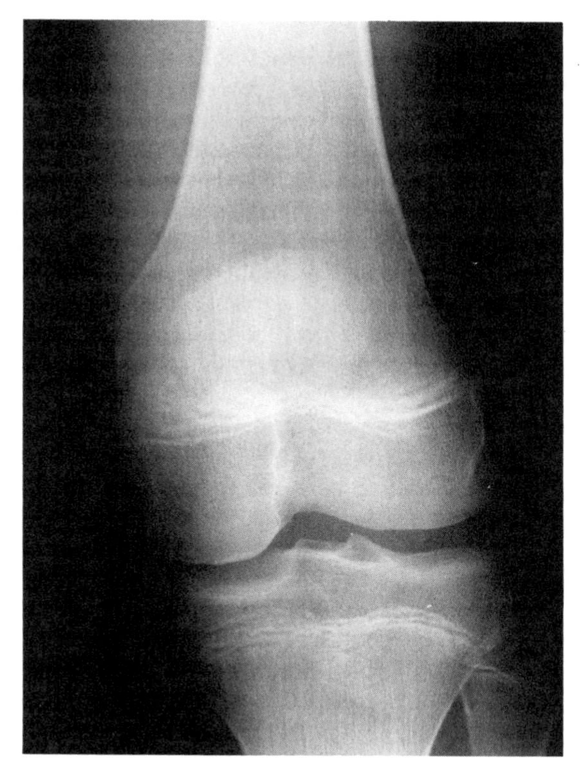

Figure 11-16. An exostosis of the lower femur that required excision. At operation, it was found to be much bigger than it appeared radiographically.

Clicking Knee

Clicking joints, extremely common in dancers, seldom lead to a medical consultation unless the click is accompanied by pain or some other symptom. Most of the clicks come from behind the patella. The articular surface of the patella has various facets that articulate with the femur in different degrees of flexion. Sometimes, as the knee is flexed and extended, the patella is held up momentarily and then moves to a new position with a faint click.

If the click is the sole problem, then the dancer can be reassured that clicking is common and quite harmless. Before giving this reassurance, the doctor should make quite sure that the clicking is not caused by a meniscus lesion, a medial suprapatellar plica, or a loose body. Fortunately, this distinction is not difficult. In many cases, a previously painless click becomes slightly painful for a time, especially if there has been an increase in the dancer's work load. If the knee is rested for a time, it will usually become painless again, although the click will persist unchanged.

Patellar Instability

The patella is a fairly unstable structure, and its position at any time is due to an equilibrium between the various forces acting on it (figure 11-17). The quadriceps tends to pull the patella upward and slightly laterally. This pull is offset by the patellar tendon, whose direction is either straight downward or down and slightly lateral. The angle between these two lines of pull is called the Q angle. When the quadriceps contracts, there is a tendency for the patella to be displaced laterally by the resultant force. Under normal circumstances, this tendency to lateral displacement is exactly balanced by the vastus medialis obliquus (VMO), and as a result, the patella runs correctly in its track.

No two dancers are built alike, and there may be one or more factors that either permit or encourage lateral displacement of the patella. These can be summarized as follows:

1. *VMO insufficiency.* In these cases, the action of the VMO is insufficient to balance the lateral pull on the patella. Dancers usually have strong, bulky quadriceps, and it is easy to overlook the fact that some of them have a very deficient VMO, despite their good overall muscle development.

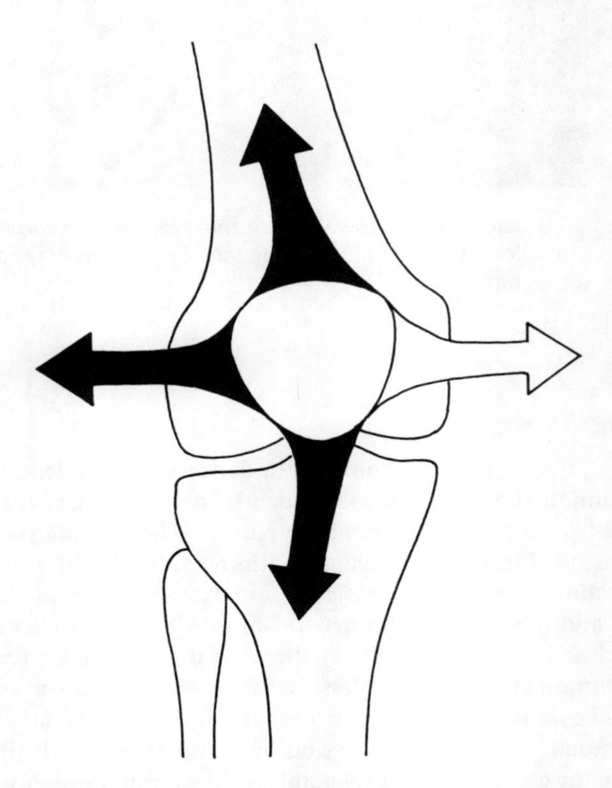

Figure 11-17. Forces acting on the patella. The upward pull of the quadriceps and the downward pull of the patellar tendon are not in line, and they produce a resultant laterally directed force on the patella. This is balanced by the pull of the VMO (white arrow).

2. *Patella alta.* The patella is partly stabilized by the trochlear notch of the femur, in which it runs. In some cases of patella alta, the patella is too high to be in the deepest part of the groove. In addition, high patellae tend to be hypoplastic.

3. *Hypoplasia.* The patella and the trochlear surface of the lower femur may be hypoplastic; frequently, hypoplasia of both is seen.

4. *Genu valgum.* The overall valgus of the knee tends to increase the Q angle, making the tibial tubercle more laterally placed.

5. *External tibial torsion.* Again, this has the effect of increasing the Q angle by making the tibial tubercle more laterally placed.

6. *Laterally placed tibial tubercle.* This can occur in the absence of genu valgum or external tibial torsion.

7. *Genu recurvatum.* This does not of itself alter the forces acting on the patella, but it contributes to general laxity of the anterior soft tissue structures and makes displacement due to other factors more likely.

8. *Soft tissue stabilizers.* Lax tissues on the medial side of the knee or tight structures on the lateral side of the knee may aggravate a tendency to lateral displacement.

More than one of these factors often will be present in a particular dancer. Thus, female dancers with anterior knee pain are frequently found to have a small, high patella, dysplasia of the femur and patella, genu valgum, and genu recurvatum. The effects of lateral patellar displacement will be considered in the next few sections.

Patellar Subluxation

For reasons given above, lateral subluxation of the patella is common in dancers. Subluxation is present when the patella is displaced laterally but some part of its articular surface is still in contact with the articular surface of the trochlear notch of the femur (figure 11-18). In a dislocation, on the other hand, the patella lies on the lateral aspect of the lateral femoral condyle, and there is no contact between the articular surfaces at all.

In a normal knee, the patella lies in the bottom of the trochlear notch, and the medial and lateral patellar facets are applied with equal force to the articular surface of the trochlea. The first stage of subluxation is an increase of pressure on the lateral facet of the patella and a corresponding decrease in pressure on the medial facet. This may not be detectable clinically or radiographically, but may have significant effects (see excessive lateral pressure syndrome).

In more severe cases, the patella rises out of the bottom of the trochlear notch and moves a little to the lateral side. Some separation now occurs between the medial facet and the medial side of the trochlear notch. Probably nothing will be detected clinically at this stage, but axial x-rays taken at 30°, 60°, and 90° may show the displacement, especially in the 30° view (figures 11-19, 11-20).

The final stage of subluxation can be observed clinically as the knee moves from flexion to extension and back. This is best observed when the patient sits with the thigh supported by the examining table, with the edge of the table at the level of the knee joint. Movement of the knee between 0-90° of

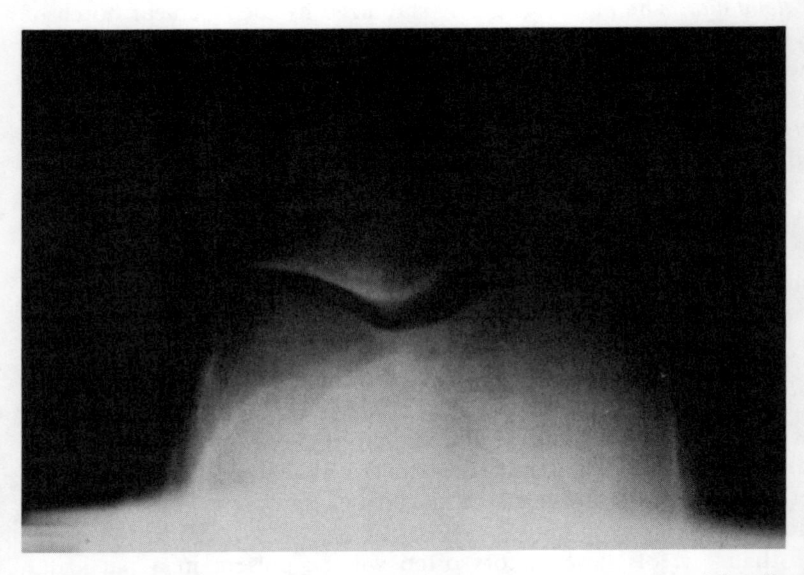

Figure 11-18. Obvious patellar subluxation is shown on an axial radiograph.

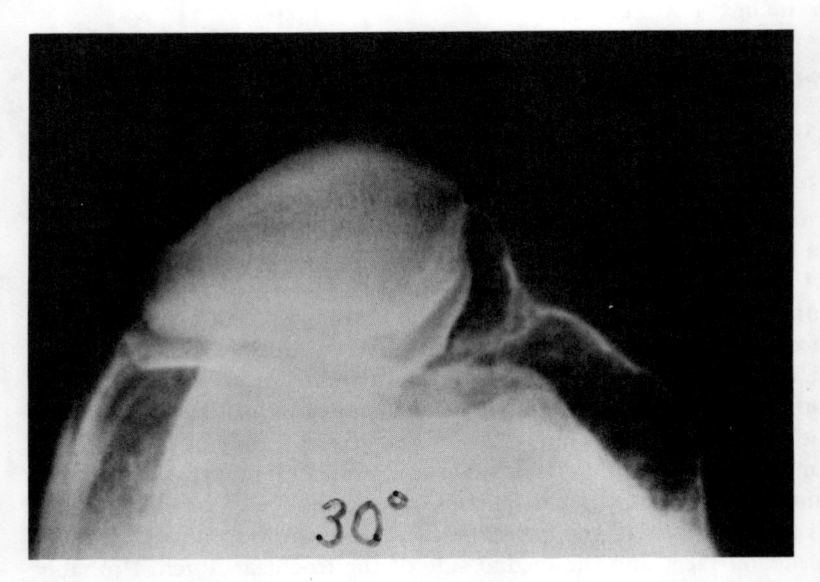

Figure 11-19. An axial view taken in the course of a double contrast arthrogram, showing marked subluxation at 30° of flexion.

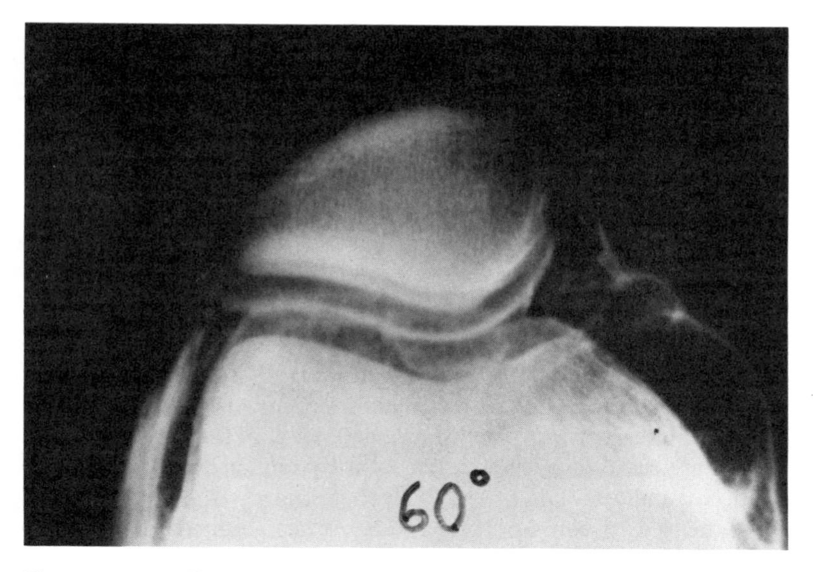

Figure 11-20. The same knee as figure 11-19. With the knee flexed to 60°, the subluxation is no longer apparent.

flexion will often disclose abnormalities in tracking of the patella due to lateral subluxation. Axial x-rays are usually helpful at this stage.

Minor degrees of subluxation are very clearly seen through the arthroscope, and arthroscopy should be employed in doubtful cases. This also gives an opportunity to assess the state of the articular surfaces. Dancers with a subluxing patella complain of anterior knee pain related to exertion, often saying that they feel the knee "go out" during certain movements. These episodes may be acutely painful.

Examination will usually disclose one or more of the causes of patellar instability listed above. The patella often can be seen to sublux. If the knee is flexed to 30° and the patella is forced laterally, the sensation may be acutely unpleasant to the patient, who often will pull the examining hand away. This is called the apprehension test, and, if positive, is almost diagnostic of significant patellar subluxation.

A remarkably high number of dancers, despite their generally good muscular development, have a very weak VMO, and most cases of patellar subluxation can be well controlled by exercises designed to develop this muscle. Other methods of improving the tracking of the patella are discussed below.

Patellar Dislocation

Dislocation of the patella, a serious injury, is not uncommon in dancers because their work is very athletic and their knees are predisposed to dislocation. Females are affected more often than males. Dislocations of the patella are customarily described as congenital, habitual, recurrent, etc., but these classifications are not of much help in treating dancers. It is far more important to know how many times the patella has dislocated and to analyze carefully the predisposing factors.

The causes of patellar dislocation are just an extension of those that cause subluxation. Typically, there is a twisting injury in which the tibia rotates laterally with respect to the femur and carries the tibial tubercle with it. Obviously, for the patella to displace so far there must be considerable disruption of the structures on the medial side of the joint, including the insertion of the VMO. A hemarthrosis is usual, and may be quite tense. Osteochondral fractures of the patella or the lateral femoral condyle may occur, and if not recognized they can give rise to loose bodies.

A dancer whose patella dislocates feels immediate and severe pain and will stop dancing at once. The knee often swells rapidly, and the tension of the hemarthrosis can be extremely painful. The dislocation sometimes reduces spontaneously within seconds, but if the patella remains dislocated it will be very obvious on the lateral side of the joint. The knee looks so "wrong" that most dislocations are reduced by the patient or a bystander immediately.

Examination usually reveals a tensely swollen knee. If the patella is still dislocated, it will be clearly seen, but if it has already been reduced, it is hard to distinguish clinically from other types of serious injury. This is why it is so very important to get a detailed and accurate history, for otherwise the diagnosis may be missed. It is sometimes possible to feel a defect in the VMO insertion, but in many cases the hemarthrosis obscures this. X-rays of the knee are essential to rule out osteochondral fractures. These do not always show well on anteroposterior lateral views, but are sometimes well seen on the axial view.

Management of this injury depends on whether it is the first dislocation or whether it is the most recent of a series. It also depends on whether there is an osteochondral fracture. A first dislocation with fracture can be managed conservatively. It is usually worthwhile to aspirate the hematoma under strictly sterile conditions, for the following reasons:

- A tense hemarthrosis is very painful.
- When the hemarthrosis has been aspirated, it is much easier to feel the defect in the VMO insertion.
- It is easier to reappose the damaged tissues by compressive bandaging when the knee is not full of blood.

The limb should be rested with the knee firmly in a compression bandage for a few days. A cast can then be applied from groin to ankle and worn for 6 weeks. Vigorous exercise under the supervision of a physical therapist should be continued until full activity is regained. If the dislocation is a recurrent one, or if there is an osteochondral fragment, surgery should be considered. Surgical techniques for realigning the extensor apparatus are described below.

Chondromalacia Patellae

Although much has been learned about chondromalacia in recent years, it remains difficult to assess and confusing to treat. The symptoms of chondromalacia are highly variable, and it can mimic quite a few other conditions within the knee. With the widespread adoption of arthroscopy, it has become clear that not all chondromalacia is painful, and that some patients have all the symptoms of chondromalacia without having any of the pathological changes.

Hughston strongly believes that chondromalacia is a secondary disorder and that in most cases, the primary cause is patellar subluxation.[6] Although in general my observations support this, I have nevertheless seen severe changes of chondromalacia in knees that bore none of the stigmata of lateral subluxation. Hughston also notes that one-third to one-half of adults have macroscopic changes of chondromalacia, but far fewer suffer from anterior knee pain. Articular cartilage has no nerve endings, so the pain of chondromalacia must come from some other tissue, but it is not clear at this stage which tissue. Our knowledge of this whole subject is still far from complete.

The pathology of chondromalacia is familiar, and it is customary to grade patellae as follows (figure 11-21):

Grade 1. Edema and softening of the articular cartilage with little or no macroscopic change. There may be a small "blister," some discoloration, or a few vertical splits. By far the majority of chondromalacia in dancers' knees presents this appearance.

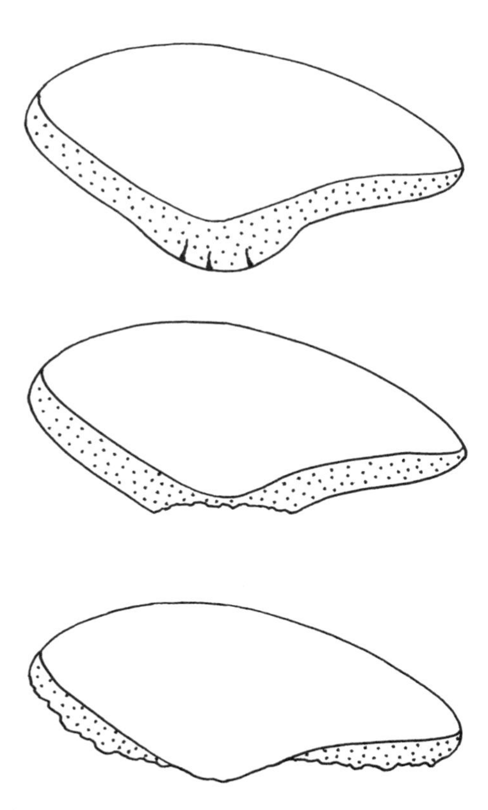

Figure 11-21. The three grades of chondromalacia. From top: grade 1 with softening and edema; grade 2 with partial thickness erosion; grade 3 with full thickness erosion.

Grade 2. Erosion of the articular cartilage with partial thickness loss.
Grade 3. Erosions down to and including bone.

Some knees, instead of showing softening, have a firm articular cartilage that is discolored and fibrillated. Short tufts or longer fronds are often seen hanging from the articular surface.

Clinically, there is no typical history, but the dancer often complains of pain when the knee is straightened under load, as in *pliés* and jumps. Pain may also be experienced on stairs or when rising from a chair. The knee may be painful after it has been flexed for a time, as at the theater or in a car. A grinding sensation in the knee is commonly complained of, and locking, catching, and giving way are sometimes a problem. Swelling is rare.

Examination often reveals some of the factors favoring patellar subluxation, and the patella may sometimes be observed to displace out of the trochlear notch. There may be tenderness behind the margins of the patella, and retropatellar crepitus may be felt on movement. This last sign is by no means diagnostic of chondromalacia; in many cases, knees that showed marked crepitus proved to be arthroscopically free of chondromalacia. Plain x-rays are of little help, although they should still be taken to exclude other conditions. It is also useful to know if the axial view shows evidence of subluxation.

Arthroscopy is often the only way to be sure whether chondromalacia is present. It is essential to remember that the articular cartilage may be macroscopically normal, and the chondral softening of grade 1 chondromalacia may be apparent only when the surface is probed. The insertion of a probe through a separate portal is an essential part of every arthroscopic examination.

The first line of treatment in most cases is to send the patient to a physical therapist for strengthening of the VMO, and often this is sufficient to relieve the pain. In more refractory cases, the two lines of treatment that seem to be most helpful are arthroscopic chondroplasty and procedures to realign the extensor mechanism. These are discussed in detail below.

The Excessive Lateral Pressure Syndrome

This condition was first described by Ficat and Hungerford.[4] The underlying defect is that the patella presses with much greater force on the lateral than on the medial side of the trochlear notch.

When the laterally directed component of the quadriceps pull overcomes the stabilizing force of the VMO, then the patella will sublux if it is free to do so. In some cases, the patella is prevented from subluxing, perhaps due to a deep trochlear notch or to capsular tethering of the lateral side, but the patella is still pulled laterally. This means that the lateral facet of the patella is pulled with increased force against the trochlear notch, whereas the load on the medial facet is reduced. If the condition persists, there is a thinning of the articular cartilage on the lateral facet, with a resulting loss of joint space. At the same time, subchondral sclerosis develops in the underlying bone (figures 11-22, 11-23). The final result of this syndrome is patellofemoral osteoarthritis.

The main symptom complained of is anterior knee pain, possibly with crepitus. This history of excessive lateral pressure syndrome hardly differs from

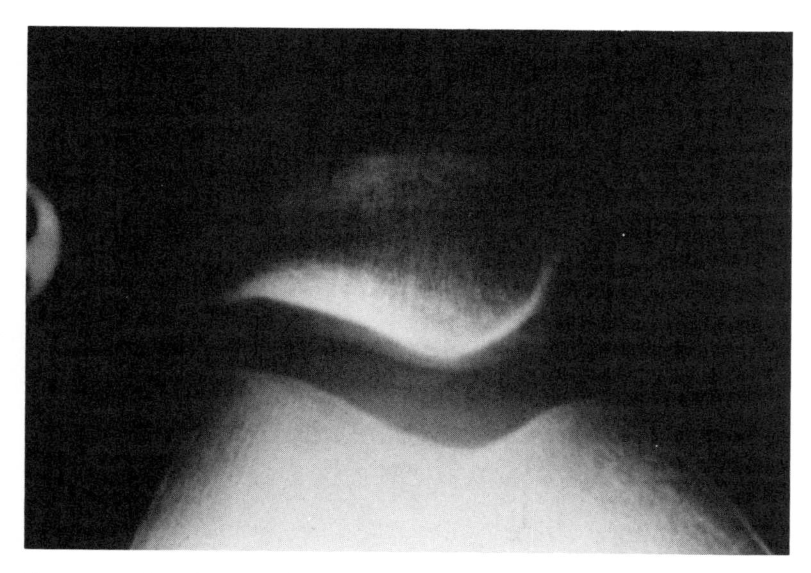

Figure 11-22. A case of excessive lateral pressure syndrome, showing marked subchondral sclerosis in the bone underlying the lateral facet of the patella.

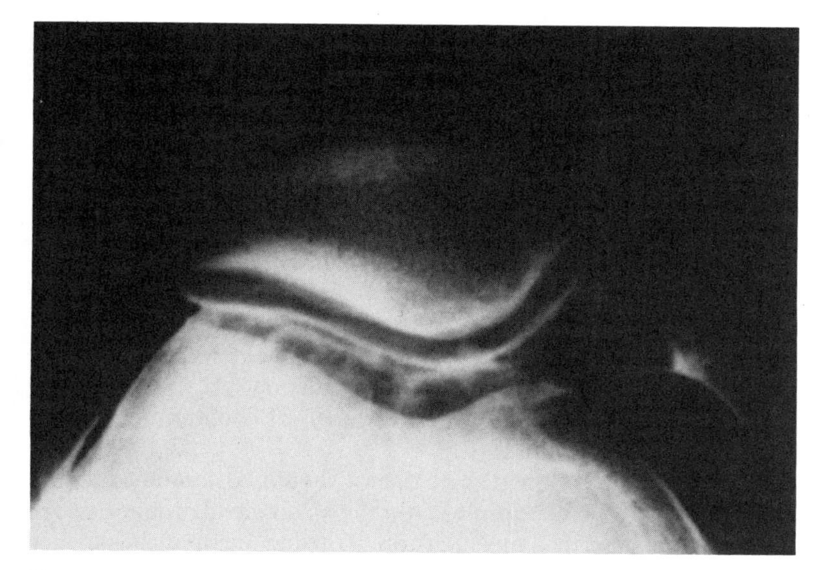

Figure 11-23. Double-contrast arthrography of the same knee as figure 11-22. There is thinning of the articular cartilage on the lateral side of the patellofemoral joint.

that of chondromalacia. Examination of the knee should include an assessment of the side-to-side mobility of the patella. In many cases of anterior knee pain, an abnormally large range of movement is found; sometimes there is a positive apprehension test. In excessive lateral pressure syndrome, however, an abnormally *small* range of side-to-side movement will usually be found.

Plain x-ray of the knee is helpful. The axial view may show tilting, but not subluxation, of the patella. There may be a diminished joint space on the lateral side and subchondral sclerosis in the same area. Ficat and Hungerford also note that in long-standing cases the trabeculae of the patella are perpendicular to the lateral facet rather than perpendicular to the equator of the patella.[4]

Treatment in the first instance is by rest, and in most cases this is sufficient. Aspirin is helpful for the pain. Quadriceps exercises in which the knee is kept straight are valuable, but exercises in which the flexed knee is extended against resistance should never be used for any patellofemoral disorder. If the knee fails to respond to conservative treatment, then surgery to divide the lateral retinaculum is recommended. This is described below.

Treatment

It may be helpful to summarize the stages of treatment for the patellofemoral disorders described above:

1. *Rest.* This can often be relative rest, in which certain injurious activities are eliminated, but the dancer continues with a fair proportion of the usual daily routine. In the early stages, most patellofemoral problems respond to rest.

2. *Physical therapy.* It is essential to maintain good quadriceps tone, and isometric quadriceps exercises and straight leg-lifting should be encouraged. Straightening of the flexed knee against resistance can only aggravate the problem and is contraindicated.

3. *Medication.* Nonsteroid anti-inflammatory medication is less helpful here than in other types of injury. Aspirin seems to have a specific effect on articular cartilage and is a useful analgesic.

4. *Open surgery.* The most frequently performed surgical procedure in this group is a lateral retinacular release. This is done through a lateral parapatellar incision of about the same length as the patella. All layers, including the synovium, are divided. Blind cutting through a short incision is not recommended. Meticulous hemostasis is essential to avoid postoperative hemarthrosis. A useful check on the adequacy of the release is to tilt the patella so that its articular surface faces the surgeon. If the release is adequate, it should be possible to stand the patella almost on its edge. Any areas of chondromalacia can be excised before closing the wound.

If lateral release alone is insufficient, then it should be combined with a medial procedure. Reefing of the capsule is usually recommended, but I prefer a VMO advancement as described by Hughston.[6] If realignment of the patellar tendon is also required, then transplantation of the tibial tubercle is required. In earlier cases I used the Hauser technique,[5] but more recently I have performed the method of Elmslie and Trillat.[11] Surgery of this type is quite compatible with a return to ballet at high levels.

I have never performed a patellectomy on a dancer, and would regard it as an absolute last resort. I have, however, been able to observe a dancer who had a patellectomy performed in England, and who subsequently danced as a soloist with the Australian Ballet without apparent difficulty for 5 years (figure 11-24).

5. *Arthroscopic surgery.* This is by far the best way of dealing with chondral erosions if no other procedure is contemplated. It is possible to perform a lateral capsular release using cutting diathermy from within, but the advantage of this over open surgery is less apparent.

Intra-Articular Injuries

Meniscus Injuries

Meniscus injuries are far less common in dancers than might be expected, and I have already explained that the nature of the dance makes unlikely the combination of forces needed to cause an acute meniscus tear. Those menisci that I have operated on tend to have a scarred degenerate area in them, suggestive of repeated minor trauma rather than a single episode of violence. For this reason, the history is seldom of a single severe injury, and the onset may be insidious. The symptoms often are vague, and it is difficult to make a diagnosis on the history alone.

Examination follows the usual methods. A positive McMurray's test is helpful, but uncommon. Perhaps the single most useful sign is localized tenderness on the joint line over one or other meniscus. The differential diagnosis

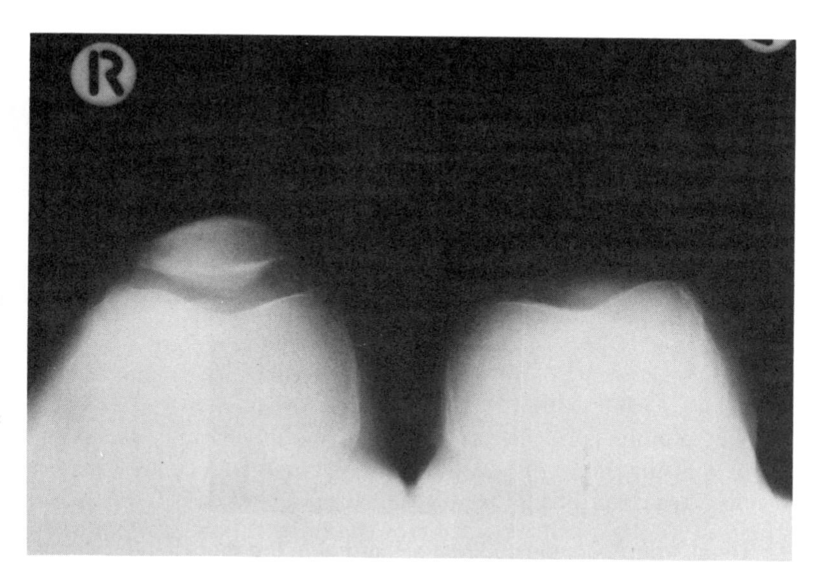

Figure 11-24. Patellectomy in a leading ballerina. This dancer continued her career for 5 years after this operation.

is from such conditions as chondromalacia, plica syndrome, fat pad syndrome, loose body, or ligamentous strain.

Arthrography of the knee frequently enables an accurate diagnosis to be made (figure 11-25). However, this is less often used nowadays, because arthroscopy offers the possibility of diagnosis and definitive treatment during the same procedure. Arthroscopic surgery for meniscus tears is greatly preferable to open surgery because the recovery period is much shorter, and the more conservative removal of meniscus tissue offers some protection against future degenerative arthritis. The prognosis for a full return to dancing following a meniscectomy is excellent.

Plica Syndrome

During embryonic life, the synovial cavity of the knee develops from three separate cavities that fuse together. Occasionally, fusion does not occur, and the suprapatellar pouch remains separated from the main cavity by a suprapatellar membrane. Much more often, however, there is incomplete fusion, resulting in a medial suprapatellar plica. This is a crescentic fold of synovial

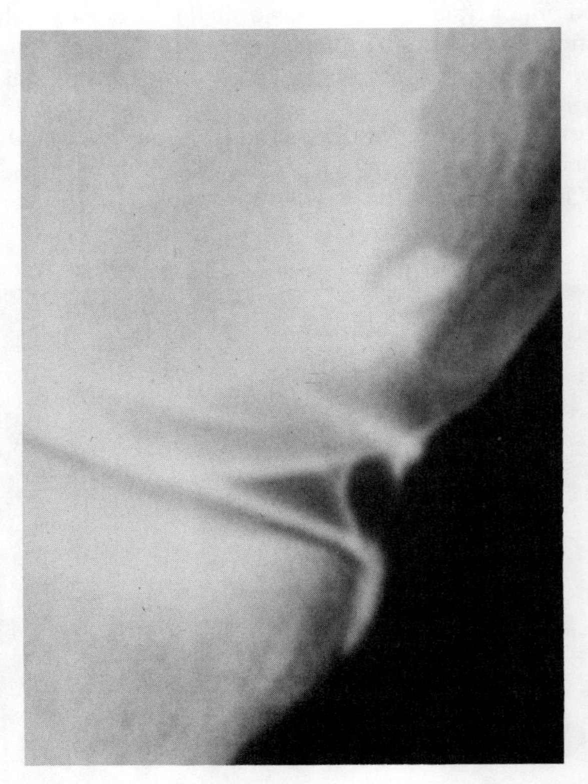

Figure 11-25. Detail from a double-contrast arthrogram. The medial meniscus is the wedge-shaped structure between the joint surfaces. The vertical line forming the base of the wedge is a tear in the meniscus.

membrane that begins in the region of the vastus lateralis insertion into the patella, passes beneath and is attached to the quadriceps tendon, and finally passes around the medial femoral condyle to the infrapatellar fat pad.

There are usually no symptoms, and the plica is noted at arthroscopy when the knee is examined for other reasons. However, the plica sometimes becomes inflamed, and there is then a complaint of pain on the medial side of the knee when sitting. When the knee is extended, there is a snap or pop, and the pain is relieved. Sometimes, there is a complaint of crepitus, swelling, and giving way.

Examination may reveal tenderness over the plica, crepitus on movement, and a small effusion. Sometimes the pop or snap can be reproduced. Arthrography usually reveals the presence of a plica (figure 11-26), but arthroscopy is generally preferred because the plica is then very clearly seen and can be removed at the same time by arthroscopic surgery. There may be fibrosis of the plica and erosion or pannus on the edges of the medial femoral condyle. Because a plica can be a cause of patellar subluxation, secondary chondromalacia may be present.

If a plica syndrome is suspected on clinical grounds, then rest and anti-

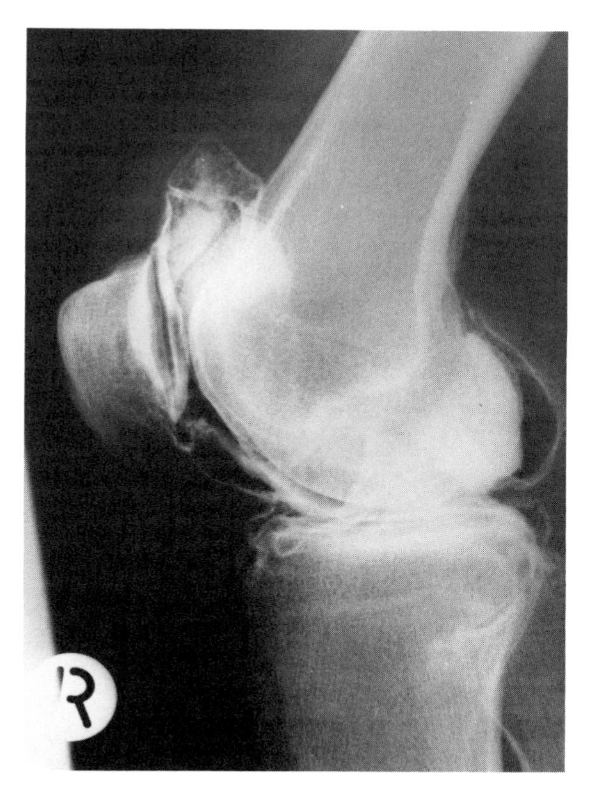

Figure 11-26. Medial suprapatellar plica. This is well shown in a double contrast arthrogram.

inflammatory medication may relieve it. However, the excision of a plica is one of the easiest arthroscopic procedures and gives good relief. For this reason, it should not be too long delayed.

Osteochondral Fractures

These fractures may occur during dislocation of the patella. The fragment may arise from the margin of the patella or from the lateral femoral condyle. If the fracture is recognized at the time of dislocation, it should be removed surgically; otherwise, it may form a loose body and require surgery later.

Osteochondritis Dissecans

This condition, seen from time to time in dancers, needs to be managed well if a good result is to be achieved. Occurring on the articular surfaces of the medial femoral condyles, it consists of a small area of subchondral bone that separates from the main part of the bone. A frequent site is the medial wall of the intercondylar notch, adjacent to the proximal attachment of the posterior cruciate ligament (figure 11-27). The area of articular cartilage involved is vari-

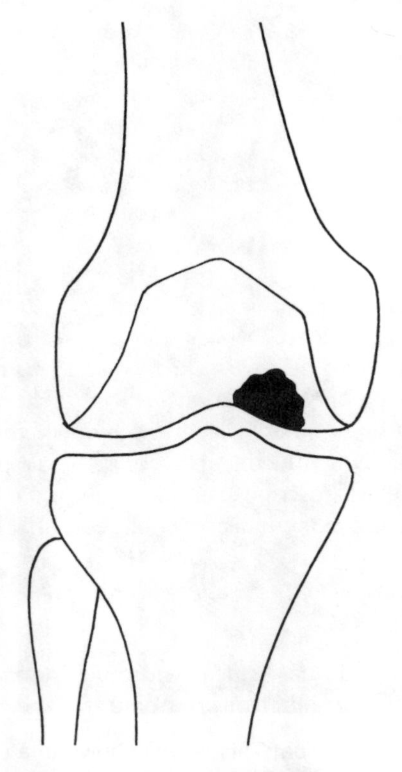

Figure 11-27. Osteochondritis dissecans. The dark area shows the most common site for the lesion.

able, but may be quite large. The etiology is not clear, but the theories revolve around (1) trauma, (2) ischemia, and (3) abnormal epiphyseal development.

In some cases there is spontaneous healing, but in other cases the bone fragment becomes detached and forms a loose body within the joint. The patient is usually an athletic adolescent male dancer. The onset is rather insidious, with a complaint of intermittent pain related to activity. Occasionally there is a slight effusion, and very occasionally the condition is bilateral. The only way to make the diagnosis with certainty is to x-ray the knee.

In young patients, rest is often the only treatment required, although it may need to be prolonged. Further x-rays may show healing within 6-12 months. If the fragment appears to have separated, arthroscopy is very helpful. It is easy to test with a probe and see whether the fragment is loose; if it is, some further procedure should be performed. If the fragment is large and involves a large part of the articular surface, an attempt should be made to pin or screw it back in place. Small fragments should be excised. A simple way to do this is to use arthroscopic instruments to divide the loose body into many small pieces, then wash these out through the arthroscope sheath. The overall prognosis for this condition is good; the younger the age at onset, the greater the likelihood of spontaneous recovery.

Loose Bodies

Loose bodies may come from osteochondral fractures or from an area of osteochondritis dissecans. Often, no site of origin is apparent. Loose bodies may be single or multiple. The dancer gives a history of intermittent pain, swelling, clicking, and locking of the knee. Sometimes a small, hard object has already been felt moving about within the knee. Examination may be rewarding, but in most cases the loose body is not palpable.

X-rays will usually show the loose body as a small opacity within the joint. Most loose bodies have a thick coating of radiolucent articular cartilage, so the radiographic appearance often gives a false impression of the total size. The fabella can sometimes cause confusion; this sesamoid bone in the popliteus tendon is a normal structure, but it can be mistaken for a loose body by those not aware of its existence.

An attempt should be made to deal with the loose body arthroscopically, as this is far less traumatic to the knee than an arthrotomy. There is usually no difficulty in finding the loose body unless it is at the back of the joint. Loose bodies that are soft can be fragmented using arthroscopic instruments and the pieces washed out through the arthroscope sheath. Larger loose bodies can be held with graspers and the arthroscopy incision enlarged until the loose body can be withdrawn.

Fat Pad Syndrome

This condition, once referred to as Hoffa syndrome, is not common, but must be borne in mind as a cause of anterior knee pain in dancers. Any condition that compresses the fat pad may irritate the overlying synovium. Examples:

- Direct trauma, as in a blow beneath the patella, or excessive kneeling

- Generalized edema, as in premenstrual syndrome
- A space-occupying lesion of the fat pad
- A bucket handle tear of a meniscus
- Genu recurvatum (which tends to cause compression of the fat pad)

The dancer will complain of pain on activity, relieved by rest. Examination reveals swelling or effusion and possible tenderness in the midline below the patella. Extension aggravates the pain, and flexion relieves it. Most cases resolve themselves without any specific treatment. Occasionally, excision of the fat pad and related synovium is required.

Chondral Softening and Erosion

The changes of chondromalacia are not confined to the patella. In a number of dancers examined arthroscopically, I have noted softening of areas of articular cartilage over the weight-bearing surfaces of the femoral condyles and sometimes the tibial condyles. Occasionally, erosions are seen. Because of this, it is desirable that all joint surfaces be tested with a probe in the course of diagnostic arthroscopy.

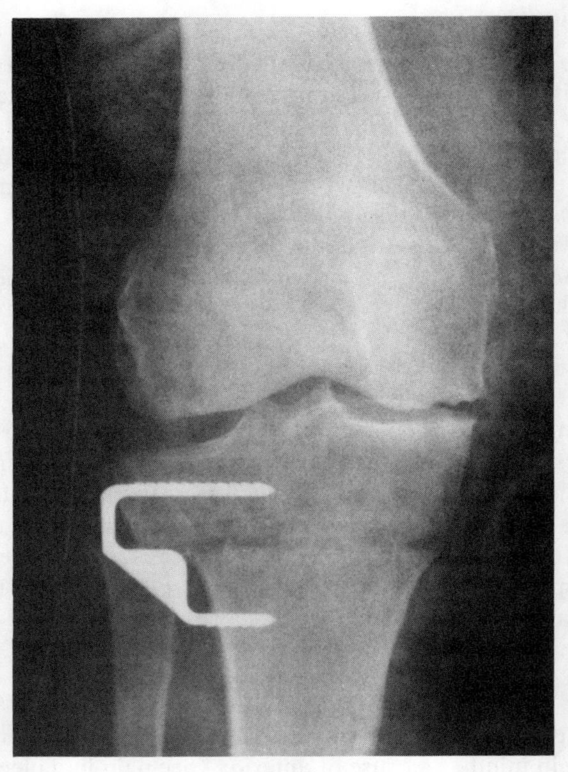

Figure 11-28. High tibial osteotomy for osteoarthritis in an elderly dancer. She remembers having pain in the knee during her years as a professional ballerina.

Osteoarthritis

The question often arises as to whether ballet causes osteoarthritis. Certainly numerous elderly dancers show quite severe osteoarthritic changes in the knees and elsewhere, but osteoarthritis is a common condition in the elderly whether they have danced or not. It is important to have some definitive view on this because it is a question often asked by parents of young students when trying to help them decide whether they should try for a professional career in ballet.

Most ballet students take relatively few classes and give up at a fairly young age in favor of other activities. There should be no significant risk to this group. Dancers who become professional members of a company should also be safe unless there is some predisposing factor such as a strong family history, a previous serious accident, or previous surgery. It would be unwise to persist in dancing on a knee that remained painful over a long period.

I recently performed a high tibial osteotomy on a retired female dancer who had been a member of Pavlova's company during the 1920s and who had had a heavy dancing schedule over a long period (figure 11-28). Her memory of pain in the knee goes back to her dancing days. Possibly if she had stopped dancing she might have avoided the operation. However, she told me that nothing at the time would have stopped her from dancing—a typical attitude of most professional dancers. It is in this dedication to their work that much of the challenge of treating dancers lies.

References

1. Beighton P, Grahame R, Bird H. Hypermobility of joints. Berlin: Springer Verlag, 1983.
2. Dandy DJ. Arthroscopic surgery of the knee. Edinburgh: Churchill Livingstone, 1981.
3. Devas M. Stress fractures. Edinburgh: Churchill Livingstone, 1975; 130-37.
4. Ficat RP, Hungerford DS. Disorders of the patellofemoral joint. Baltimore: Williams and Wilkins, 1977.
5. Hauser EDW. Total tendon transplant for slipping patella. Surg Gynecol Obstet 66:199, 1938.
6. Hughston JC, Walsh WM, Puddu G. Patellar subluxation and dislocation. Philadelphia: WB Saunders, 1984.
7. Kennedy JC. The injured adolescent knee. Baltimore: Williams and Wilkins, 1979.
8. Muller W. The knee. Berlin: Springer Verlag, 1983.
9. Quirk R. Ballet injuries: the Australian experience. Clin Sports Med 2:2. Philadelphia: WB Saunders, Nov 1983; 507-14.
10. Thomasen E. Diseases and injuries of ballet dancers. Denmark: Universitetsforlaget I Arhus, 1979.
11. Trillat A, Dejour H, Puddu G. Recurrent subluxation of the patella. Ital J Orthop 1:209, 1975.
12. Wieberg G. Roentgenographic and anatomic studies on the femoropatellar joint with special reference to chondromalacia patellae acta orthop scand. Acta Orthop Scand 12:319-410, 1941.

12

THE DANCER'S HIP

G. James Sammarco, M.D., F.A.C.S.

ALL VISION IN DANCE concentrates on a pivot between the torso and the lower extremities. High visibility of the hip is important because it is at this joint that the torso and lower extremities can combine to show intent, motion, and purpose without actually moving. Yet when moving, the hips connect the seemingly fixed torso to dynamic action of grace and elegance.

Flexibility is extremely important whether the dance is of a formal, regimented nature or a highly stylized, asymmetric form. Because the hip is the prime connector, essentially dividing the body into equal portions, it is the area upon which the audience concentrates as the dancer moves.

Turn-out

Turn-out is required in all forms of dancing, including modern dance with its asymmetry and very personal choreographic styles; folk dance; jazz, which is based on folk rhythms and traditional dance steps from a particular area or ethnic origin; and variety dance, which includes all of the above elements (figure 12-1).

An important difference in training for dance in Western cultures is first apparent in the beginning dance classes. The female dancer starts training at about the age of 5 years.

Girls are not permitted to dance on their toes (*sur les pointes*) before they have developed balance, coordination, maturity to understand the dance steps, and appropriate strength. Periods of concentration for the young dancer are as much as 1 hr. The young dancer often does not have this concentration ability

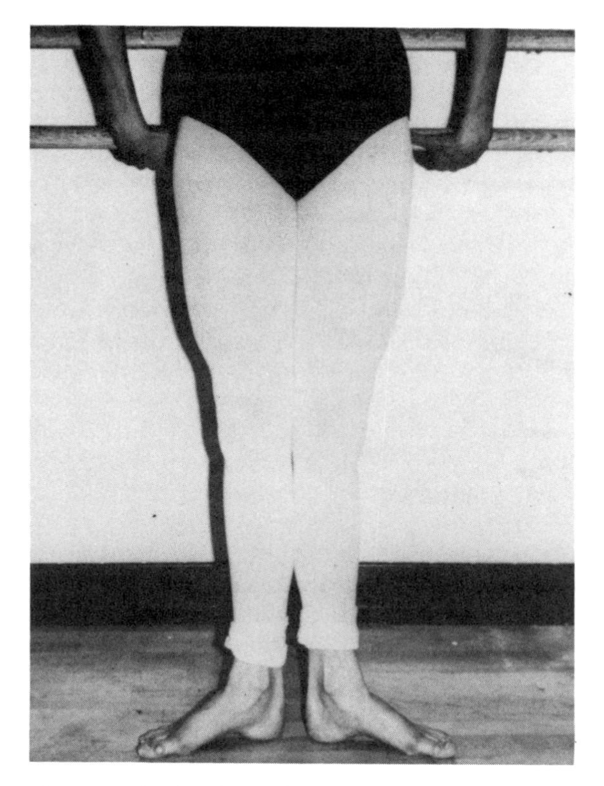

Figure 12-1. Photograph of a dancer's hips and legs in first position demonstrating turn-out. The entire lower extremity is externally rotated from the hip. (From: Sammarco GJ. The foot and ankle in classical ballet and modern dance. In: Jahss MH, ed. Disorders of the foot. Philadelphia: Saunders, 1982; 1626–59.)

before the age of 11. The muscles about the hip have not developed sufficiently, nor is their strength sufficiently developed prior to that time. It takes about 3 years to adequately develop these qualities before going on *pointe*.

Boys, on the other hand, often begin training for dance as a career late in adolescence. By this time, they may have participated in contact sports for several years. When beginning dance, previous trauma to the hip from football or basketball becomes apparent.

Turn-out, which occurs at the hip (figure 12-2), allows the dancer to face the audience while having the leg appear in profile.[14] It is external rotation of the entire lower extremity beginning at the hip, but including the knee and leg. It develops an aesthetic line of the lower extremity so as to imply position, intent, and movement without actually having the extremity move.

If a child has retroverted hips, turn-out is all the easier to achieve, since retroversion permits a child to walk in external rotation. Femoral anteversion might seem less desirable than retroverted hips in a child first learning to dance, but this is not the case. Newborns have hips in a significant amount of

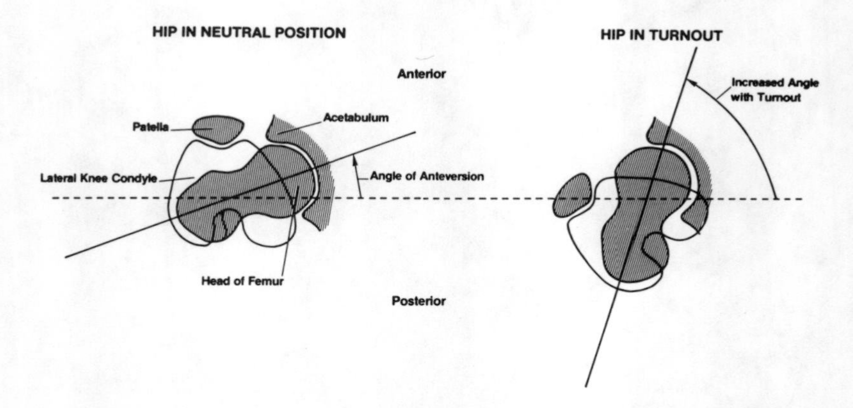

Figure 12-2. Diagram of left hip in transverse section demonstrating that turn-out involves external rotation of the hip without subluxation. The knee is superimposed to show the position of the patella with relation to the acetabulum. The head of the femor remains within the acetabulum. Left—neutral; right—externally rotated. (From: Sammarco, GJ. Clin Sports Med 1983; 2:485.)

anteversion. This anteversion decreases until about the age of 11, when bony changes cease and change of the anteversion angle no longer occurs at the femoral neck.

Children beginning to dance between the ages of 6 and 12 have the benefit of maintaining their turn-out through a stretching process by externally rotating the hips and holding them in that position, as during dance class. After the age of 11, the femoral neck can no longer be altered to the molding process of continual pressure, such as lying on the floor with the hips flexed, abducted, and externally rotated—the so-called "frog position." Subsequent development and maintenance of external rotation must be achieved by stretching the soft tissues about the hip. Although there is some elasticity in the collagen fibers that comprise the capsular structures of the hip, microscopic ruptures of these fibers do occur as the hip capsule matures, and subsequent scarring allows some increase in external rotation during the adolescent and young adult years.

All serious dancers perform a regular routine of warm-up and flexibility prior to dance class and rehearsal.[2] The classical ballet dancer performs a more formalized warm-up and flexibility program, which is then followed by a formal dance class and rehearsals. This routine permits the dancer to maintain the flexibility and full range of motion required to stretch the hip capsule and thus develop the external rotation in a slow, steady manner so that the microinjury is kept to an absolute minimum. Natural flexibility in a dancer is also an advan-

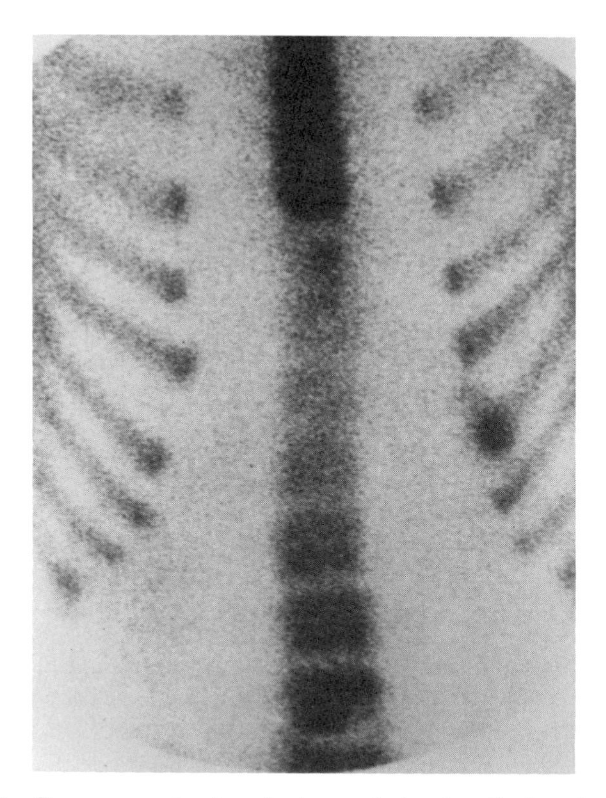

Figure 12-3. Bone scan of a female dancer in her fourth decade. Increased uptake is noted in the lumbar spine in the absence of other disease, reflecting her high activity level. (From: Sammarco GJ. Contemp Orthop 1984; 8:15.)

tage, since dancers with more flexibility tend to have less difficulty in their adult years, even when they have begun dance late in adolescence, as with males (figure 12-3).

Because dance is a fine-art form, the shape of the dancer's hip is as important as its flexibility, and acceptable body type is then a product of the contemporary attitudes of the audience, as well as the artistic license of the director who chooses dancers representing his own aesthetic taste. Thus, the ideal shape for a dancer has changed over the years. Dancers with a minimal amount of fat are preferred. The current standard for a classical female dancer is a small head, long neck, slightly shortened torso, and long, thin legs. Because of this, the percentage of fat to body weight in the female dancer tends to be below the tenth percentile.

Males beginning dance in adolescence must have natural turn-out, either through retroverted hips or flexible joints, or they must achieve this by stretching the soft tissue structures about the hip, including the capsule and muscles.

In the zeal to increase turn-out, the dancer can create problems, both at the hip and elsewhere. If the hips are forced into abduction for several hours a day with the dancer in a single position, stretching at the hip capsule can cause chronic strain resulting in calcification at the acetabular attachment of the capsule. Straining at turn-out and forcing the hips into the externally rotated position causes tension over the medial internal capsular attachment and compression at the superolateral acetabulum. Such chronic minitrauma also contributes to the formation of osteophytes on the femoral neck. Fortunately, problems directly associated with turn-out tend to be minimal; through a regular program of daily training, stretching, and standardized movements, the range of motion of the hip can be kept at its maximum range.

The professional dancer spends up to 6 hr./day dancing, often 6 days a week. Although this level of activity maintains flexibility of the hip, such stress may also lead to overuse syndromes. Degenerative changes that occur in the hip can sometimes limit motion, particularly in the older dancer, and contribute to loss of turn-out.

Male dancers tend to be taller and heavier than their female counterparts. Their leaps are often higher and the forces that develop within the hip are higher. Osteoarthritis can develop, and this, combined with starting to dance at a later date, can be a significant problem in the fourth or fifth decade. Because dance is an art form and total body flexibility is maintained, the charisma that the dancer has developed with considerable skill and talent over the years, as well as a highly motivated, goal-oriented personality, can easily mask a stiff and painful hip joint until arthritis reaches an advanced stage. Some dance careers are cut short by an arthritic condition that might have been slowed or prevented if a proper flexibility program and rehearsal schedule had been followed.

Stiff Hip

In an effort to increase turn-out, the dancer may abuse the hip. Part of auditioning for ballet companies requires the dancer to be viewed by the company director, the so-called "meat show" in which dancers are observed for their body shape and style. Because turn-out is desirable, there is concern by many companies about a lack of this, or "stiff hips." Increasing turn-out in the mature hip by forcing abduction and external rotation can lead to capsular strain with calcium deposition. In addition, forcing external rotation can cause problems in the medical ligaments of the knee and in the medial foot. To force the hip outward, both the leg and the torso must be braced against a hard object. It is, therefore, helpful for a male dancer to have a natural turn-out.

Males and females differ in the development of turn-out. Both use the full range of motion of the hip daily, but because males begin dancing years later than females, their bodies are more mature and their joints tend to be less flexible. In adolescence, the anteversion angle of the femoral neck is fixed in the adult position. To increase turn-out, the male dancer stretches the hip capsule, leading to microtrauma.

The so-called "stiff hips" have a maximum range of motion within the normal limits, but this is less than desirable for dance that uses a range of motion at the upper limits of normal. Tight hips are often found in dancers who have not participated in regular sports activities prior to choosing dance.

Flexibility Program

The dancer's schedule varies, both with the dancer and with the type of dance being pursued. In Western dance, classical ballet has the strictest schedule. In professional dance companies, the schedule often runs 6 days per week. Although the dance day begins with barre exercises and a dance class for warming up and developing flexibility, most dancers perform a flexibility program prior to the barre.[4] Barre exercises are a precise set of exercises performed while holding onto a rail. After the barre exercises and dance class comes a scheduled rehearsal, after which the dancers are excused. However, many dancers go through a "cool-down" stretching routine that avoids the abrupt stoppage of physical activity.

The very style of modern dance, with its barefooted, asymmetrical character and its fall and recovery style, often gives the appearance of a less regimented schedule. Likewise, jazz, tap, variety, and folk dance tend to appear less regimented, lulling dancers into feeling that they are adequately warmed up when, in fact, their joints are stiff. It is important to develop a flexibility program in order to prevent injuries, as well as to concentrate on muscles and joints that have been previously injured or that are in some stage of rehabilitation (table 12-1).

The dancer should do certain stretching exercises related to the trunk, upper back, neck, hips, thighs, knees, legs, and feet. It is important to teach children this concept early in their training. When the young dancer enters a dance style other than a well-structured dance class such as modern or ethnic dance, the highly technical steps required can predispose to injury if warm-up has not been adequate.

Dance is not an endurance sport. Observation during rehearsal and in performance reveals that the dancer dances with great intensity over a short period of time, often 3-4 min., and cardiac output may approach maximum only during that period. These short periods of maximum effort lasting a few minutes are followed by periods in which the dancer performs at a considerably lower activity level.

Overuse Syndrome

Several factors contribute to preventing the development of an overuse syndrome. The dancer must be properly conditioned and have proper nutrition and rest. A regular schedule of stretching and dance class should be followed. The dancer should not advance too rapidly or beyond his or her training and ability level. The right psychological attitude about study is necessary. Proper rest between dance classes is also important because injuries frequently occur toward the end of class and toward the end of the day.

When an overuse syndrome does develop, the search for the cause must include the environment, the type of shoes the dancer wears, and the type of flooring on which dancing is performed. The dance surface is important, since it is the reactive forces through this surface that can be the deciding factor in the development of an overuse syndrome. Hardwood floors with springs beneath seem to offer the best dance surface.[19,20] There is a damping mechanism

Table 12-1. Dance Flexibility Program

Joint/Muscle Group	Objective	Position	Description
Lower back and hp	Flexibility	Standing	Stand with feet 2 ft. apart and hands on hips. Make a circle with the upper torso, keeping hips motionless. Repeat with upper body, still making a figure 8 with hips.
Groin	Stretch	Sitting	Sit on floor with soles of feet in contact with each other. Pull feet toward buttocks while pressing outside of knees to floor. Relax. Repeat. Then, with legs spread apart as far as possible, reach with both hands to grasp right foot while leaning out over right leg. Hold. Relax. Repeat with left leg.
Lateral hip	Flexibility	Sitting	Right Hip: Sit on floor, bend left knee beneath hip. Put right foot on left side of left knee. Turn body to right and pull right knee to chest with left arm. Hold.Relax. Repeat for the left hip.
Hamstring and thigh	Stretch	Standing	With legs straight, try to touch toes with fingertips; then bend knees and put palms on floor. Slowly straighten legs. Hold. Relax. Repeat.
Hamstring	Flexibility	Standing	Cross right foot over and in front of left foot. Bend at waist to touch toes with fingertips, keeping legs straight. Hold. Relax. Repeat. Repeat, crossing left foot in front of and over right foot.
Quadriceps	Stretch	Sitting	Sit on floor with right leg straight ahead and toes pointed upward. Bend left leg and place left foot behind hip. Lean backward and hold. Lean forward, trying to touch toes. Relax. Repeat. Repeat with the other leg.
Quadriceps	Stretch	Standing	Bend left knee and grab ankle with left hand, pulling left foot toward buttocks. Hold. Relax. Repeat. Repeat exercise with right leg.
Calf	Flexibility	Standing	With feet together and facing a wall, lean body at a 45° angle, keeping heels flat on floor and holding stretch. Relax. Repeat.
Soleus and Achilles tendon	Flexibility	Standing	With feet together and facing a wall with heels on floor, lean into the wall, bending knees. Stretching will be felt lower down leg and in Achilles tendon area. Hold.
Ankle	Flexibility	Standing	Rotations: Keep leg straight and make circles with foot moving first clockwise, then counterclockwise. Repeat. Flex and point: Keep leg straight. Bring foot toward face. Hold. Next, point the toes. Hold. Repeat.

NOTE: Stretching movements are slow and smooth and are performed without bouncing. Hold each stretch for 10 sec., relax,and stretch further the next time.

and an elasticity to this type of flooring that provide an optimal cushioning effect, absorbing energy at a proper rate in order to help prevent overuse syndrome.

The dancing surface should not be overly springy, yet it should be resilient enough not to absorb all the energy when the dancer lands from a leap. Synthetic floor coverings are available that are stored in rolls and used mainly by touring dance companies. The covering is laid across the stage and rehearsal hall to provide smooth, consistent friction characteristics, along with some resiliency. If this type of flooring is placed over concrete, however, the slight cushioning effect cannot absorb enough energy to prevent stress fracture.[9] No dance company should be misled into feeling that such a thin floor covering will prevent overuse syndromes.

Stress Fracture

Stress fracture is an incomplete fracture caused by fatigue of bone in areas where high, normal, compressive, and tensile loads occur. In the hip, it occurs most commonly in the neck.[3,14,17,23] It is the result of a normal activity performed for an abnormal number of repetitions over a prolonged period. When this occurs, the normal breakdown of the bone exceeds the rate at which the normal repair of bone occurs. The small microinfractions of bone develop along the femoral neck and begin to progress. The dancer may feel vague pain in the groin. At first, pain is of a nondescript character and is relieved by rest. Pain tends to increase with beginning of class, decrease during class, and increase again after class. The pain stops during layoff periods, only to start again when classes and rehearsals resume.

The fracture begins at the superior lateral aspect of the femoral neck and tends to propagate medially and inferiorly. Physical examination reveals no limitation of motion of the hip, but occasionally groin tenderness is present. As symptoms progress, pain is present at the limits of motion in flexion, abduction, and external rotation in the "heel to knee" test. Adduction and internal rotation—Gaenslen's sign—are positive as well. Standard x-rays fail to show a fracture. If symptoms have been present for many months, a small fracture line may be seen at the superior neck, with characteristic sclerosis surrounding it. A bone scan is necessary, however, to locate the area of increased bone activity (figure 12-4). Computerized axial tomography (CT) scans, although useful in finding stress fractures in other structures, namely the foot and the ankle, are less effective in the hip unless the particular cut of the scan passes directly through the fracture. The differential diagnosis includes early arthritis without evidence of bony changes, chronic synovitis, chronic infection, and tumor.

When treating a stress fracture of the hip, weight bearing by the hip must be decreased dramatically. Performances and rehearsals are curtailed. The patient is prescribed crutches and nonsteroidal anti-inflammatory medication. The water barre, a complete barre exercise program done in a pool, with the dancer submerged to the nipple line, is instituted. The injured part is used as the working leg to perform a particular dance step. The sound leg is used as the leg of support, the leg in contact with the floor. Air-filled wraps ("water wings") are applied to the ankle to provide resistance in the water.

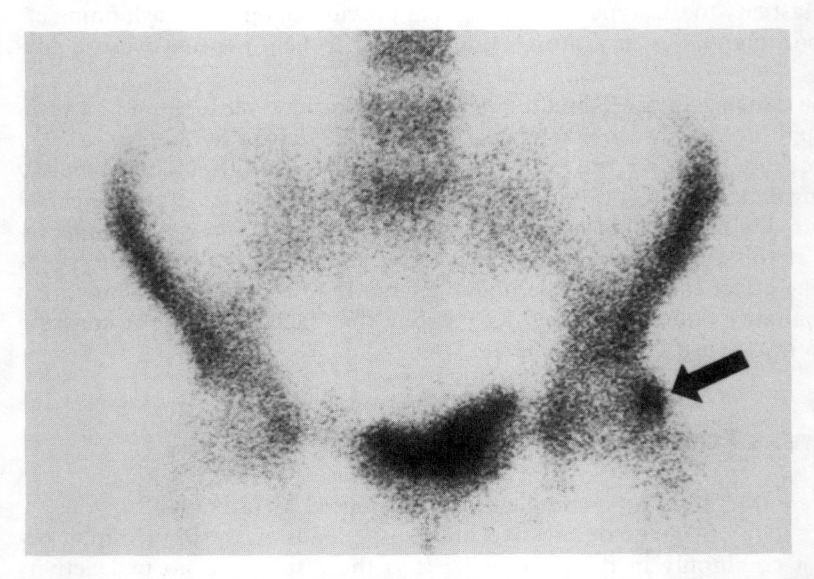

Figure 12-4. Bone scan of a dancer with stress fracture in the left femoral neck. Symptoms were present for 3 months. Routine x-rays were negative. (From: Sammarco GJ. Dance Injuries. In Nicholas JA, Hershman EB, eds. The lower extremity in sports medicine. St. Louis: AJ Mosby, 1986; 1406–39.)

When symptoms subside, a rehabilitation and flexibility program is begun. Nonweight-bearing floor exercises are performed first. A minimum of 2 months of such treatment is necessary before the dancer is able to return to class. It may take considerably longer for the fracture to heal, up to 6 months.

If surgical intervention is necessary, a closed hip pinning through a small lateral incision, with multiple pins into the femoral neck and head, is performed with the aid of an x-ray image intensifier. In the author's experience, it has not been necessary to perform such surgery in the dancer.

Muscle Injury

The employment schedule of a dancer is not always full time. In large companies, a dancer may be employed on a full-time basis, but some companies have seasonal employment only. Many companies employ dancers for a single performance. Because of the inconsistent nature of rehearsals and performances, the dancer is naturally at risk of losing that highly tuned strength and coordination during long periods of layoff. Accordingly, the dancer must be highly disciplined to maintain a flexibility and power-building program during periods when not dancing. Maintained conditioning is important as an injury preventive measure. Dancers have a saying, "If I miss a day of rehearsal, I know it. If I miss 2 days, the director knows it. If I miss 3 days, the audience knows it." In a general sense, there is truth to this.

In addition to an adequate conditioning program, diet is also important. Young dancers are often swayed by fad diets that are nutritionally inadequate, concentrating on a particular vitamin or food. Such a diet leads to mild, chronic, and progressive malnutrition, predisposing muscles to injury and prolonging recovery time. If a dancer is chronically malnourished and poorly conditioned, fatigue occurs earlier in the rehearsal day, thus increasing the risk of injury.

In the high-performance athlete, poor discipline and irregular employment often lead to stiff joints, tight muscles, and loss of muscle mass and strength. Dietary habits may change when the dancer is not in a rehearsal schedule, allowing weight gain. Such layoffs, as well as irregular periods of unscheduled dance activity, contribute to muscle injury. Muscle injury is also caused by a dramatic change in dance technique. When a new step is introduced, a muscle group is suddenly overused and is at risk of fatigue and tearing.

The hip is controlled by four major muscle groups: adductors; extensors, including the hamstrings; abductors; and flexors, including the quadriceps and iliopsoas. Several muscles within each of these groups are diarthrodial or polyarthrodial in nature, passing over two or more joints. This characteristic of muscles about the hip and elsewhere in the body permits the strongest contracting length of the muscle to be shifted as the joint moves so that larger muscle bulk is not required to achieve the same strength necessary to move that joint as it would be if the muscle were fixed across a single joint.

Muscle injury occurs most commonly at its origin. Occasionally, injury occurs in the upper third of the muscle belly, particularly in the adductors, and also at the musculotendinous junction (figure 12-5).[1,13,17,21] Diagnosis includes differentiating such an injury from an apophyseal avulsion from its origin. The immature skeleton of a young dancer makes diagnosis difficult, inasmuch as the ischial apophysis may be absent or unfused. X-rays, therefore, may be of limited usefulness. In 2 weeks, periosteal reaction at the site of bone injury will aid in diagnosis. Still later, myositis ossificans may be visible on x-ray, but does not prevent return to a full dance routine.

On physical examination, tenderness is located over the specific area of the injury. Ecchymosis may often be present, but this is not a constant finding. Swelling and muscle spasm are also signs of acute muscle injury. Rarely will a muscle defect be palpable. If a complete rupture of the muscle has occurred, a palpable, tender soft tissue mass is present. The voluntary contraction of the muscle causes the mass to become firm and move. Pain in an injured region produced by active resistive motion confirms the diagnosis and localizes the muscle group. The most common area involved is the ischial tuberosity. The adductor attachments and the origins of the gracilis and adductor longus from the pubis are also common areas to be injured.[22]

Treatment of muscle injury includes rest for 3 to 5 days, with anti-inflammatory medication and hot packs to the area of tenderness. As pain subsides, a water barre and general flexibility program is begun. Therapy modalities under supervision, including ultrasound, may be instituted. The rehearsal schedule is reduced until a full, painless range of motion has returned. If complete muscle rupture has occurred, and an unaesthetic tender mass is vis-

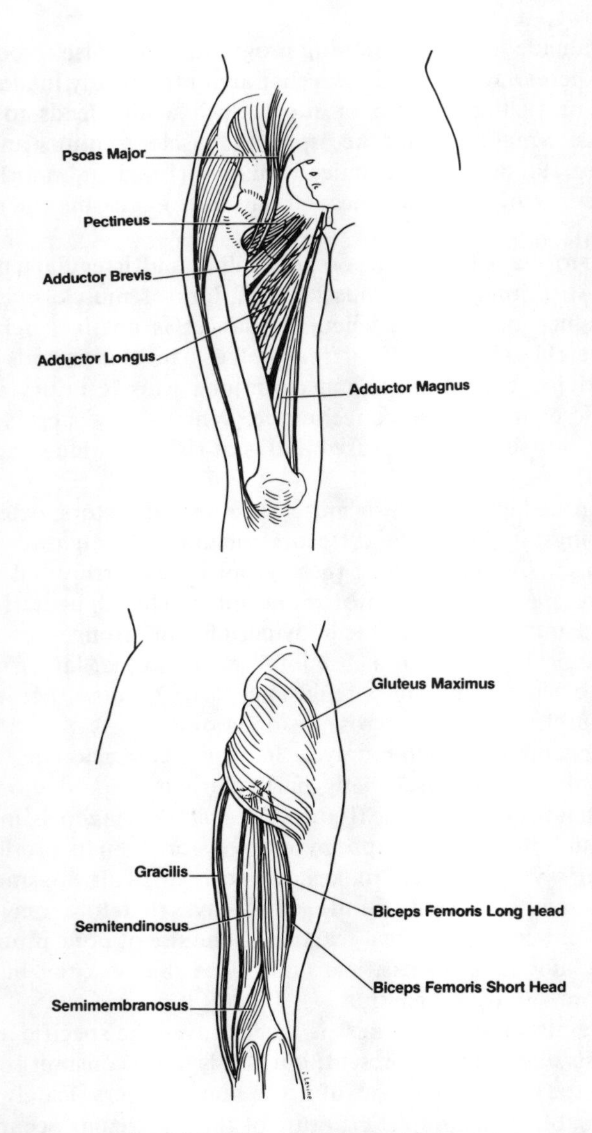

Figure 12-5. Diagram of hip and thigh musculature showing anterior view (top) and posterior view. (From: Sammarco GJ. Clin Sports Med 1983; 2:485.)

ible, complete excision of the muscle belly is indicated. Otherwise, dancing should not be restricted completely, since inactivity is often the cause of acute muscle injury.

Iliacus Tendinitis

The anatomy of the hip is such that the psoas muscle combines in a conjoined tendon with the iliacus muscle as it exits the pelvis, passing over the anterior inferior iliac spine and anterior hip capsule to insert on the anterior and medial portions of the lesser trochanter. The iliacus portion of the muscle passes beneath the inguinal ligament as it courses through the inguinal canal. This is the strongest flexor of the hip; accordingly, as the hip rotates, it changes so that it still maintains the function of flexion even in external and internal rotation.

The muscle and tendon are in close contact with the lateral attachment of the inguinal ligament as the hip is brought into flexion, external rotation, and abduction—the dance step *développé* (figure 12-6). This step, part of the basic barre exercise, is also widely used in classical ballet and in modern and ethnic

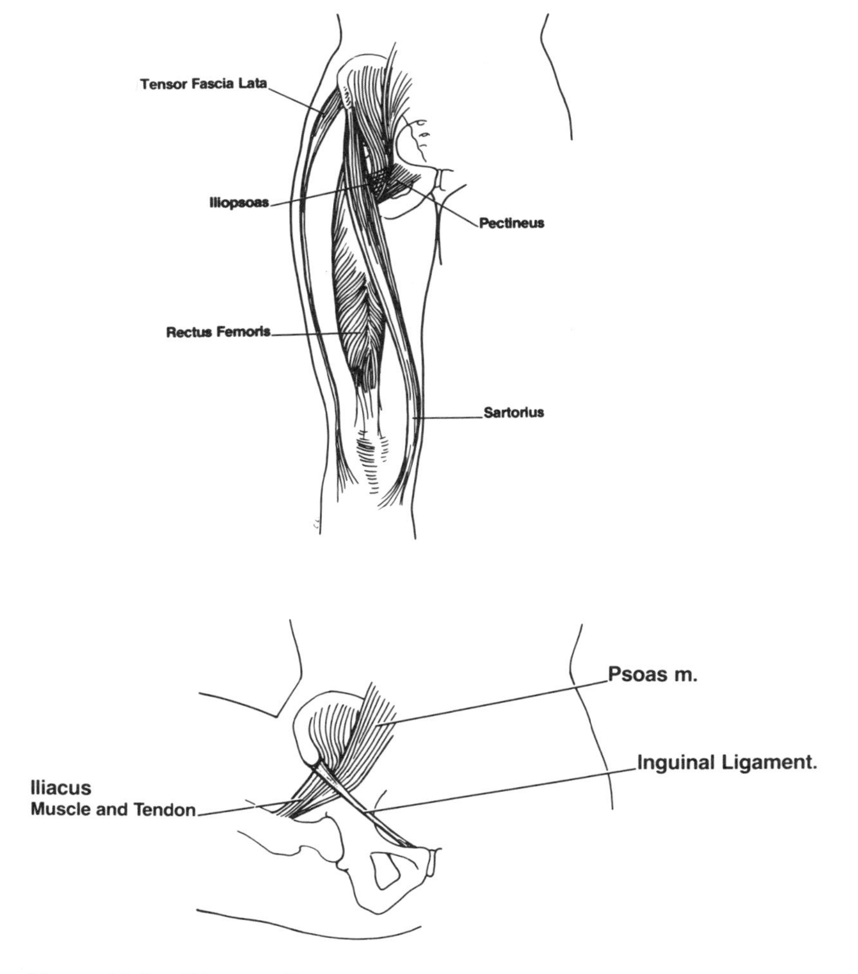

Figure 12-6. Diagram illustrating the position of the iliacus muscle and tendon as it passes beneath the inguinal ligament to combine with the psoas muscle and insert on the lesser trochanter. Shown in first position (top) and during développé, showing "U" in the muscle that gives rise to symptoms.

dance. During this step, the tendon turns in a "U." It is here that irritation of the tendon occurs as it passes beneath the inguinal ligament.[14,17] This disorder is most frequent in females late in their second and early third decades. Crepitus is palpable in the groin, and an audible sound may be noted. Although this sound may be asymptomatic, it is a cause of concern to the dancer. In addition, symptoms of pain can occur in the groin, along with stiffness. Pain is present when beginning barre exercises, after which the pain subsides during dance class and rehearsal, only to be followed by an ache subsequent to these activities. Diagnosis is made by palpating the iliopsoas tendon as it exits the pelvis in the lateral portion of the inguinal canal while the dancer performs a *développé*. Tenderness is noted in the same region. When symptomatic, treatment consists of anti-inflammatory medication, perfecting dance technique (which often is the subtle offender), and prescribing a good flexibility program. Occasionally, an injection of corticosteroid about the tendon sheath may be necessary. This tendon has not been known to rupture in the dancer here or at its insertion on the lesser trochanter; therefore, impending rupture is not of concern.

Myositis

Overuse can also cause a myositis in the muscles about the hip. This characteristically follows periods of layoff. It is usually bilateral and mild, but occasionally is progressive. Crepitus is noted at the start of the class, usually on the medial side of the thigh; this tends to disappear with class activity, only to reappear. Diagnosis is made by palpating the specific muscle group. Treatment includes anti-inflammatory drugs, flexibility and stretching exercises, water barre, and physical therapy modalities such as ultrasound. This problem is seldom totally disabling.

Bursitis

Bursitis is a common and disabling condition. Of the several bursae present about the hip joint, the most common one to be affected is that overlying the greater trochanter (figure 12-7). The patient experiences a painful, grating sensation, and palpation over the greater trochanter may elicit crepitus. The iliotibial band passing over the trochanter causes an irritation that inflames the bursa.[8,15,18] The dancer feels sharp pain with motion over the greater trochanter and slightly posterior to it. The pain is accentuated when landing from a leap. Tenderness can be elicited if the dancer does such barre exercises as *rond de jambe*. X-rays usually show no abnormalities; however, on occasion, calcification can be seen within the bursa. When this is present, treatment includes aspiration of fluid with amorphous calcium from within the bursa, using an 18-gauge needle, and injection of a corticosteriod preparation, i.e., 1 cc of intra-articular betamethasone mixed with 1 cc of 1% lidocaine in the same syringe. A heating pad is helpful prior to warming up before the barre exer-

TROCHANTERIC BURSITIS

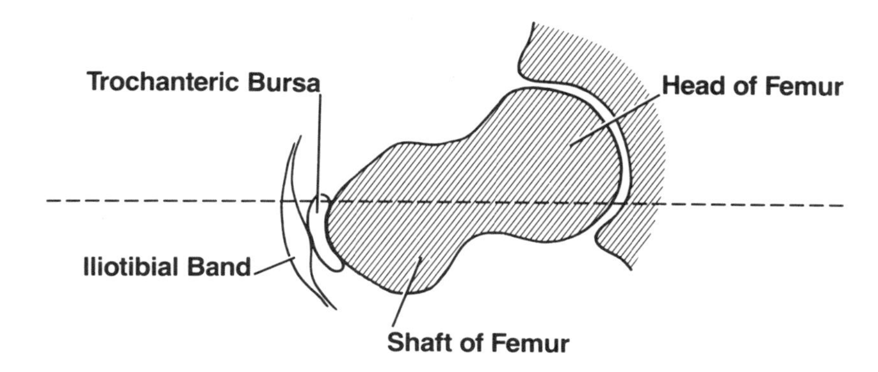

Figure 12-7. Diagram of the left hip in transverse section showing the relationship of the trochanteric bursa to the iliotibial band and greater trochanter. (From: Sammarco GJ. The hip in dancers. In: Medical problems of performing artists, vol. 2. Philadelphia: Hanley and Belfus, 1987.)

cises. Perfecting dance technique and strengthening abductors and extensors of the hip are also of benefit.

Occasionally, persistent symptoms and lack of absorption of calcium by the body may necessitate surgical excision. A small lateral incision is made directly over the painful bursa. The iliotibial band is split in the direction of its fibers, and the bursa is excised sharply, including its attachment to bone. Hemostasis is achieved with electrocautery. Meticulous closure of the iliotibial band and subcuticular closure of the skin are necessary. Rehabilitation is begun when the dancer is able to tolerate weight bearing (about 10 days).

Bursitis of the anterior hip capsule occurs when the bursa lying between the capsule and iliopsoas tendon becomes inflamed. Groin pain is characteristic of this condition, but crepitus is generally not palpable. Symptoms may be persistent and chronic, being present for several weeks or months. Pain occurs when motion begins, decreases during class, and returns toward the end of the day as the dancer rests. Treatment of this condition includes general stretching exercises, use of anti-inflammatory medication, use of the water barre, and refinement of dance technique. Occasionally, injection of a corticosteroid preparation with lidocaine may be beneficial (figure 12-8). This author has not found it necessary to perform surgery for anterior hip bursitis.

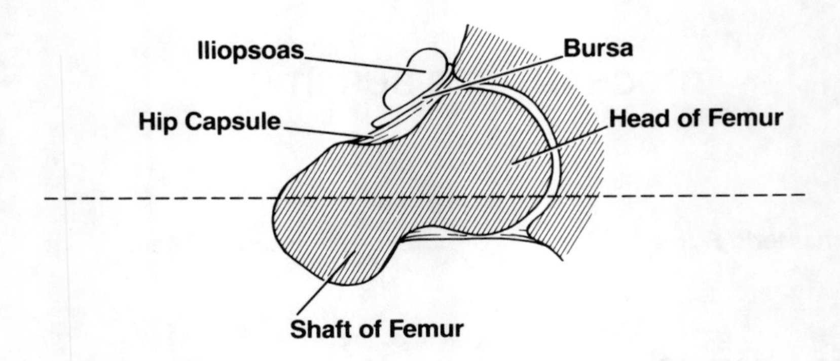

ANTERIOR HIP BURSITIS

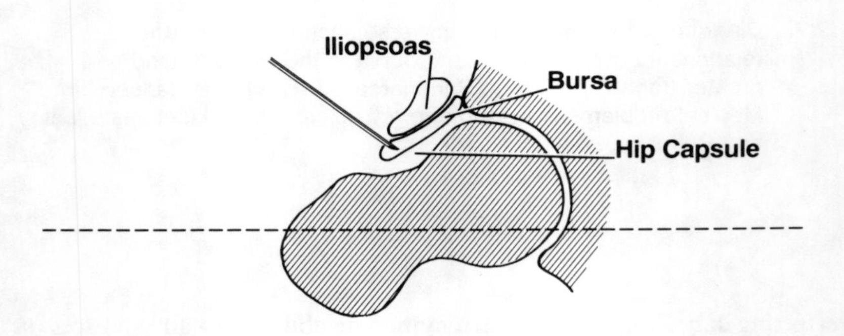

Figure 12-8. Diagram of the left hip in transverse section showing (top) the relationship of the bursa to the hip capsule and iliopsoas tendon. Treatment may include injection of corticosteroid into the bursa (bottom). (Source: same as figure 12-7.)

Clicks and Snaps

Anterior Click

The anterior hip click is caused when the iliopsoas tendon passes across the anterior hip capsule as the hip moves. When the hip is brought from flexion abduction and external rotation to the ballet first position, a characteristic click is felt and occasionally heard.[6,10,12,14] The noise itself is of no consequence; asymptomatic noises in joints of the body are considered normal phenomena. The strong flexors of the hip and the relatively thick anterior hip capsule are tented up by the externally rotated femur as the femoral head is rotated anteriorly. The insertion of the iliopsoas is moved laterally, allowing the tendon to

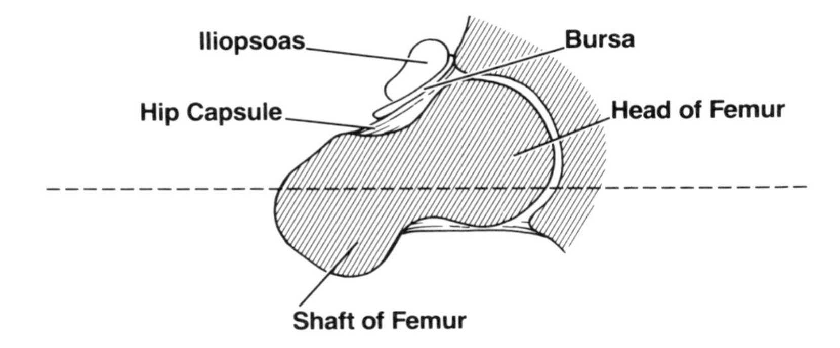

EXTERNAL ROTATION OF HIP

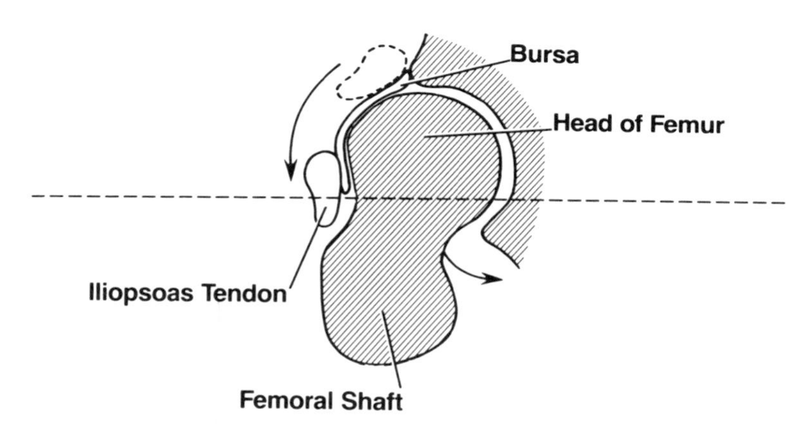

Figure 12-9. Diagram of the left hip in transverse section showing (top) the relationship of the iliopsoas tendon to the anterior hip capsule. When externally rotating and flexing the hip, the tendon rides over head of femur causing a click (bottom). This also occurs when the hip is brought back to neutral. (Source: same as figure 12-7.)

slip laterally over the anterior hip capsule (figure 12-9). As the hip is brought back to neutral, the tendon rides back over the capsule, causing a click. The anterior hip click is palpable in the groin at the capsule and may occur both in flexion and extension; it commonly occurs in young dancers, but is rarely disabling.

Examining the hip may be done with the dancer supine or standing. The groin is palpated as the hip is flexed, abducted, externally rotated and then brought back into the neutral position with the leg slightly internally rotated again until neutral position is reached. When symptomatic, treatment includes a dancer's flexibility program, anti-inflammatory medication, use of the water

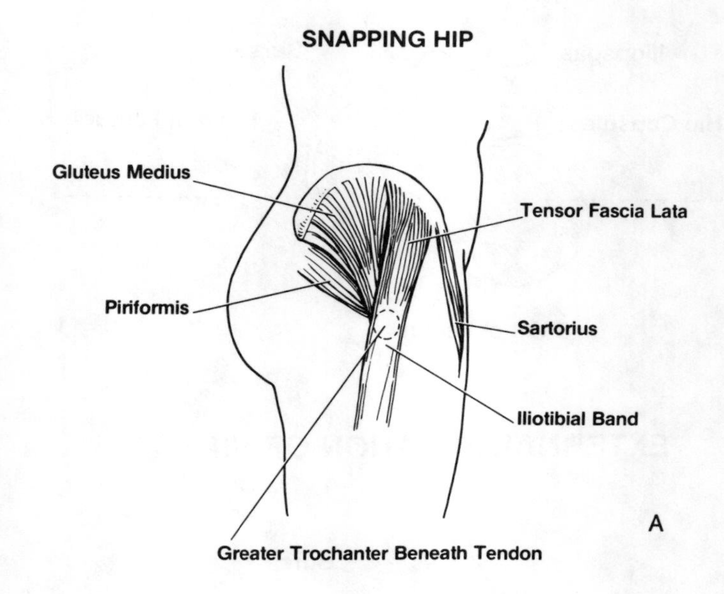

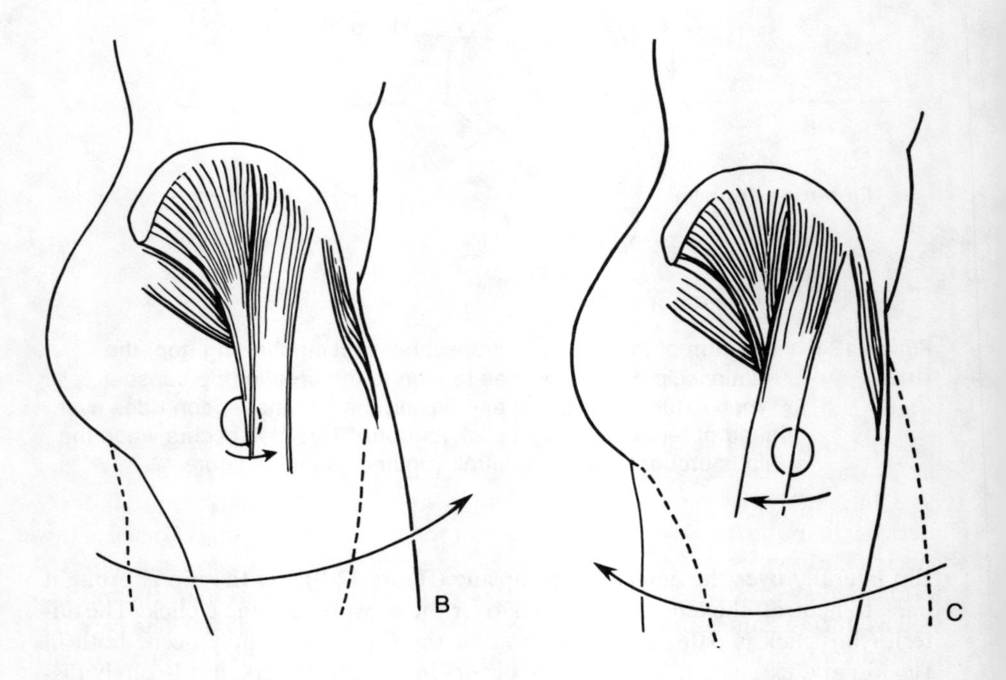

Figure 12-10-A, 12-10-B, 12-10-C. Diagram of the right hip showing the relationship of the tensor fascia lata and iliotibial band to the greater trochanter. A—lateral view; B—The tendon snaps forward as the dancer flexes the hip when landing from a leap; C—The tendon snaps backward as the dancer recovers and extends the hip. (Source: same as figure 12-7.)

barre, and perfecting dance technique. Occasionally, injection of corticosteroid preparation deep into the bursa and reducing the dance schedule are necessary. Surgery has not been necessary.

Snapping Hip

Snapping hip occurs laterally as the iliotibial band passes rapidly across the greater trochanter. This may be caused by inadequate conditioning of the dancer, particularly in the abductor muscles. As the dancer lands from a leap, the load rapidly increases across the hip joint. As the tensor fascia femoris muscle contracts, its tendon, situated posterior to the greater trochanter, snaps forward, jerking the pelvis into flexion (figure 12-10-A, 12-10-B, 12-10-C).[18] This sudden movement, which is unaesthetic in appearance,[7,16] is usually present unilaterally. The dancer feels the sensation of the hip "going out of place." A palpable snap is present, and occasionally it is audible. Diagnosis is made by palpating over the greater trochanter as the dancer performs a *rond de jambe* or *grand plié*. X-rays of the hip show no abnormality. Treatment includes the development of the abductor and extensor muscle groups, a good flexibility program, water barre, and anti-inflammatory medication. Symptoms may be persistent and annoying.

Occasionally, surgical intervention may be required.[24] A small incision, 2 cm long, is made over the lateral trochanter under local anesthetic. Tissue dissection is developed down to the tight iliotibial band. A small transverse incision is made with a no. 11 blade through the area of the band that is snapping, and the wound is closed with subcutaneous 3–0 absorbable suture and 4–0 subcuticular absorbable suture. A flexibility program is initiated as soon as the dancer is able to tolerate motion, and a power-building program is resumed.

Posterior Hip Syndrome

A dancer may occasionally develop pain over the posterior hip capsule. Although it is localized to the buttocks overlying the capsule itself, its specific origin is difficult to determine. Symptoms may develop in the dancer's second decade. The high flexibility of dancers predisposes them to stretching of the hip capsule. Many young dancers also participate in gymnastics and cheerleading. Such activities may include such maneuvers as the "split," which traumatizes the posterior hip. In addition, "straddle" injuries from gymnastics or specialty dances using large props may cause capsular injuries, resulting in posterior pain as a residual.[5] Pain can be elicited on external rotation of the hip as well as during dance steps requiring hyperextension and *grand plié*. The pain is nonradicular in character. The piriformis muscle exits through the sciatic notch from the pelvis to insert at the superolateral base of the femoral neck (figure 12-11). This short tendon is closely aligned with adjacent muscles, and it is unlikely that a tendinitis solely of this tendon is the cause of pain. Chronic strain of all the external rotators may contribute to symptoms. Moreover, the sciatic nerve has a variable relationship with the piriformis muscle as it leaves the sciatic notch from the pelvis; with hypertrophy of that muscle, the nerve may be entrapped by the muscle belly.

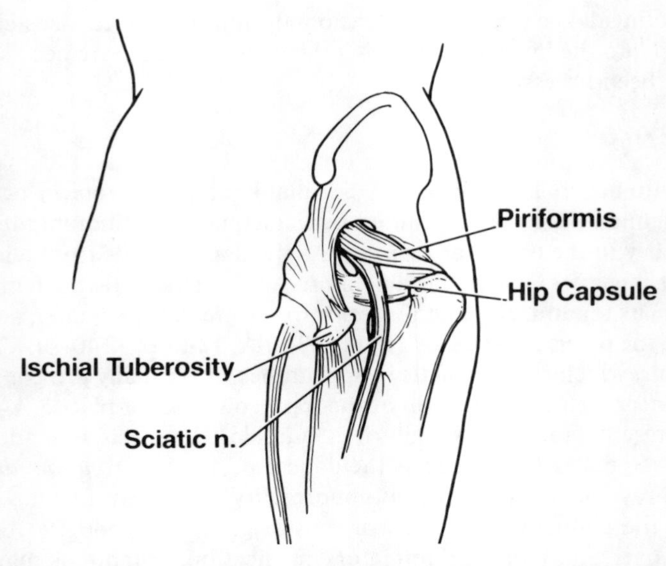

Figure 12-11. Diagram of significant structures in the region of the posterior hip. (Source: same as figure 12-7.)

Physical examination reveals tenderness specifically over the posterior hip capsule, away from the insertion of the gluteus maximus and hip abductors. There is no Tinel's sign present over the sciatic nerve. Rectal examination usually fails to elicit tenderness over the muscle belly of the piriformis within the pelvis. If the rectal examination is negative, the piriformis is not the causative factor. Symptoms are often vague and chronic, and are occasionally disabling. A bone scan is indicated to determine whether a synovitis or a stress fracture is present. Treatment includes the water barre, perfecting dance technique, a program of dance instruction for flexibility, anti-inflammatory medication, physical therapy modalities, including ultrasound, and hot packs prior to rehearsal. This condition may be disabling, and as with chronic synovitis elsewhere, can even terminate a dancer's career. The dancer should be advised of the prolonged nature of the symptoms and that patience is required to "work through" the problem.

Neurological Conditions

Sciatica

Trauma to the sciatic nerve can occur if the dancer performs dance steps or gymnastics that permit trauma directly to the nerve as it lies adjacent to the hip.[14] Pain may be of a radicular nature, and paresthesias may occur in the leg. There are anatomic variations in the path of the sciatic nerve as it exits from the sacral plexus. The nerve may be divided as it exits the pelvis, with portions of the piriformis muscle passing between its tibial and peroneal divisions. In addition to repeated trauma, applying direct pressure to the nerve for prolonged periods in unusual postures can cause symptoms. Physical examination may reveal a positive Tinel's sign over the area of entrapment or trauma.

A differential diagnosis includes either tendinitis at the gluteus maximus insertion, posterior hip syndrome, sacral plexopathy, or herniated disk syndrome. An electromyelogram is helpful in differentiating these entities. Deep palpation at the ischial tuberosity will differentiate pain at the origin of the hamstrings. Treatment includes slow, gentle stretching exercises; anti-inflammatory medication; avoiding contact of the nerve with hard surfaces as performed during special dance steps or gymnastic maneuvers such as the "split"; perfecting technique; and the water barre.

Femoral Neuritis

Pain in the anterior thigh can result from unusual posturing during certain dance steps. This uncommon traction injury often occurs in inexperienced dancers when they perform dance steps with hyperextension of the hips and lumbar spine associated with acute hyperflexion of the knees.[11] Weakness develops in the thigh muscles over a period of weeks. A dancer who is not properly warmed up or who has not achieved the appropriate flexibility to perform such steps can also develop associated hip pain. A positive Tinel's sign may be present as the femoral nerve exits the inguinal canal. Weakness of the quadriceps muscles can also occur. Differential diagnosis includes meralgia paresthetica and other anterior hip syndromes. An electromyelogram is a helpful diagnostic aid. Treatment includes anti-inflammatory medication and, until symptoms subside, avoiding dance steps and those postures that put traction on the femoral nerve. Improving flexibility and close adherence to a dance routine schedule are of benefit in preventing recurrence. Although symptoms may be present for several months, permanent injury has not been reported.

Referred Pain to the Hip

Several organ systems present symptoms that refer pain to the hip. Pain referred to the hip can originate in the right or left lower abdominal quadrants, groin, medial thigh, hamstring origins, testes, labia, and flanks. The dancer may complain of pain and discomfort, generally located in the hip region but without localizing signs. The menstrual cycle in female dancers is often altered due to low body weight and physical stress. Conditions such as premenstrual syndrome may also manifest themselves with symptoms referable to the hip. Disease of the genitourinary system is one of the most common systems referring pain to the groin and medial thigh area. Kidney stones and ureteral stones occur, even in dancers in their second decade. Symptoms of excruciating pain and cramping may vary considerably from the lower abdominal quadrant to the medial thigh. Findings in examination of the hip are completely within normal limits. Referred pain to the groin and medial thigh prompts diagnostic studies such as an x-ray, CBC, and urinalysis. A standard K.U.B. examination often reveals a characteristic radiopaque stone, and urinalysis shows hematuria

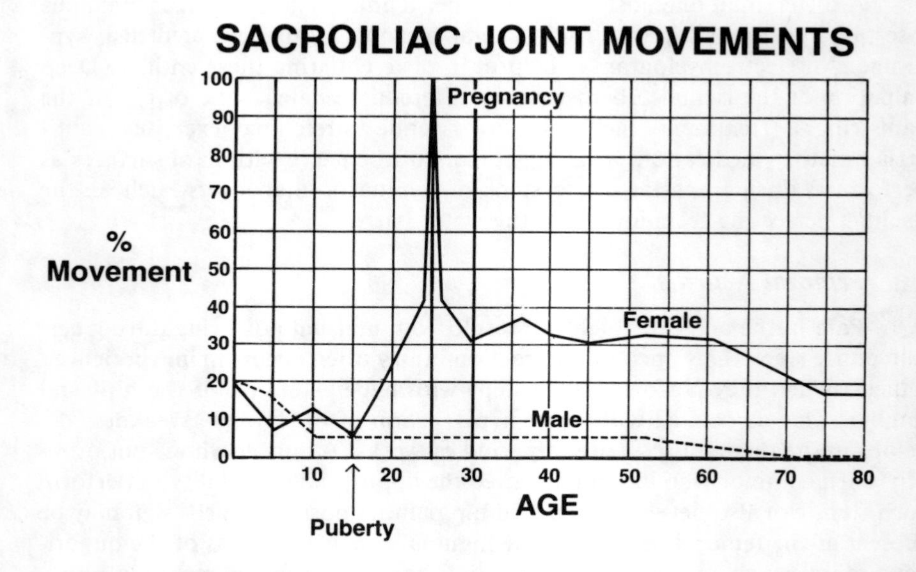

Figure 12-12. Diagram illustrating that little motion is achieved at the sacroiliac joints except in the last trimester of pregnancy. (From: Brooke, R.: J. Anat. 58:299, 1924.)

with an elevated WBC. The pain occurs either in the left or right lower abdominal quadrant.

Cystitis commonly occurs in young adolescent and juvenile females. Symptoms of groin pain associated with suprapubic pain, urinary frequency, dysuria, and nocturia are common. The medical history and urinalysis, however, will confirm the diagnosis. Appropriate antibiotics, as well as counseling the young dancer not to take prolonged tub baths, are indicated.

In males, urethritis is less commonly referred to the hip, but kidney disease, including pyelonephritis, can refer pain to that region. In the male, inflammation of the urethra and prostate, abscess formation, orchitis, epididymitis, and abscess of the iliopsoas tendon must be considered as part of the differential diagnosis. Gastrointestinal conditions (such as appendicitis) and those of the colorectal region include proctitis, cryptitis, perirectal abscess, and symptomatic hemorrhoids. Because multiple muscle origins and insertions occur about the hip, abscess or tumor in any one of these regions must be considered.

Additional gynecologic problems of the female often include delayed menarche. The reasons for this include low body-fat-to-weight ratio and the increased performance level of a young female athlete, often on a poor diet. Occasional pain in the right or left lower quadrant may be misinterpreted as hip disease. Ovarian cysts and endometriosis can have similar symptoms. If the hip examination findings are within normal limits, consideration should be given to the above conditions. If indicated, pelvic examination should be performed. In the young female, rectal examination is substituted. If the findings are normal, the dancer should be given an appropriate diet that includes a vitamin supplement and counseling against fad diets. The dancer should also be informed that the dance life-style often leads to menstrual abnormalities.

Symptoms of herniated disk may be referred to the posterior hip. Because of the highly motivated, goal-oriented artistic personality of the dancer, pain may be of less importance; accordingly, symptoms referable to the hip may draw attention to atrophy of the calf muscles, pain being of secondary importance. Physical examination, of course, will reveal depressed reflexes in the tendo Achilles region and sensory abnormalities in the lower extremity. However, positive straight-leg raising and Lasègue's sign may not be present. CT scan and magnetic resonance imaging both are helpful when confirming a diagnosis of herniated disk disease.

Inflammation of the sacroiliac joint, including early symptoms of ankylosing spondylitis or rheumatoid arthritis, can often be misrepresented as hip disease, along with infection and osteoarthritis of the sacroiliac joint.

Flexibility of sacroiliac joints is quite limited in both male and female dancers. In the female dancer, it is increased only in the last trimester of pregnancy (figure 12-12). However, such are the stresses about the dancer's hips and pelvis that osteophytes form as early as the second decade. The pain is usually posterior, located over the joint, and characteristically is mistaken for hip pain. X-ray of the pelvis and views of the sacroiliac joint often reveal osteophyte formation at the inferior limit of the joint. Treatment for this condition is symptomatic.

References

1. Backhouse KM. Medicine and ballet. Trans Med Soc Lond. 1980–81; 97:51–53.
2. Como W. Raoul Gelabert's anatomy for the dancer with exercises to improve technique and prevent injuries. New York: Danad, 1964; 51–57.
3. D'Ambrosia R, Drez D Jr, eds. Prevention and treatment of running injuries. Thorofare, NJ: Charles B. Slack, 1982.
4. Flexibility program for the dancer. Cincinnati: Clin for Performing Arts, 1986.
5. Garrick JG, Requa RK. Epidemiology of women's gymnastics injuries. Am J Sports Med 1980; 8:261–64.
6. Howse AJ. Orthopaedists aid ballet. Clin Orthop Rel Res. 1972; 89:52-63.
7. Jacobs M. Snapping hip phenomenon among dancers. Am Corr Ther J 1978; 32:92–98.
8. Krout RM, Anderson TP. Trochanteric bursitis: management. Arch Phys Rehabil. 1959; 40:8–14.
9. Laws K. Physics and the potential for dance injury. Med Probl of Performing Artists. 1986; 1:73–79.
10. Lyons JC, Peterson LFA .The snapping iliopsoas tendon. Mayo Clin Proc. 1984; 59:327–329.
11. Miller EH, Benedict FE. Stretch of a femoral nerve in a dancer: a case report. J Bone Joint Surg. 1985; 67:315–317.
12. Quirk R. Ballet injuries: the Australian experience. Clin Sports Med. 1983; 2:507–514.

13. Rovere GD et al. Musculoskeletal injuries in theatrical dance students. Am J Sports Med. 1983; 11:195–198.
14. Sammarco GJ. The dancer's hip. Clin Sports Med 1983; 2:485–98.
15. Sammarco GJ. Diagnosis and treatment in dancers. Clin Orthop Rel Res. 1984; 187:176–187.
16. Sammarco GJ. Treating dancers. Contemp Orthop. 1984; 8:15.
17. Sammarco GJ. Dance injuries. In: Nicholas JA, Hershman EB, eds. The lower extremity in sports medicine. St. Louis: CV Mosby, 1986; 1406–39.
18. Sammarco GJ. The hip in dancers. In: Medical Problems of Performing Artists, vol 2., no. 1, 5-14. Philadelphia: Hanley and Belfus, 1987.
19. Seals J. A study of dance surfaces. Clin Sports Med. 1983; 2:557–61.
20. Seals J. Dance floors. Med Probl Performing Artists. 1986; 1:81–84.
21. Stojanovie S, Marenie D, Ikropina D. Diseases in ballet dancers. Srp Arch Celok Lek. 1963; 91:903.
22. Thomasen E. Diseases and injuries of ballet dancers. Arhus, Denmark: Universitetsforlaget i. Arhus, 1982.
23. Tountas AA, Waddell JB. Stress fractures of the femoral neck: a report of seven cases. Clin Orthop Rel Res. 1986; 210:160–165.
24. Zoltan DJ et al. A new operative approach to snapping hip and refractory trochanteric bursitis in athletes. Am J Sports Med. 1986; 14:201–204.

13

INJURIES TO THE DANCER'S SPINE

Richard M. Bachrach, D.O.

THE VAST MAJORITY OF injuries incurred by dancers, like those sustained by athletes in noncontact sports and participants in fitness programs, are primarily microtraumatic in origin. Solomon and Micheli, in a study of modern dancers in the Boston area, concluded that preponderance to be about 2 to 1.[1] The causes for these cumulative microtraumata are clear. As long as the body is able to compensate or adjust, the result of overload will be adaptation and increased strength and/or flexibility. It is the breakdown of the adaptive mechanism that results in stress-related injury, and this breakdown may be facilitated by a series of factors that, working together or alone, create an atmosphere conducive to injury. These include: technique inappropriate to the dancer's body, overuse on nonresilient floors, cold studios, overly demanding choreography, abrupt changes in style, and duration or intensity of dance activity. These problems may not be under the control of the dancer.

By far the greatest source of overload, however, is inappropriate biomechanical usage or defective technique, most of which is attributable to maladaptive alignment. This is particularly applicable to injuries to the dancer's back and neck. Factors causing maladaptive alignment may be physiologic or anatomic, such as leg length inequality, foot pronation, discrepancies and/or deficiencies in degree of external rotation at the hip, etc., but most are due to muscular imbalances involving hip flexors, erector spinae, abdominals, hip rotators, gluteals, and hamstrings. Whatever the cause, maladaptive alignment is not beyond the dancer's control. The difficulty is in recognition and acknowledgment, then finding the appropriate source of help.

In this respect, it is important to note that most dancers coexist with constant low-level back pain, something they accept as "coming with the territory." It is my contention, however, that this pain often has more profound significance. In many cases, it is the result of malalignment caused by musculotendinous imbalances or may signal more obvious and perhaps more emergent conditions involving the lower extremities. This concept will be explored later.

Most dance-related injuries involve the foot, ankle, or knee. In addition to being microtraumatic, these injuries are profoundly interrelated not only to one another but, more often than not, to dysfunction of the lower back.

The most common site of spinal or paraspinal injury in dancers is the lower back, and the muscles of the lower back are the most commonly injured muscle group. Indeed, symptoms referable to the cervical and thoracic spine usually have their ultimate source in derangements or dysfunctions of the lower back. This applies to all forms of dance and to both men and women, young or old.

Anatomy of the Lower Back

Consideration of the osseous structures must, of course, begin with the five lumbar vertebrae, but because of the complex musculotendinous connections related to the biomechanics of the lower back, we must also include the twelfth thoracic vertebra; the last ribs; the pelvis, including the fused ilium, ischium and pubis; the sacrum and coccyx; and the proximal femorae (figure 13-1).

These vertebrae are connected to one another above and below posteriorly by the apophyseal joints, which arise from the articular processes. Anteriorly, they are connected by the intervertebral disks. The spinal nerves exit the spinal canal between the vertebrae through the foramina formed by the junction of the articular processes, the bodies of the vertebrae, and the intervening intervertebral disks (figure 13-2).

These intervertebral disks are hard, fibrocartilaginous rings surrounding a soft, jellylike center. They facilitate movement between vertebral segments and serve as shock absorbers. The result of acute or chronic disturbance in their functioning is disruption of normal intervertebral biomechanics; this affects all segments, particularly the apophyseal joints. These are true arthrodial joints, and like the ankle and the knee, have the same essential makeup, i.e., articular cartilage, synovial membrane, and joint capsule. Of those structures, only the joint capsule has nerve endings (nociceptors) sensitive to painful stimuli.

The vertebrae are further connected throughout the length of the spinal column by ligaments: the ligamentum flavum, the intertransverse ligaments, the interspinous and supraspinous ligaments, and the anterior longitudinal and posterior longitudinal ligaments. These are presented in ascending order of sensitivity to painful stimuli; there are virtually no nociceptors in the ligamentum flavum, but the posterior longitudinal ligament is replete with them. Nociceptors are also present in the cancellous bone of the spinous processes and the articular facets, as well as in the intramuscular perivascular tissues and in the thoracolumbar fascia (figure 13-3).

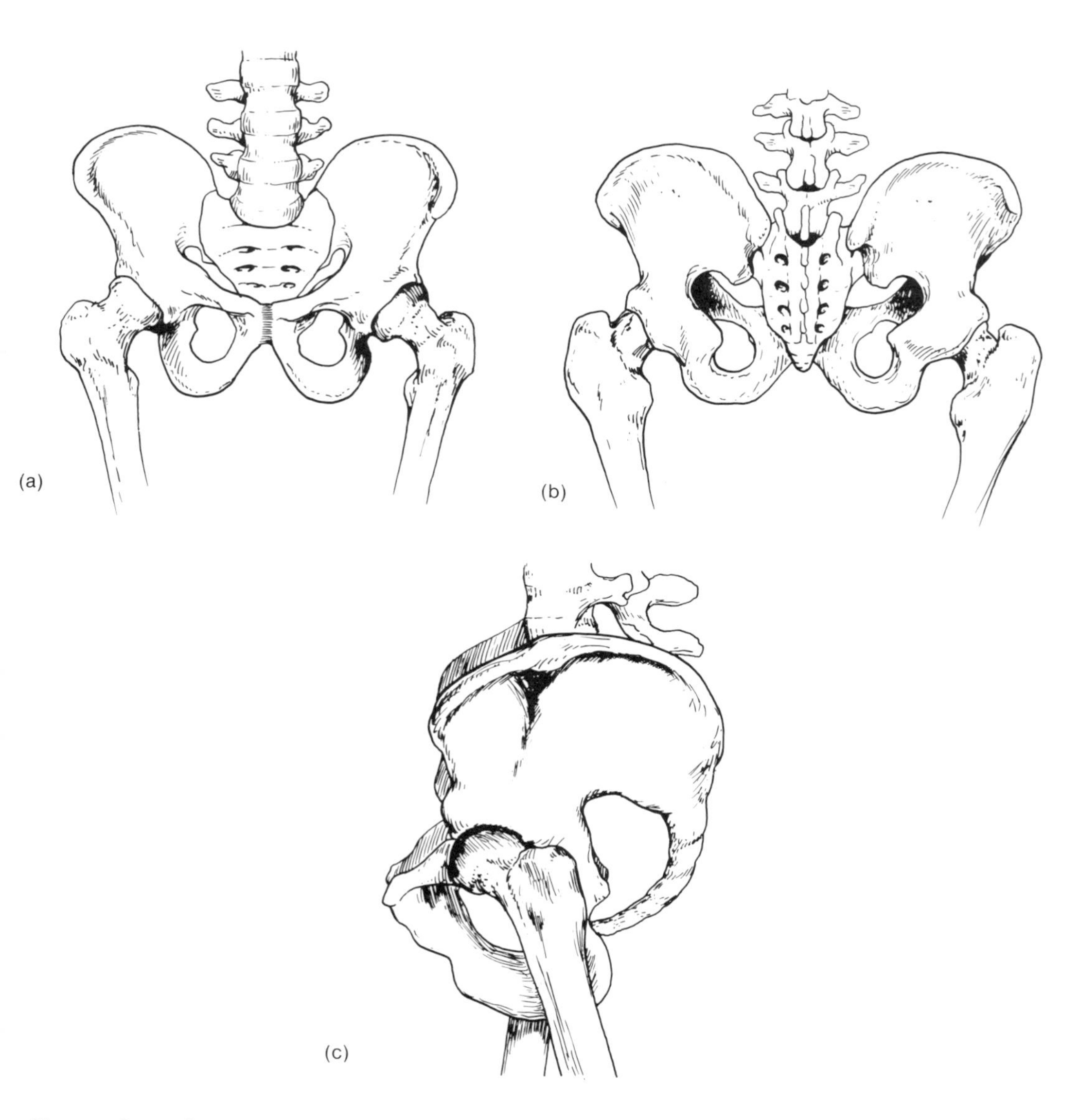

Figure 13-1. Anterior (A), posterior (B), and lateral (C) views of the skeleton showing the lower lumbar spine, pelvis and proximal femurs.

Viewed from the side, the normal lumbar spine exhibits a curve, concave posteriorly (figure 13-4). This lordosis is a response of the developing body to weight bearing. It is associated with a similar curve in the cervical region, and one in the opposite direction (kyphosis) in the thoracic region. Maintenance of the normal lordosis in both the lumbar and cervical spine is essential to the maintenance of flexibility and strength of the vertebral column. The admonition to keep the back flat, attributed to dance teachers and physical education instructors in the past, runs counter to good vertebral biomechanics. The "flat

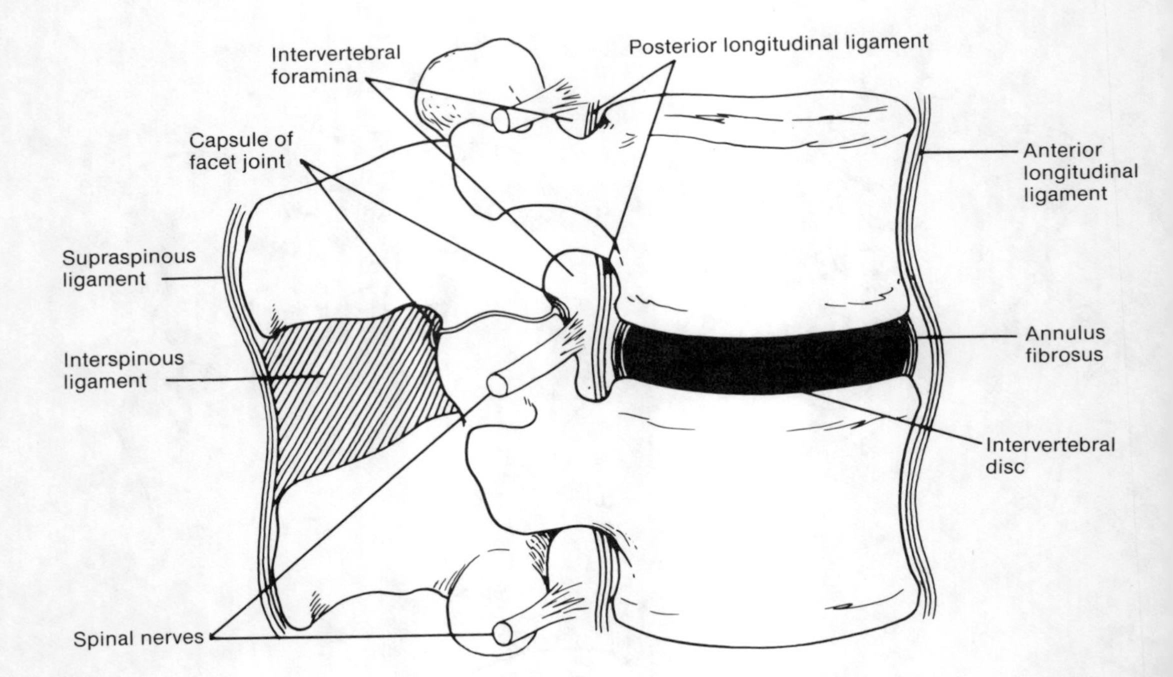

Figure 13-2. Lateral aspect of two adjacent lumbar vertebrae showing the anterior and posterior articulations, the intervertebral disk, the intervertebral foramina, and the spinal nerves.

back" as well as the hyperlordotic back predisposes to injury and early development of spinal osteoarthritis.

In the erect position, the major possible movements in the lumbar area (most of which occur between the fifth lumbar vertebra and the sacrum) are flexion (forward bending), which results in a decreased lumbar lordosis, and extension (backward bending), which increases it.

The range of extension exceeds that of flexion because of the relative tautness of the posterior longitudinal ligament, which narrows as it descends to terminate at the sacrum, thereby allowing for some increase in forward flexibility of the spine in the lower lumbar area. The narrowing, however, weakens the posterior lateral support of the intervertebral disks, predisposing this area to disk protrusion or herniation, particularly between the fourth and fifth lumbar vertebrae and between the fifth lumbar and the sacrum.

Multiplanar movements, however slight, occur at both the pubic and sacroiliac joints. Maintenance of that motion is essential to the functional integrity of the lower back and pelvis. Dysfunction of either sacroiliac articulation, produced by muscular imbalances, is a major source of lower back pain in dancers.

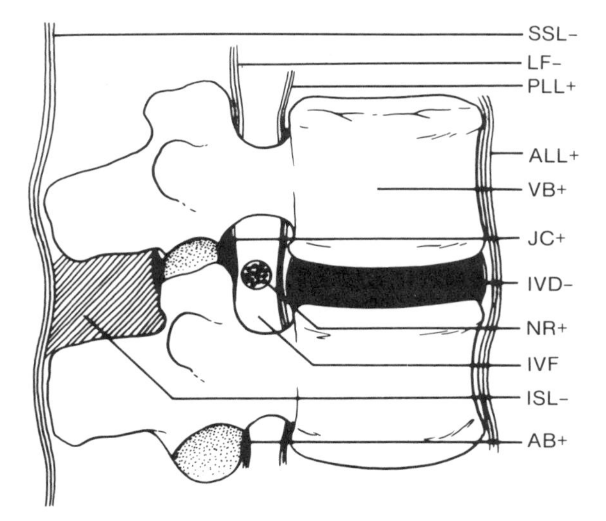

Figure 13-3. Two adjacent lumbar vertebrae showing pain-sensitive tissues of the functional unit. The tissues labeled + are pain sensitive in that they contain nerve endings that evoke pain when stimulated. Tissues labeled – have little or no nociceptive receptors.
IVF = Intervertebral foramina
NR = Nerve root
LF = Ligamentrum flavum
PLL = Posterior longitudinal ligament
ALL = Anterior longitudinal ligament
IVD = Intervertebral disk with annulus librous
ISL = Intraspinous ligament
SSL = Supraspinous ligament
JC = Joint capsule
AB = Articular process cancellous bone
VB = Vertebral body cancellous bone

Musculature of Spinal Movement

The musculature responsible for movement of the back is divided into three groups—intrinsic, extrinsic, and superficial. The intrinsic (or paraspinal) group, the erector spinae, is situated on the dorsal surface of the vertebral column (figure 13-5). It maintains erect posture by straightening or extending the spine, and when acting unilaterally, assists in bending the spine to the side of contraction. The erector spinae are invested by two layers of fibrous connective tissue, the thoracolumbar fascia, which serve as the origin for the superficial back muscles and those of the abdominal wall.

The extrinsic muscles are located anterior to or in front of the vertebral column; thus, in general, their contraction flexes the spine forward or bends

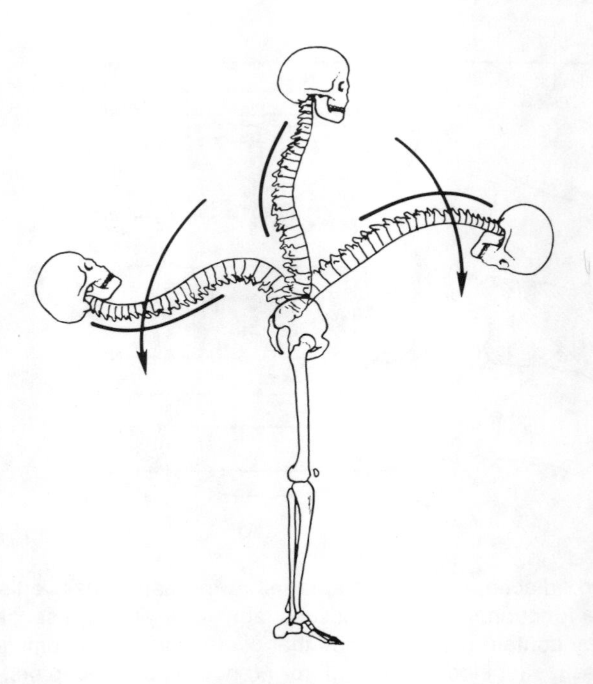

Figure 13-4. Normal curvatures of cervical, thoracic, and lumbar spines with ranges of motion.

the torso forward on the pelvis. Unilaterally, their contraction pulls the spine to the side of the contraction.

The abdominal muscles consist of three basic groupings: the deep; the lateral, including the external and internal obliques and the transversus abdominus; and the medial, including the rectus femoris and pyramidalis. Essentially, the lateral and medial groups form the anterior wall of the abdominal and pelvic cavities, thus supporting the abdominal contents. They lower the ribs and elevate the anterior pelvic rim. They also aid in flexing the trunk on the hips, in side-bending or twisting the trunk, and in rotating the trunk with the lower extremities fixed. Their contraction during respiration elevates the intra-abdominal pressure, thus assisting the erector spinae and vertebral column in supporting the erect body. Weakness of these muscles associated with hyperlordosis is the cause of most lower back injury.

The quadratus lumborum is a triangular sheet arising from the iliac crest and extending upward to insert into the twelfth rib and into the transverse processes of the lumbar vertebrae. Its bilateral contraction will extend the spine, while its contraction will lower the twelfth rib and/or flex the body to the side of contraction. It, along with the psoas, is further classified as a deep abdominal muscle (figure 13-6).

The superficial back muscles, including primarily the latissimus dorsi, serratus anterior and posterior, and trapezius, function to attach the trunk to the upper extremities and to aid in their movements.

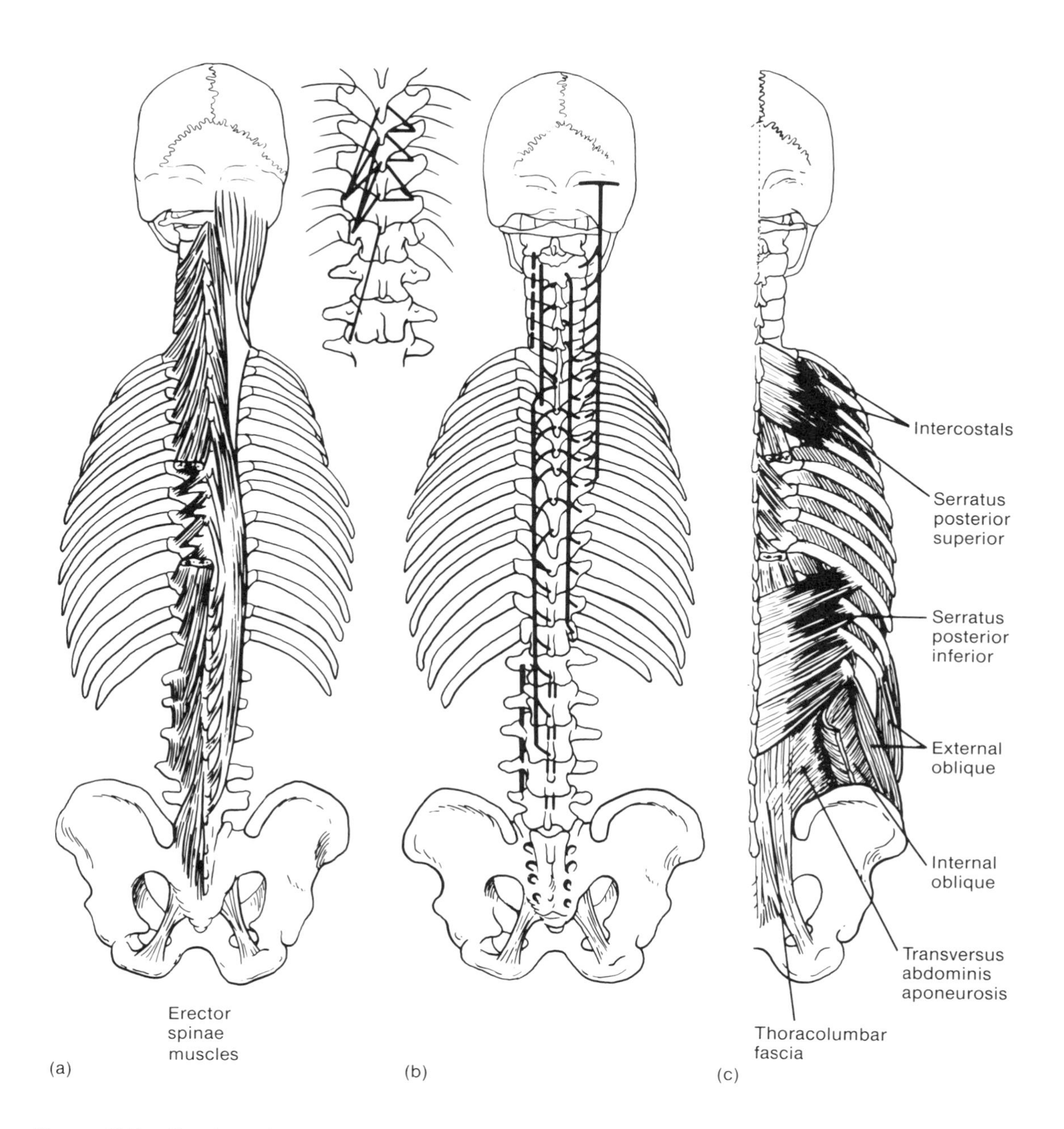

Figure 13-5. Erector spinae.

The hip flexors include the rectus femoris, pectineus, sartorius, the adductors of the thigh, the tensor fascia lata, the anterior fibers of the gluteus medius and minimus, and most important, the psoas, and to a lesser extent its companion, the iliacus (figure 13-7).

The hip flexors function principally in flexing the thigh on the trunk and

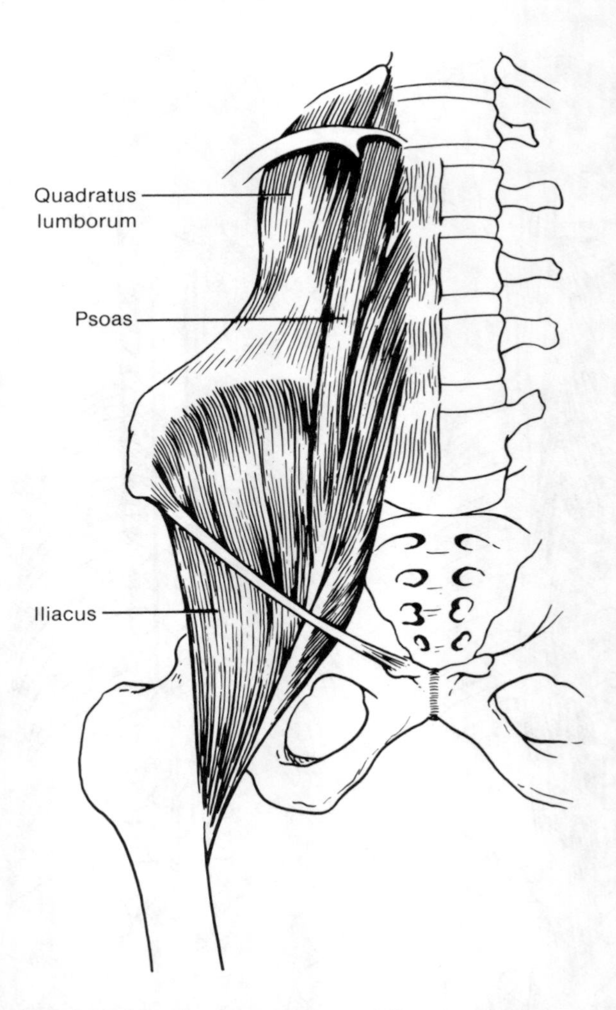

Figure 13-6. Quadratus lumborum, psoas and iliacus muscles.

acting from below up in flexing the trunk on the thigh. Because they are vitally involved in postural and movement mechanics, they are of prime concern not only in injuries to the lower back but in all overuse-related dance injuries.

The hamstrings (semimembranosus, semitendinosus, and biceps femoris), by virtue of their connection from the ischial tuberosity to the proximal tibia and fibula, cross two major joints, the hip and the knee. In addition to being knee flexors, they act as extensors of the thigh on the pelvis, and pulling in the opposite direction bring the posterior aspect of the pelvis downward. In this latter action, the hamstrings complement the action of the abdominals in flexing the pelvis on the lumbar spine while opposing that of the psoas, which extends the lumbar spine, thereby extending the pelvis (figure 13-8-B).

The gluteus maximus is an extensor of the thigh on the hip, and in the extended position, the most powerful external rotator of the thigh (figures 13-8-A, 13-8-B). Like the hamstrings, it acts from below upward to pull down the

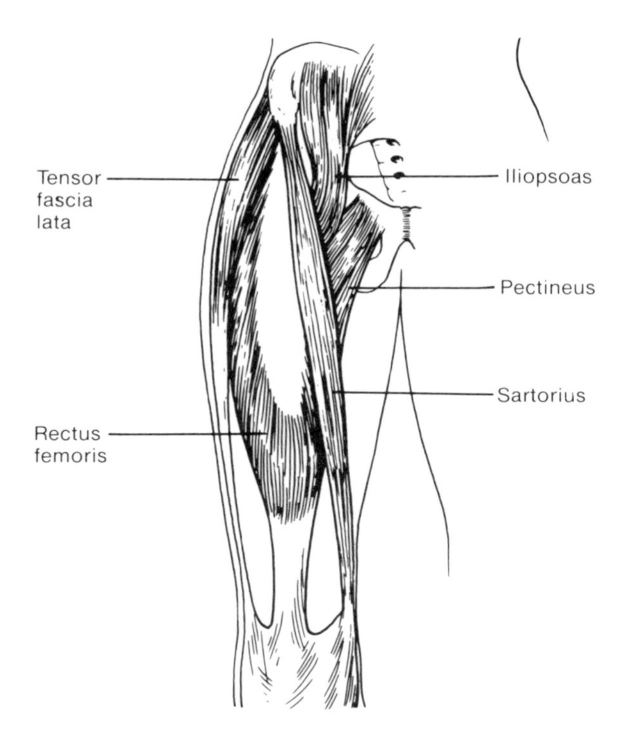

Figure 13-7. Hip flexor muscles.

posterior pelvis, thereby flexing it on the lumbar spine. It also acts as an abductor of the thigh and, through its attachment to the iliotibial band, as a stabilizer of the pelvis.

The gluteus medius and minimus are the muscles of primary importance in maintaining the pelvis close to horizontal with the weight on one leg. They are, with the tensor fascia lata and to a lesser extent, the semitendinosus, semimembranosus, and the posterior fibers of the adductor magnus, the only internal rotators of the hip.

The external rotators, in addition to the gluteus maximus, are the adductors longus and brevis and the anterior fibers of the adductor magnus. These latter are of primary importance in maintaining turn-out in *plié*. Fine tuning of external rotation is through the short, deep lateral rotators: the piriformis, obturator internus and externus, the gemelli, and quadratus femoris. The addition of the iliopsoas, pectineus, gracilis, and sartorius makes the sum of the power of the external rotators much greater than that of the internal rotators; with the limb free, the total effect is external rotation.

The rectus femoris is one of the quadriceps group of knee extensors on the front of the thigh. By virtue of its proximal attachment to the anterior inferior iliac spine, it may act as an extensor of the pelvis on the lumbar spine as well as a flexor of the thigh on the pelvis. Therefore, a tight rectus femoris will act in concert with a shortened psoas to pull the pelvis into hyperextension (figure 13-9).

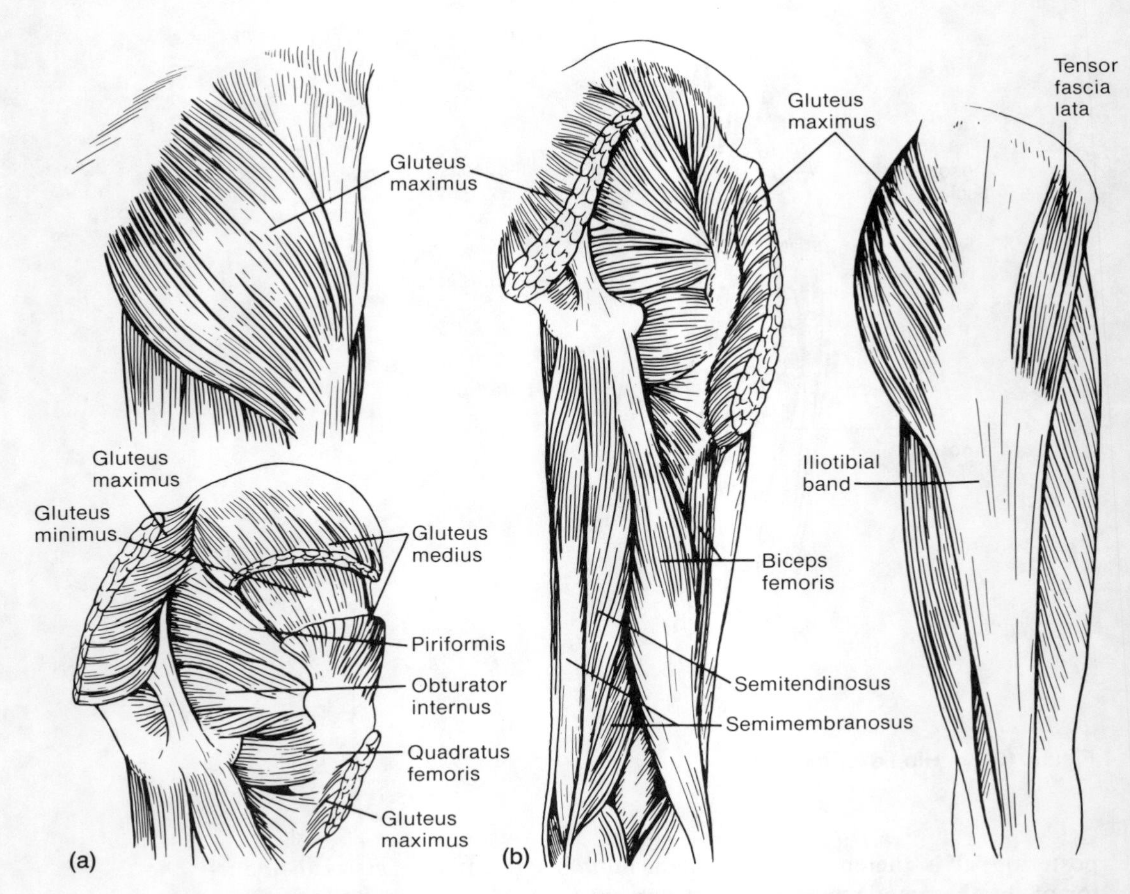

Figures 13-8-A, 13-8-B. Hamstring, gluteus maximus, medius and minimus, and deep external rotator muscles.

Injuries to the Lower Back

As indicated earlier, most dance injuries are the result of repetitive microtraumatic overloading, with consequent failure of the body's adaptive mechanisms. The underlying pathology of almost all dance-related lower back pain is hyperlordosis, which subjects the vertebral column to inappropriate and excessive strains.

One of the best illustrations of this phenomenon is the stress fracture of the vertebral articular pillars, spondylolysis. It is caused by the repeated lower back hyperflexion and hyperextension found in dance and gymnastic movements. Whereas spondylolysis occurs at a rate of 3% in the general population, some authorities* believe the rate to be as high as 10% among adolescent female dancers and gymnasts. Spondylolysis occurs more frequently in female

*In particular, William Hamilton, A.J.G. Howse, and Arthur Michele.

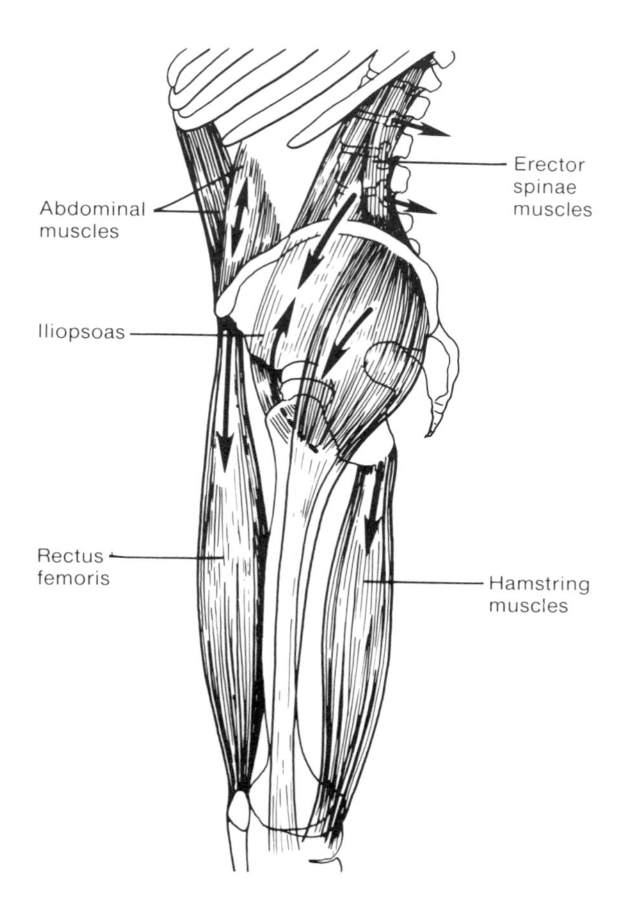

Figure 13-9. Interrelationships between erector spinae, abdominal, iliopsoas, rectus femoris, and hamstring muscles.

dancers primarily because they usually begin their dance training earlier than men—prior to epiphyseal union, when the developing connection is fibrous and thus more vulnerable to trauma. The hyperlordosis associated with forcing turn-out at the hip predisposes to this type of lesion (figure 13-10).

During adolescent growth spurts, when rapid bony elongation occurs without concomitant lengthening of muscle and fascia, there is a relative increase in frequency of hyperlordosis and compensatory thoracic kyphosis. This results in tightness of the thoracolumbar fascia, hamstrings, and calf muscles, predisposing to lower back injury. Hyperlordosis is also a concomitant of idiopathic scoliosis,the incidence of which seems disproportionately high in the dance population.

Warren et al suggest that hyponutrition (particularly with regard to calcium and vitamin D intake) and hypoestrogenism, related to delayed menarche

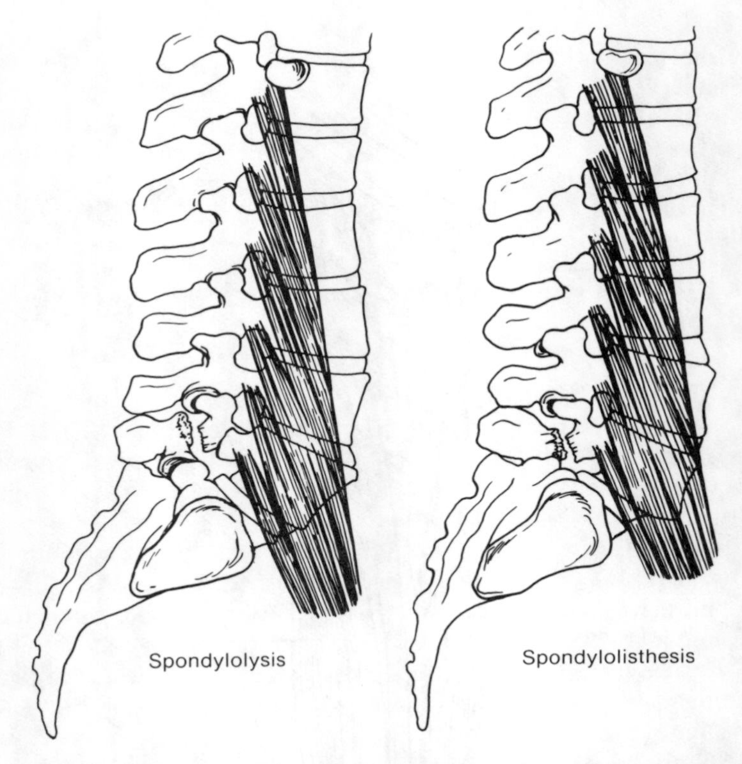

Figure 13-10. Spondylolysis associated with lordosis and spondylolisthesis.

and increased frequency and duration of amenorrhea, both prevalent in the female dance population, may be at the source of both the increased frequency of scoliosis and of stress fractures in that group.[2]

With articular pillar stress fracture, the dancer typically complains of unilateral "pinching" lower back pain occurring consistently with *arabesque* or any extension of the back on the affected side. In the more mature dancer, this type of complaint signals apophyseal impingement (or facet syndrome), to which the dancer is predisposed by the aforementioned hyperlordosis. Differentiation between the facet or apophyseal impingement syndrome and spondylolysis may be difficult, particularly in the more mature adolescent dancer who may have an old, asymptomatic lysis. Radionuclide bone scan is of value in distinguishing these conditions. A "cold" scan, even in the presence of plain film evidence of spondylolysis, rules out active stress fracture. On the other hand, a "hot" spot, even in the absence of other radiographic indications, demands treatment as a stress fracture. All pain-producing activities must be avoided. An antilordotic brace should be applied and all hyperflexion and hyperextension movements avoided. The psoas should be kept at rest, but abdominal strengthening exercises are an essential part of the program. The duration of treatment is 3-6 months or longer.

Spondylolisthesis may be due to a progression of bilateral spondylolysis, in which actual forward slippage of the vertebral body is assisted by a forward pull of the shortened and tight psoas muscle. This condition is only rarely a cause of disability in itself, and treatment of lower back pain, when present, is that indicated for the presenting clinical problem, which may range from disk disease to psoas insufficiency. The presence of spondylolisthesis in an adolescent dancer does not mitigate against professional training or performance status, but rather indicates the necessity for monitoring every 6 months during the period of active growth.

Psoas Insufficiency Syndrome

By far the greatest number of injuries to the lower back are muscular, although these may not be the most serious from the standpoint of lost work time. Most, if not all, are the result of the failure of compensatory mechanisms for contracture, shortening or failure of adaptive lengthening, and usually, weakness of the psoas.

The psoas arises from the bodies, intervertebral disks, and transverse processes of the twelfth thoracic and fifth lumbar vertebrae. It courses distally, anteriorly, and slightly laterally to cross the front of the hip joint, where it dips posteriorly and joins the tendon of the iliacus to be inserted into the lesser trochanter of the femur (figure 13-11). It receives its innervation from the first to the third lumbar nerves, which pass through its substance.

These paired muscles act from below up to flex the trunk at the hip and to pull the lumbar vertebrae anteriorly, increasing the lordosis and thus hyperextending the pelvis. Acting on the free lower limb in the opposite direction (from above downward), psoas contraction flexes the thigh at the hip, adducts it, and slightly rotates it outward. When fixed as the standing leg, however, working in concert with the internal rotators, the psoas externally rotates the pelvis and therefore the trunk, on the ipsilateral femur, to advance the opposite side in walking, becoming in effect an internal rotator of the femur. Thus, a tight psoas restricts external rotation of the fixed lower extremity, particularly at the end range. The body weight is shifted not only posteriorly but toward the midline. The dancer is thus required to force turn-out at the ankle, resulting in pronation of the feet. This, in turn, causes internal femoral rotation and, consequently, a paradoxic increase in lordosis and further psoas shortening.

Unilateral or predominately one-sided psoas pull on the thoracolumbar spine will produce a list and a scoliosis in the direction of the pull, with rotation of the vertebral bodies to the opposite side. The same muscle action on the pelvis will produce anterior torsion and consequent dysfunction at the sacroiliac joint; accompanying pain is caused by depolarization of the ligamentous and joint capsule nociceptors secondary to stretching and/or twisting of those fibers.

With optimal alignment in the erect position, only the psoas and, to a lesser extent, the calf muscles demonstrate significant electrical activity (figure 13-12).

However, in the presence of hip flexor tightness, principally due to tightness and weakness (i.e., insufficiency) of the psoas, the following scenario en-

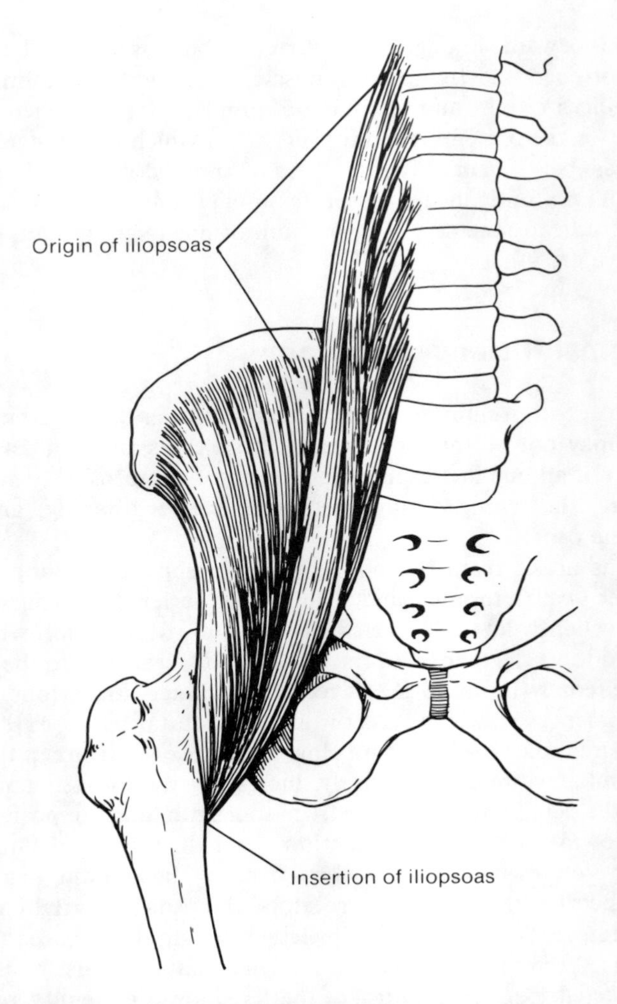

Figure 13-11. Origin and insertion of the iliopsoas muscle.

sues: The thighs are slightly flexed at the hips, the lumbar lordosis is increased, and the pelvis is extended on the lumbar spine, resulting in anterior displacement of the center of gravity at this level (figure 13-13). The abdominal muscles are stretched and weak. This impairs the purchase of the hamstrings and gluteals on the bony pelvis, reducing the effectiveness of both as flexors of the pelvis on the spine, and—more important—the effectiveness of the gluteus maximus as an external rotator of the femur.

In order to compensate and maintain verticality, the posterior compartment of the lower extremities (including the hamstrings and the calf muscles) is contracted, throwing the weight not only back on the heels but toward the midline. Because external rotation at the hip is restricted by psoas tightness, the dancer is obliged to turn out at the ankle, with resultant foot pronation. This produces internal rotation of the femorae, with consequent further increase in

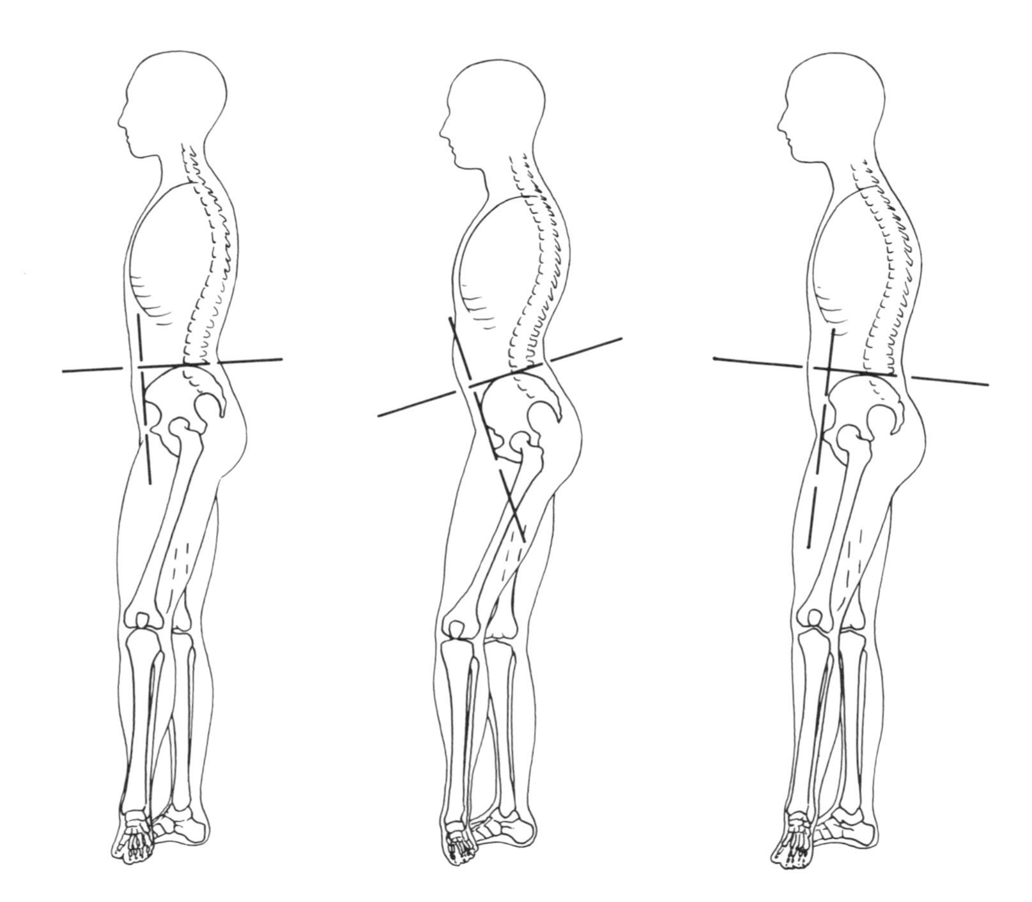

Figure 13-12. Facilitative alignment of the skeleton with parallel levels of the shoulder, hip, knee, and ankle.

lordosis. Thus: Psoas tightness = restricted turn-out at the hip = forced external rotation at the ankle with resultant pronation and internal rotation of femur = increased lordosis and increased flexion at the hip.

Tightness of the back extensors and hamstring muscles decreases the range of forward motion at the hips, further stressing the hip flexors, including the psoas and rectus femoris. Other compensatory changes, including tightening of the thoracolumbar fascia and shortening of the erector spinae, also limit forward movement.

The thoracic kyphosis is increased with forward position of the head and neck, resulting in predisposition of these areas to muscular and ligamentous strains, the principle types of upper back and neck injuries.

Lumbar hyperlordosis causes approximation of the spinous processes and apophyseal joint surfaces, thereby restricting movement posteriorly, as in *arabesque* and *port de bras* back. This will be perceived by the dancer as a feeling of tightness or pinching in the lower back (centralized, across the back, or unilateral) upon execution of movements to the rear. This may be particularly ap-

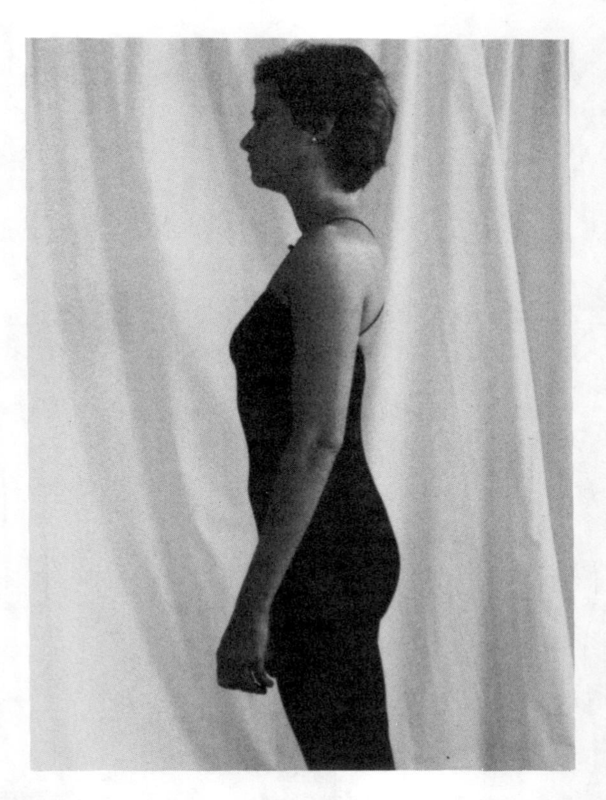

Figure 13-13. Lateral view of dancer with psoas insufficiency showing hyperlordosis that approximates the lower spinous processes and stresses the apophyseal articulations.

parent with the introduction of a torsional component. X rays may demonstrate stress changes at the apophyseal joints due to chronic musculotendinous imbalances or intervertebral disk pathology.

About 40-45% of lower back pain is due to activation of joint capsule nociceptors, while 30-35% is muscular, the result of activation of the intramuscular perivascular nociceptive receptors through stretching of tight or contracted muscles.

Diagnosis of Psoas Insufficiency Syndrome

Typically, the dancer with psoas insufficiency, either acute or chronic, complains of lower back pain uni- or bilateral, often alternating sides, present on forward-bending, extension, or side-bending away from the painful side. There may be radiation to the hip, usually anteriorly, or to the anterior or posterior aspect of either or both thighs, but never below the knee.

The major physical criteria include sacroiliac or iliosacral somatic dysfunction, usually right-sided, with an anterior innominate and positive forward flexion test on the side of dysfunction. Tightness and weakness of the psoas will be noted bilaterally, but this will be more pronounced on the side of primary dysfunction. Both psoas motor points will be tender and there will be decreased range of both hip flexion and extension on the dysfunctional side. Iliotibial band tightness, often bilateral, will consistently be noted on the side opposite the primary dysfunction; it may be the cause of more prominent symptoms involving the contralateral posterolateral thigh and knee. This may or may not be accompanied by piriformis contracture. Hyperlordosis is a constant finding, except in the rare case in which the trunk is pitched forward and flexed at the hips, with flattening or reversal of the lordosis.

The abdominals will be weak and the hamstrings unduly tight. There may be an apparent or actual longer leg on the dysfunctional side. Bilateral foot pronation resulting from the restricted hip external rotation is a frequent concomitant. Perhaps the most important single criterion is the relief of pain and increased range of motion, however temporary, following psoas stretching.

Treatment of lower back pain resulting from psoas insufficiency and its sequellae obviously must finally depend on restoring normal alignment, using the appropriate stretches and strengtheners, along with manual therapy and visualization techniques (figures 13-14-A, 13-14-B, 13-14-C). Selective rest and the adjunctive use of nonsteroid anti-inflammatory medication during the acute phase is of particular value in the management of these problems.

Fortunately, intervertebral disk injuries in dancers are less frequent than conditions discussed previously. However, the eventual evolution of psoas insufficiency-related hyperlordosis into disk disease later in life is fairly common. The pathology usually involves bulging or actual herniation of disk material into the neural foramina or into the posterior longitudinal ligament, producing pain due to stretching of that ligament and pressure on the dural sleeve or on the nerve root itself. In long-standing cases of disk derangement, pain may be caused by alteration in the mechanics of the apophyseal joint, thereby depolarizing the nociceptors in the joint capsule or those in the cancellous bone of the articular pillars. Osteoarthritis of these joints, with hypertrophic changes and narrowing of the intervertebral formina and spinal canal, may be the end result.

Discogenic syndromes are much more common in male ballet dancers, undoubtedly due to lifting. Further support for this concept comes from the fact that the incidence of intervertebral disk pathology and indeed, lower back injury in general, is much lower in modern dance, which involves fewer and different types of lifts.

Treatment of disk disease in dancers is basically no different from that in the nondancing population. Selective rest is essential in the early, acute phases with or without sciatica, when all but the most moderate activity must be avoided. Bed rest, however, is to be reserved for the most severe cases, and unless there is pain, movement even while at rest must be encouraged. Ice, rather than heat, is indicated for topical analgesia. If required, narcotic analgesia should be given around the clock rather than on an as-needed basis, in order to discourage habituation. As soon as feasible, narcotics should be replaced by nonsteroid anti-inflammatory medication. Physical therapeutic modalities and judicious osteopathic manipulation or other manual therapy may be of great help in all phases.

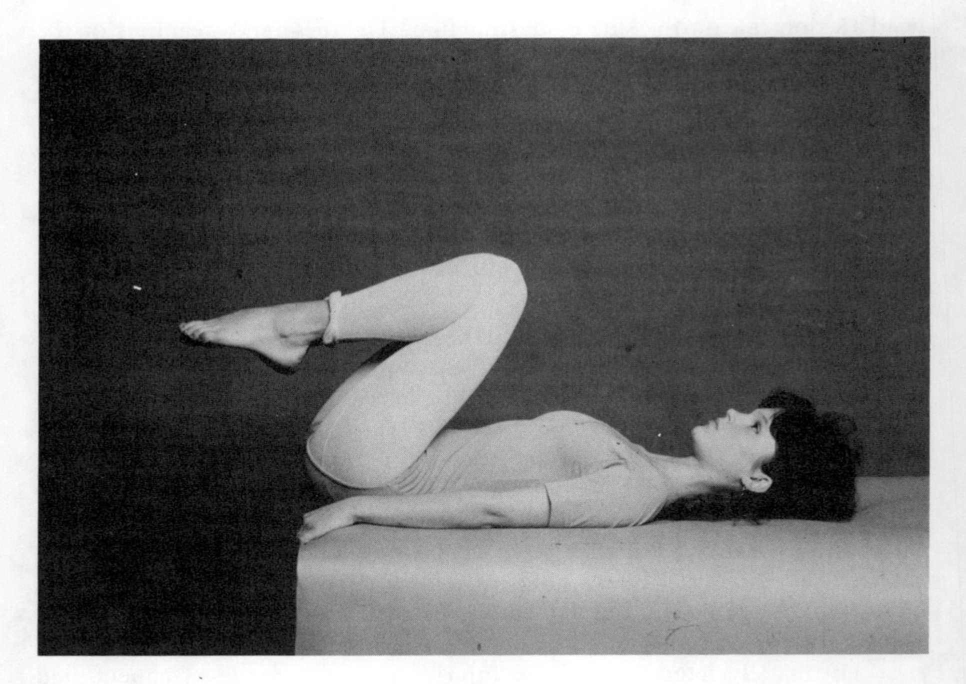

A.

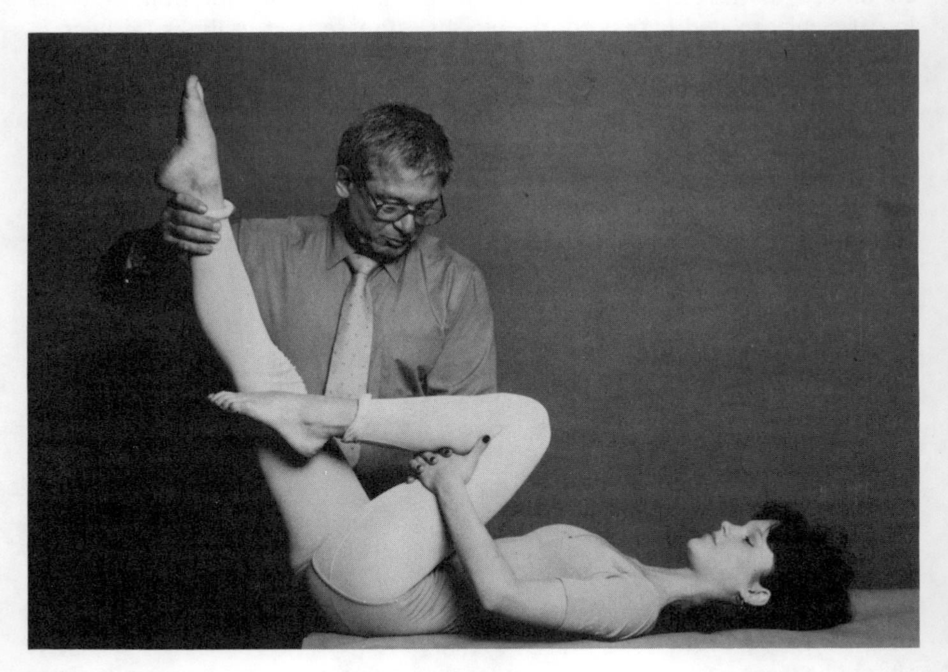

B.

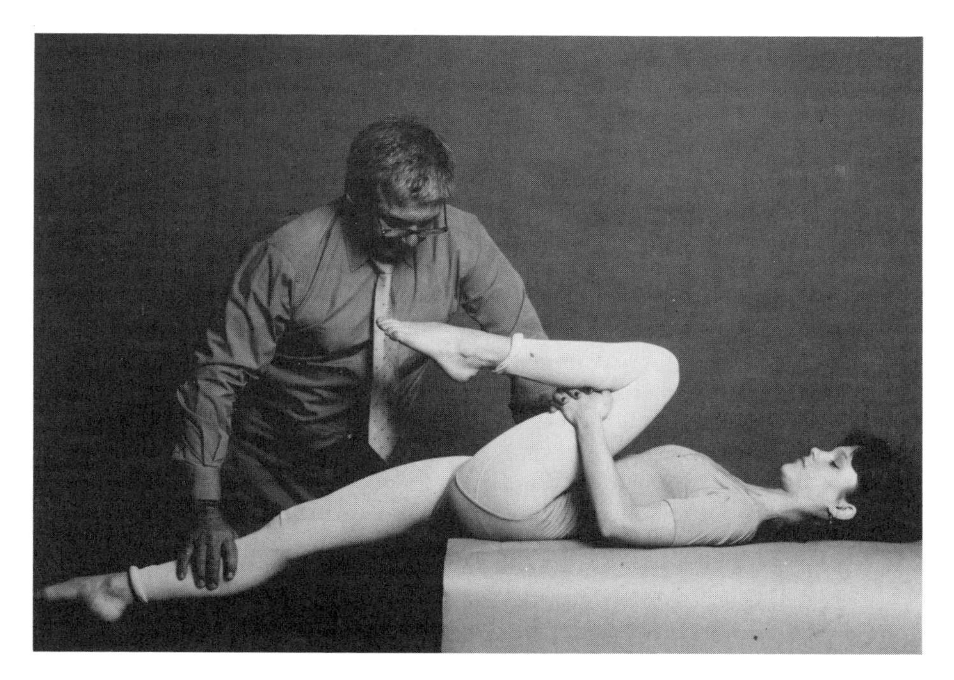

C.

Figures 13-14-A, 13-14-B, 13-14-C. Dancer lying supine shows elevation of the buttocks with thighs flexed on the hips indicating tight psoas muscles. The therapist stretches these muscles and the hamstrings to allow relaxation.

Weight bearing, when indicated, may be facilitated by the use of a lumbosacral support, which will also be of value upon resumption of dance training. As soon as possible, a program of abdominal strengthening, psoas stretching and strengthening, and piriformis and hamstring stretching exercises should be instituted. Lifting and other movements producing pain should, of course, be proscribed.

The persistence of disabling pain or the presence of progressive motor or sensory deficits mandates early intensive diagnostic inquiry, including computerized axial tomography or magnetic resonance imaging and neurosurgical consultation. Although certainly a last resort, surgical intervention, preferably microsurgical discectomy, must be considered for the refractory case. The value of chymopapain injection is still questionable, the indications being strictly limited, the postinjection rehabilitative period extensive, and the efficacy equivocal.

Following surgery, whether laminectomy or microsurgical discectomy, recovery is slow, and rehabilitation is intensive. Return to full dance activity may take a year or more, with the strong possibility that return to the preinjury level of artistic competence will not be feasible.

Another less common cause of back pain in dancers is the phenomenon known as "kissing spines." This is an essentially benign condition resulting from the impingement of larger spinous processes at the end range of extension. Tenderness is localized to the tips of the involved spinous processes (usually lower thoracic or thoracolumbar) and their supraspinous ligaments. Pain is produced by passive or active extension, and the condition is usually self-limiting. The pain may, however, be incapacitating when it is provoked.

In the presence of disk space narrowing, kissing spines may result in posterior displacement of the axis of rotation in extension of the lumbar spine. This stresses the apophyseal joints, and the consequent adventitious motion may result in osteoarthritis with or without subluxation. Treatment consists primarily of avoiding repetition of the etiologic movement, but recovery may often be facilitated by the injection of a local anesthetic—a long-acting corticosteroid mixture into the area of maximum tenderness. This can be done with relative impunity because it is neither a weight-bearing structure nor one subject to tensile stresses.

Injuries to the Cervicothoracic Spine

Injuries to the cervicothoracic spine in dancers are of considerably less severity and importance (except to the dancer suffering from them), but they can be quite painful and threatening nonetheless. They are usually closely related to maladaptive alignment, and therefore to psoas insufficiency, i.e., lumbar hyperlordosis, increased thoracic kyphosis and/or scapular retraction, forward-craning head position, and flat cervical lordosis. The center of gravity at the head is displaced anteriorly, thereby increasing the work requirements of the cervical paravertebral musculature in order to support the 15–20-lb. head. There is decreased range of motion, particularly in extension and rotation.

The net effect is increased susceptibility to muscular strains, which may produce a wide variety of symptoms and signs when the dancer is subjected to some of the more rigorous modern choreographic demands. These include percussive modern/jazz movements requiring shoulder and neck "contractions" and "isolations," quick "head drops" to the back, and "whiplash" rotations.

Head drops to the back, for example, must be executed with an arching and lengthening motion rather than a compressive one. To accomplish this with the erector spinae muscles already contracted to keep the head from falling off is almost impossible. At best, movements such as these can be safely executed only from a position of near-perfect alignment.

It should be noted at this point that the slightest deviation from optimum alignment in one part of the body has profound effects on the rest of the body. Restriction of elevation of the shoulders will—in lifting, for example—necessitate increased hyperextension of the lower back, increasing lordosis and predisposing to lumbosacral strains and stress fractures.

Unfortunately, modern choreography (modern, jazz, and even some ballet) often calls for movement that, performed incorrectly, may cause injury to the cervical and thoracic spine and upper extremities. Supporting the body on the head, neck, and arms can easily precipitate injury if the dancer is physically unequal to the task or unaware of how best to perform the movement kinesthetically. Choreography of this type often demands a strength in the upper body that dancers have not developed in traditional training, which emphasizes strength and flexibility in the lower extremities. The choreography of classical ballet, on the other hand, rarely involves breaking the line of the neck. With the exception of male roles, ballet demands little upper body strength and rarely calls for support on the back. Additionally, many teachers of ballet, modern, and jazz either neglect posture and alignment or teach them incorrectly.

The dancer with a cervicothoracic muscular injury typically complains of pain that appears to arise from one or the other interscapular areas, radiating to the neck and often into the ipsilateral arm. The pain may be associated with numbness and tingling, possibly following nerve root distribution. There may be weakness of the involved extremity. Radiation may also take place into the head and/or face. Headache may be a prominent feature. The dancer complains of an inability to turn the head fully to either side, particularly away from the pain. Side-bending is similarly affected, as is extension.

It is important to distinguish this condition from cervical disk disease with foraminal encroachment, which has a much more serious prognosis. The latter syndrome is characterized by restricted motion in the direction of the pain and an increase in pain with or without radiation to the upper extremity upon forward flexion of the neck. There may be neurologic changes, both sensory and motor in either situation, but the diagnosis can usually be made from the history, physical examination, and x-ray studies. With respect to the history, it is important to note that most often, there is a clear stress relationship to this type of musculoskeletal pain syndrome. Treatment of this posture-injury- stress-related musculoskeletal dysfunction includes selective rest, i.e., the avoidance of pain-producing movements; osteopathic or other manual therapy; temporary immobilization with a soft cervical collar during the acute phase, with early but gradual weaning; ice massage to levator scapula, rhomboid, and trapezius trigger points; nonsteroid anti-inflammatory agents; and in severe cases, anxiolytics and, for brief periods, narcotic analgesics. Ultimately, successful treatment depends on resolution of the underlying psychological and/or alignment pathology.

Psychological or emotional as well as physical stress attributable to postural malalignment or injury is, over a prolonged period, capable of producing degenerative changes in the intervertebral disks and apophyseal joints. These changes, in turn, can cause nerve root impingement, with dire orthopedic and neurologic consequences. It is of major importance, therefore, to effect changes in posture and movement mechanics wherever possible, in order to prevent serious problems (figure 13-15).

In discussing dance alignment, it is important to note that this term carries a variety of connotations, depending upon the educational level of the dancer.

Alignment, both good and poor, facilitative or maladaptive, exists in both stillness and movement. One's biomechanical and neuromuscular patterns

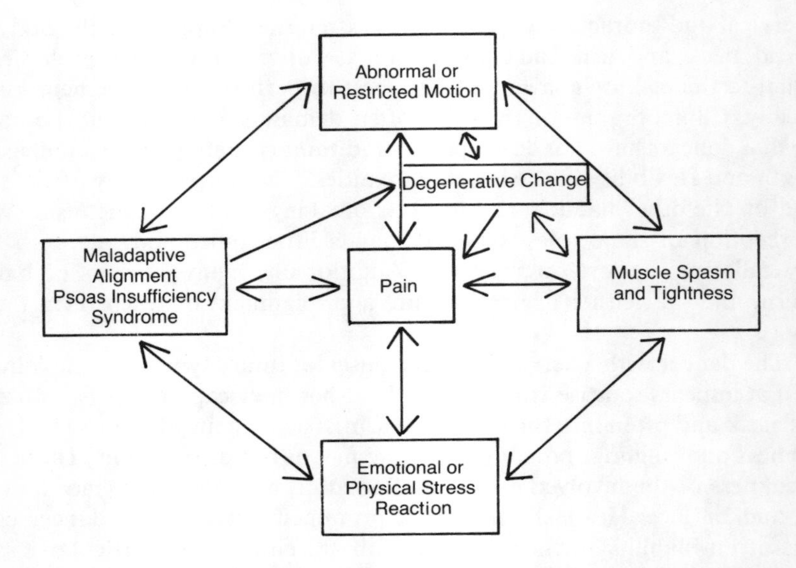

Figure 13-15. Interrelationships between abnormal motion, posture, muscle tightness, stress reactions, and pain and degenerative change.

do not get better or worse moving from one state to another. True "perfect alignment," when present in stillness, translates into movement as well, the body moving efficiently with minimal physical exertion and tension. Conversely, poor static alignment—lumbar hyperlordosis, for example—continues to manifest itself, and even increases, under the stress of movement.

Often realizing that they have postural defects, dancers try to compensate through a variety of muscular tricks. Some of these include tucking the pelvis under in an attempt to reduce the lumbar spine hyperextension, flexing at the hip to increase turn-out, pulling the jaw back into the neck to reduce the forward thrust of the head, and pulling up on the arches to correct pronation. The attempt to exert conscious control over subcortical movement patterns is extremely inefficient, requiring an incredible expenditure of effort and energy just to remain vertical. And, unfortunately, as soon as the dancer moves, the old patterns reappear. Such holding only creates more bad habits and predisposes the dancer to injury.

In correcting a postural defect, it is important to emphasize that there are two phases to the process: (1) the release of old, inefficient neuromuscular response patterns and (2) the development of more efficient new patterns. This is not achieved by conscious holding of muscles and body, but may be effected on a subcortical level through working with a certified movement analyst or kinesiologist sophisticated in dance anatomy, biomechanics, and neuromuscular facilitation and reeducation.

Summary

Most dance and athletic injuries are due to cumulative microtraumata. These, in turn, are due to inappropriate usage, training errors, or defective technique. Most injuries, particularly in dancers and involving the back, are the result of maladaptive alignment. Although back pain to some degree is part of the life of the dancer, it often has great significance and relevance to injuries of the lower extremities and thus deserves close attention. Most lower back pain in dancers is related to the maladaptive alignment resulting from hyperlordosis, which in turn is related to psoas insufficiency, abdominal muscle weakness, and tightness of the hamstrings and gluteals. Spondylolistchesis, spondlylothesis, apophyseal impingement syndromes, and intervertebral disk syndromes are conditions commonly affecting dancers, but muscular strains resulting from psoas insufficiency are the most frequent source of injuries of the lower back. Injuries to the cervical and thoracic spine are much less frequent, but underlying alignment defects secondary to hyperlordosis and psoas insufficiency are their principal source. Early and comprehensive management of stress- and posture-related musculoskeletal dysfunction is essential to avoid later degenerative changes involving the intervertebral disks and arthrodial joints. This management includes modification of posture and movement mechanics as well as conventional treatment methods.

References

1. Solomon R, Micheli L. Concepts in the prevention of dance injuries: a survey and analysis. 1984 Olymp Sci Cong Proc, vol 8. Champaign: Human Kinetics Publishers.
2. Warren MP, J. Brooks-Gunn J, Linda Hamilton L, Fiske Warren LF, Hamilton W. Scoliosis and fractures in young ballet dancers. New Engl Med 314:21; 1348–53, May 22, 1986.

Bibliography

Bachrach RM. Diagnosis and management of dance injuries to the lower back. The dancer as athlete. 1984 Olymp Sci Cong Proc, vol 8. Champaign: Human Kinetics Publishers, 1986.

Bachrach RM. A Physician's primer of dance injuries. Osteo Med News, vol. 2, 1985; 1-5.

Bachrach RM. The relationship of low back pelvic somatic dysfunction to dance injuries. Kinesiol For Dance, 1986; 8:4.

Clanin DR, Davison DM, Plastino JG. Injury patterns in university dance students. 1984 Olymp Sci Cong Proc. Champaign: Human Kinetics Publishers, 1986.

Dowd I. Taking root to fly: seven articles on functional anatomy. New York: Contact Collaborations, 1980.

Hamilton W. Personal communications, 1980-86.

Howse AJG. Lectures and personal communications, 1982-84.

Howse AJG. Alignment and dance injuries. Phys Sportsmed (audiotape). Chicago: Teach 'em, 1984.

Garrick J. The dancer's spine. Phys Sportsmed (audiotape) Chicago: Teach 'em, 1984.

Meglin J. Ideokinesis as it applies to injury prevention. 1984 Olymp Sci Cong Proc. Champaign: Human Kinetics Publishers, 1986.

Meyers M. Perceptual awareness in integrative movement behavior: the role of integrative movement systems (body therapies) in motor performance and expressivity. 1984 Olymp Sci Cong Proc. Champaign: Human Kinetics Publishers, 1986.

Michele AA. Iliopsoas: development of anomalies in man. Springfield: Charles C. Thomas, 1962.

Micheli LJ. Back injuries in dancers. Clin Sportsmed. 2:3. W.B. Saunders, 1983.

Nixon JE. Injuries to the neck and upper extremities of dancers. Clin Sportsmed 2:3. W.B. Saunders, 1983.

Quirk R. Ballet injuries, the Australian experience. Clin Sportsmed 2:3. W.B. Saunders, 1983.

Solomon R, Micheli L. Concepts in the prevention of dance injuries: a survey and analysis. 1984 Olymp Sci Cong Proc, vol 8. Champaign: Human Kinetics Publishers, 1986.

Sparger C. Anatomy and ballet. Great Britain: J.W. Arrowsmith, 1957.

Sparger C. Ballet physique. Great Britain: J.W. Arrowsmith, 1958.

Stevens A. Personal communication, 1986.

Thomasen E. Diseases and injuries of ballet dancers. Denmark: Universitetsforlaget I Arhus, 1982.

Warren MP, Brooks-Gunn J, Hamilton L, Warren LF, Hamilton W. Scoliosis and fractures in young ballet dancers. New Engl J Med 314:21, 1348-53.

Wyke B. General principles of articular neurology; Clinical neurology of lumbosacral pain. (audiotapes). 2nd Annu Meeting and Semin Am Assoc Orthop Med, 1985.

14

INJURIES TO THE NECK AND UPPER EXTREMITY

Anthony P. Millar, M.B., B.S., F.R.A.C.P., F.A.C.R.M.

INJURIES TO THE NECK and upper limb in ballet have received little attention in the past. Sparger,[4] in an excellent book, did not mention the problem, and Dunn[2] and Arnheim,[1] in their respective publications, devote only a few pages to the subject.

A 20-year review of ballet injuries at the Lewisham Hospital, Petersham, New South Wales, showed no injury to this area in the first 5 of those years. A slow, steady increase has been noted in the intervening years, and in the 1985-86 period, injuries to the neck and upper limb represented 4% of all ballet injuries.

For explanation, it is necessary to review the dancer's life. Originally, all dancing was classical in type, but the past 2 decades have seen an increasing interest in modern dance, dance drama, jazz ballet, and similar activities. These new forms require different attitudes of the body to meet the choreographer's needs. These attitudes place greater stress on the cervical spine and its support structures and also require greater use of the arm, not only as a method of expression of feeling but also to support the dancer's body or that of another dancer. The male dancer is required to catch the ballerina from a leap. Some movements require the dancer to fall gracefully on an outstretched arm and then rise again from the prone position.

Practice and rehearsal times have been maintained at 8 hr./day as a minimum, but the approach of performance dates sometimes increases the working hours, leading to overload. An increasing number of dancers compete for places in companies, adding a dimension of emotional pressure to practice sessions. Paradoxically, the number of dancers available for the less attractive companies has decreased, so that less well-trained applicants are required to cope with dances for which they do not have adequate technical ability. This leads to bad performance and injury.

Weight training has been popularized in sport in general, and male dancers have used it to develop their arm strength for lifting. As in other sports, poor technique, overloading weight, and too frequent repetitions lead to shoulder and neck injuries, particularly when added to long rehearsal periods.

It has been generally recognized that there has been an increase in the level of emotional stress in the community at large. This influences the ballet community as well, and will increase the likelihood of injury. Added to this are the interpersonal stresses present in any company that performs over a long period; as Nideffer has shown, injury is a likely visitor to the stage under these circumstances.[3]

This discussion focuses on the injuries occurring in ballet and dance as a particular facet of the technique rather than injuries resulting from falls and inappropriate movements. Accidents as such will be mentioned only when there is a problem related to the management of the disability that can be affected by the particular needs of the dancer.

Cervical Injuries

The most common ballet injury in the cervical region is the so-called cervical strain. This is an injury to the ligamentous tissue in the region of the facet joints due to excessive and repeated movement beyond the range obtainable by the dancer under normal circumstances. It is brought on by too rapid a progression and too frequent repetition of a given movement.

The dancer complains of aching and soreness along the side of the neck extending down along the upper border of the trapezius out toward the shoulder joint. As the condition worsens, the aching and soreness extends down along the dorsal spine and into the rhomboid muscles along the medial border of the scapula. It is sometimes described as being in between the scapula and the chest wall "just where my hand cannot reach." It does not usually extend down the arm unless the disability has been present for a long time. Occasionally, the ache will spread anteriorly around the base of the neck to the upper pectoral region. The condition is not accompanied by the paresthesias or muscular weakness, but is accompanied by an inability to maintain a strong contraction for very long.

Examination of the cervical spine will reveal restriction and pain in one or more movements of the neck. The opposite movement is characteristically unaffected. There is no evidence of involvement of the reflex, motor, or sensory systems. Shoulder movements are full. Movements of the dorsal spine are unaffected, although palpation will reveal tenderness along the side of the neck and down over the upper dorsal spines just lateral to the midline. X-rays are not necessary for diagnosis, and if taken rarely show a significant abnormality.

Treatment of the condition is to mobilize the neck and upper dorsal spine on several occasions some days apart. This should be done by a physician knowledgeable and experienced in manual manipulation or by a qualified physical therapist. The dancer is encouraged to perform movements of the neck and head that involve the total range of pain-free movement. In this way, the range regained as a result of mobilization will be maintained. The dancer should not perform those ballet movements that cause pain. The mobilization will need to be performed on several occasions, and within 2 weeks the condition should have fully cleared.

To prevent recurrence, the dancer should be advised to resume the offending attitudes gradually, to increase the repetitions slowly, and to avoid emotional stress. This last factor is a frequent cause of poor technique, as it is often accompanied by lack of concentration and fatigue.

Shoulder Injuries

Shoulder injuries are most commonly represented by rotator cuff strains, particularly in male dancers. This injury, more frequent in modern ballet, can be precipitated by the weight training necessary to develop the appropriate strength for lifting the ballerina (figure 14-1).

The history is one of pain and aching in the shoulder region extending down over the deltoid. The pain does not extend in toward the neck. Initially, the pain is present after effort, and as the condition progresses, it begins to occur during the activity. It is not uncommon for the patient to complain that it is

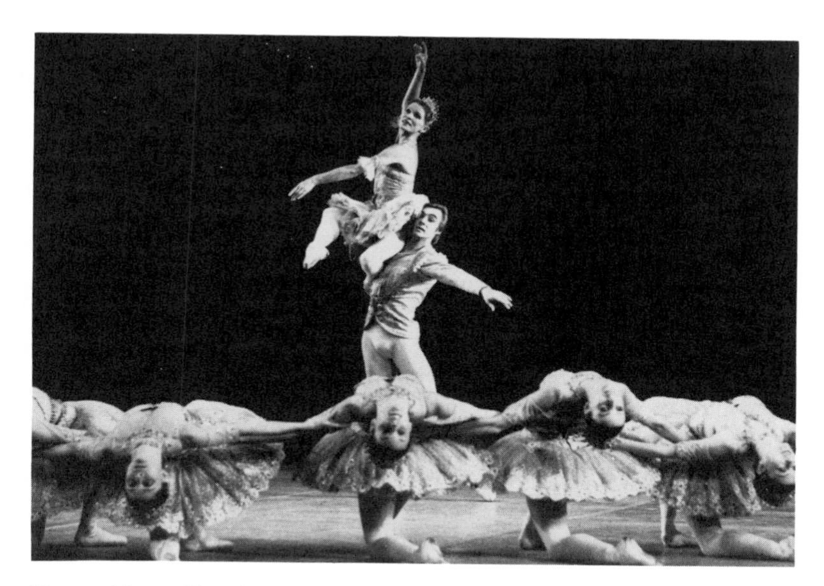

Figure 14-1. Shoulder injuries, most commonly represented by rotator cuff strains among male dancers, can be precipitated by the weight training necessary to develop the appropriate strength for lifting the ballerina. (Galina Samsova and David Ashmole, Sadlers Wells Ballet.)

impossible to lie on the shoulder at night because of the discomfort experienced.

Findings in the examination of the shoulder vary, depending upon the particular tendon involved. In the case of the supraspinatus, abduction may be possible only to 80° in a marked case. Occasionally, a painful arc is present from 80-120°, but the range is complete. Resisted abduction of the arm, with the arm by the side, will be painful in a supraspinatus lesion. In the case of the infraspinatus tendinitis, resisted external rotation of the arm is painful. Tenderness in these cases is present over the lateral and posterior parts of the humeral head, respectively, with the arm lying in the neutral position by the side. When the shoulder ache extends down the anterior aspect of the arm, bicipital tendinitis is the likely diagnosis. There will be tenderness over the bicipital groove and a positive straight arm-raising test; resisted forward movement of the arm at 80° with the elbow extended is painful.

Rotator cuff injuries will respond to rest over a period of time. Physical therapy, which provides relief over a period of 2-3 weeks, must include mobilization of the joint by a qualified therapist to ensure that all accessory movements are full. A progressive resistance exercise program should be incorporated in the regime with a view to protecting the shoulder when full activity resumes. Local corticosteroid injection may produce a cure if relief is not obtained by physical therapy, but it is important that it be injected directly into the cuff just proximal to its humeral attachment. Adding local anesthetic to the injection will allow resisted movement to be tested; if it is painless, the injection has been placed correctly. The injection may need to be repeated in a few weeks. In young dancers, the results are quick and satisfactory, and no long-term problems arise.

Pain and aching at the shoulder, or just slightly internal to it, occurs in chronic acromioclavicular joint sprain. This can be detected by the presence of tenderness over the acromioclavicular joint, with pain on abduction of the arm above 120° (rotation of the clavicle occurs at this point). Resisted abduction of the arm is painful; forcing the arm into abduction across the body also may produce pain. The acromioclavicular joint is tender to the touch.

Treatment of the condition consists of diminishing or eliminating, if possible, the activity causing the pain and discomfort. When this is not possible, physical therapy, associated with a diminution in the intensity and frequency of effort, will often provide a satisfactory result. To prevent a recurrence, it is important that full movement at the joint be obtained by careful therapeutic manipulation. Injection of local corticosteroid into the joint and its ligaments is effective, but does make the area sore and painful for a few days. This treatment would preclude a performance until pain is relieved or markedly diminished.

For the dancer who has a generalized ache around the shoulder and no specific findings on examination, or in whom examination findings vary on retesting, there is often an area of tenderness over the anterior and lateral aspects of the shoulder joint due to a subdeltoid bursitis. The condition itself can be treated with rest, physical therapy, or local corticosteroid injection. The last treatment is probably best, because the condition is chronic. Because this lesion is frequently associated with a heightened emotional tension, this factor should be evaluated if recurrence is to be avoided.

Contusions of the Upper Arm

Dancers are subject to blows to the upper arm during performance or practice, but because they are usually not severe blows, no specific treatment generally is required for any resulting bruises. In the case of repeated blows over a given area that do cause a problem, it is important that treatment be gentle. There should be no forced extension of the elbow joint to try to stretch the muscle fully, for this will likely lead to myositis ossificans. Should the contusion not disappear within 3 weeks, and if the elbow is not fully extensile at that time, x-ray of the upper arm should be performed to determine whether calcification associated with myositis ossificans is present. If calcification has developed, an extended period of 3-6 months' rest is indicated. No curative treatment is available, and surgery will not improve the rate of recovery.

Elbow Joint Injuries

Lateral epicondylitis, the most frequent injury to the elbow, is related to the performance of handstands and the raising and lowering of the body in the press-up mechanism. Medial epicondylitis is less frequent.

The dancer complains of pain over the lateral or medial aspect of the elbow that is related to activity and relieved by rest. Pain gradually extends down the forearm if activity is continued; in the case of medial epicondylitis, possible involvement of the ulnar nerve may cause paresthesia along the medial forearm and hand.

Examination shows that resisted wrist extension is painful in lateral epicondylitis and wrist flexion in medial elbow pain. Tenderness is present at the epicondyle and over the adjacent ridge.

The conditions can be treated by the cessation of the activity causing the discomfort and the infiltration of the affected area with corticosteroid. One or two injections are usually adequate. The steroid should be mixed with local anesthetic so that resisted extension, in the case of lateral epicondylitis, or resisted flexion of the wrist, in the case of medial epicondylitis, can be tested after the injection to ensure that the material has been placed correctly. At that time, the resisted movement should be painless. Following recovery, it is advisable that the dancer undertake a redevelopment program for the forearm musculature to try to prevent a recurrence.

Wrist Injuries

Overuse injuries to the wrist occur mainly at the ulnar and radial borders of the wrist, although the centrally placed lunocapitate joint is at times damaged by too frequent hyperextension in a wrist that is a little less mobile than normal.

The dancer complains of aching in the wrist after a performance. This subsides with rest, but recurs progressively earlier in subsequent efforts. Clinically, the wrist shows a full range of movement. With lunocapitate strains, forward flexion is painful at the end of range, particularly when forced. The capitate can be seen subluxed from its lunate cavity, and the area is tender. When abduction is painful, tenderness is present from the tip of the radial styloid to the scaphoid along the line of the radial collateral ligament. Adduction pain is associated with tenderness over the ulnar collateral ligament due to strain in that ligament. Tenderness anterior to the ligament would involve the flexor carpi ulnaris tendon or, if bony, the hamate bone. In the latter case, an x-ray should be taken with a "tunnel" view to rule out a fracture of the hook of the hamate.

Treatment of these strains consists of infiltrating the affected area with local corticosteroid and reducing the overall work load. One or two injections, 3 weeks aparts, provides relief. Following this, every effort should be made to restore any lost range and to rebuild muscle strength. Care should be taken to maintain good technique if weights are being used.

Prevention

Prevention of injury involves many factors, of which overuse and poor technique are the main offenders. This is true not only in the dance but also in

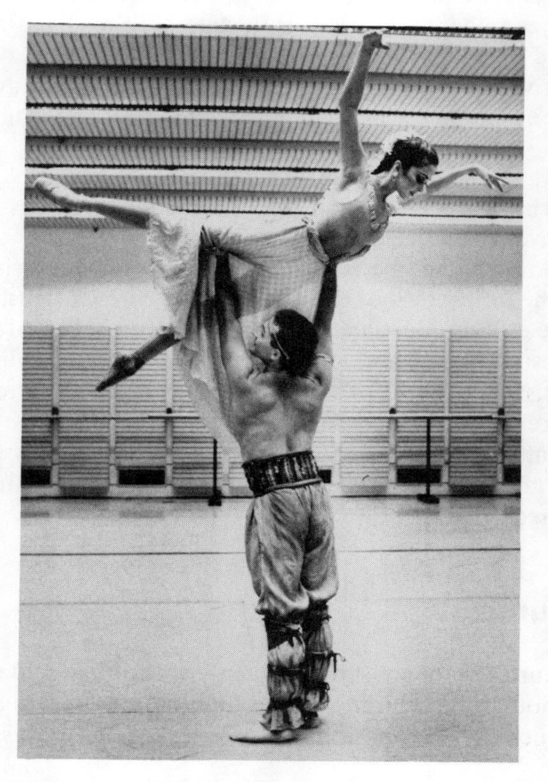

Figure 14-2. The dancer needs full range in the joints and full power; both factors are easily maintained with careful programming. (Stephen Morgante and Margaret Illman, Australian Ballet.)

training programs performed away from the studio to improve strength. The presence of emotional tension, which is easily detected in most cases, should be appropriately treated with relaxation programs. Even in dancers where it is not readily apparent, some search for evidence of tension should be made to resolve conflicts that lead to injury and slow recovery. The dancer needs full range in the joints and full power; both factors are easily maintained with careful programming (figure 14-2). Any disability is better prevented than cured; with an injury prevention program, there is less loss of fitness, less stress, and a more rewarding career.

References

1. Arnheim DD. Dance injuries: their prevention and care. 2nd ed. Toronto: CV Mosby, 1980.
2. Dunn B. Dance therapy for dancers. London: Heinemann Health Books, 1974.
3. Nideffer R M. The ethics and practice of applied sport psychology. Ann Arbor: Movement Publications, 1981; 142-50.
4. Sparger C. Anatomy and ballet. London: Adam & Charles Black, 1970.

15

MUSCULOSKELETAL PROBLEMS IN MODERN, JAZZ AND 'SHOW BIZ' DANCERS

Ernest L. Washington, M.D.

Introduction

ALL DANCERS REGARDLESS OF the style and type of dance they engage in, all dancers subject their bodies to physical demands, both musculoskeletal and physiologic, far beyond those of the nondancer performing "everyday" nondance activities.

The type and frequency of musculoskeletal problems does vary, however, among the various theatrical dance forms, depending upon the type and style of movement and the type of (and absence or presence of) various items of wearing apparel, particularly shoes.

The classical ballet dancer is much less likely than the modern dancer to develop "floor burns" (abrasions) over the bony prominences of the lower extremities because of the shoes and tights covering the lower extremities used by classical ballet dancer. The classical ballet dancer also is less likely to perform movements while sitting, kneeling, or lying on the dance surface. The modern dancer, on the other hand, engages in a great many movements while sitting, kneeling, or lying on the dance surface and may not wear shoes or tights covering the feet and ankles. But modern dancers are not as likely to develop the special problems associated with the use of *pointe* shoes by the classical ballet dancer.

The female jazz dancer required to work for prolonged periods in very high heels may develop a posterior impingement syndrome because of the position of extreme equinus of the ankles required in wearing very high heels. Essentially, the foot of the female jazz dancer in very high heels is in *demi-pointe* position.

Ethnic dancers who perform barefoot may develop foot problems similar to those seen in modern dancers.

Modern dance, also known as contemporary dance, had its origins in America and to some extent in Europe, particularly in Germany, in the early part of this century. It was born out of a desire to develop a freer form of dance that would allow the expression of a broader spectrum of feeling and emotion than was possible within the "artificial" confines and rigid rules and structure of the classical ballet. Early modern dancers such as Isadora Duncan shocked the dance world by dancing barefoot, free of the rigid, "unnatural" confines of the *pointe* shoe worn by the female classical ballet dancer.[1] The absence of footwear, however, exposed the modern dancer's foot to adversities not encountered by the classical ballet dancer. The style of movement developed by the early modern dancers was also quite different from that seen in classical ballet in that much "floor work" was involved in the various modern dance techniques. The floor work required the dancer to sit, kneel, or lie on the dance surface in various positions. A modern dance class often begins with exercise and movement on the floor, whereas the classical ballet class begins with barre work, progresses to work standing in the center of the floor, and finally consists of allégro movements across the floor. It is unusual in a classical ballet class to be presented with "floor work."

Jazz dance, which also appears to have originated in America, is characterized by sharp, percussive, angular movements. It is very often seen in Broadway productions and other types of "show-biz" dance. The jazz dancer does wear shoes, either the special jazz shoe that laces up and has a small raised heel and a thin sole, or tennis shoes, high heels, or whatever other type of footwear a particular piece may require. Other types of "show-biz" dance are combinations of classical ballet, modern jazz, jazz dance, and various ethnic forms, depending upon the style and mood that the choreographer wishes to create.

These differences in style and type of movement with the use of various types of footwear produce variations in the types of musculoskeletal problems seen in the various dance forms.

The material that follows is based upon the author's 34 years of experience as a modern and African ethnic dancer and as an orthopedic surgeon treating and observing musculoskeletal injuries related to dance activities. During this 34-year period, the author has treated and observed hundreds of injuries in various types of dancers. The material presented is obtained from the medical files of dancer/patients and from the recollections of the author.

The Foot

Floor Burns

Floor burns are abrasions, usually sustained by modern dancers on the dorsal, lateral, and medial aspects of the foot while performing slides on the floor without the protection of shoes or tights. The affected area is usually "shiny," erythematous, and painful, and a small amount of bleeding may also be present. Treatment consists of cleansing with an antiseptic solution and application of protective coverings such as adhesive bandages or tape. Of course, the maneuver that caused the injury must either be eliminated or performed with better technique in order to avoid repeated damage to the area.

Bone Bruises

These are contusions to the bony prominences of the lower extremities, primarily of the lateral malleolus and, to a lesser extent, the medial malleolus, the dorsal aspect of the toes, and the tibial tubercles. These injuries are most frequently sustained by kneeling on the floor or by other movement that result in traumatic impact of the bony prominence against the dance surface. Bone bruises are best treated by the use of protective coverings such as an elastic wrap, adhesive bandages, or tape, and variation in the movement pattern or improvement of the technique that caused the injury.

Skin Crease Lacerations

Most of the modern dancers and other barefoot dancers seen over the years have complained of lacerations in the skin creases on the soles of the feet, plantar aspect of the toes, and interdigital areas. These small lacerations in the skin creases of the toes and feet may bleed slightly; they are best treated by cleansing with soap and warm water, application of antiseptic solutions, and protection with tape or adhesive bandages. The simple act of good foot hygiene, which can be accomplished by showering before and after dance class, will prevent the lacerations from becoming infected.

Plantar Calluses

Many modern dancers complain of calluses over the plantar aspects of the first, second, and, to some extent, the third and fifth metatarsophalangeal joints. This is thought to be due to the fact that modern dancers do a great deal of work on *demi-pointe* without the protection of shoes or other types of foot coverings. Helpful in preventing these calluses are commercially available sandals that cover and protect the plantar aspect of the metatarsophalangeal joints and the anterior sole of the foot (figure 15-1). Because the posterior aspect of the foot is not covered, the use of this sandal gives the illusion that the dancer is bare footed.

Case Example

A female dancer past 60 years of age had engaged in various free-style dance forms since childhood. The patient was a member of the Katherine Dunham dance company for 3 years, and for about 25 years had headed her own dance company, which performed various types of stylized ethnic dance forms and "show-biz" dancing. She gave a history of having had many floor burns, bruises, and contusions to her feet over the years. She also received a puncture wound to the medial aspect of the arch on the right foot when she stepped on a nail protruding from a stage floor many years before. This patient was seen because of a growth on the dorsal aspect of the left foot that had been present for many years and, according to patient, had not increased in size re-

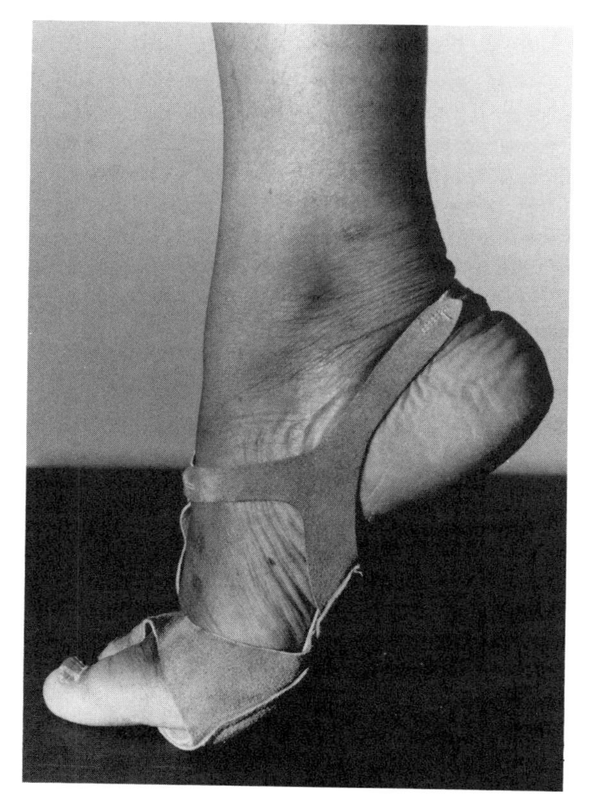

Figure 15-1. The SandaSol® foot protector for modern dancers protects the anterior aspect of the foot with a strap passing between the first and second toes and another strap passing behind the ankle. It gives the illusion that the dancer is barefooted, but provides protection to the forefoot, particularly the ball of the foot while the dancer is working on half-toe.

cently. It measured 1 × 1.5 cm and was nontender to palpation. It was slightly pedunculated. She felt that this growth was the result of many years of engaging in dance activity that required kneeling and sliding on the floor, from which she received trauma to the dorsal aspect of her foot. She requested that the mass be removed surgically.

Splayfoot

Badnin and Sammarco have described in dancers a falling of the longitudinal and transverse arches of the feet causing an increase in the shoe size over a period of years.[2,3] This is said to be due to the fact that dance requires a great deal of weight bearing on the feet, with an increased amount of stress on the transverse and longitudinal arches of the feet, causing them to flatten. The author has encountered many dancers over the years who indicate that as they have grown older, their shoe size has increased by one-half to a full size.

Fractures of the Phalanges

Fractures of the toes occur in modern dancers because the female dancer does not have the protection of the toe shoe used in classical ballet. On the other hand, the female modern dancer seldom develops the dorsal digital calluses and onycholysis seen in the female classical ballet dancer who uses the *pointe* shoe. Fractures of the sesamoid bones have been seen in tap dancers as a result of "slam" movements in which the plantar aspect of the foot repeatedly strikes the dance surface. Fractures of the sesamoid bones may also occur in Far East dancers, who perform a great many activities in the *demi-pointe* position with the knees flexed.

The Ankle

Impingement Syndromes

The posterior and anterior impingement syndromes have often been described in the dance medicine literature,[4,5,6] with the posterior impingement syndrome seen primarily in classical ballet dancers. The author has, however, seen one case of posterior impingement syndrome that became a problem for a jazz or "show-biz" dancer.

The anterior impingement syndrome may be present in both classical ballet and modern dancers because both of these dance forms require *demi-plié* and *grand plié*. The syndrome is caused by the impingement of the anterior lip of the tibia on the neck of the talus. If osteophytes develop in the area, they may require surgical excision and may recur even after excision. The dancer's *grand plié* may be permanently limited.[5]

Case Example

A 23-year-old female's dance activity at the time of evaluation required the use of very high heeled shoes. Examination revealed that she had asymmetry of the point of the left foot as compared to the right; that is, she was able to flex the right foot plantarward 15-20° more than the left foot. She demonstrated tenderness to palpation of the posterior aspect of the left ankle and complained of pain upon attempting to flex the left foot and ankle plantarward beyond a certain point. She indicated that this was a problem for her because it was difficult for her to wear heels (requiring extreme plantar flexion of both feet and ankles) and perform the many strenuous movements required during a specific dance. X-rays of both ankles revealed no evidence of an os trigonum. We therefore concluded that this patient had a pinching of the synovium and capsule in the posterior aspect of the left ankle, probably brought on by the use of the left lower extremity as support during turns and other maneuvers done on one leg. Conservative management was begun, consisting of avoidance of high heels, a physical therapy program, and use of oral anti-inflammatory medications. We had initially expected to find an os trigonum because of the clinical presentation of the problem. She responded well to conservative treatment and did not require surgical intervention.

Ankle Sprains

Ankle sprains have been described as the most common acute injury in dance, and this is certainly true in classical ballet. Ankle sprains are also seen in modern dancers, but to a lesser extent, possibly because the female is not on *pointe* or *demi-pointe* as much as the classical ballet dancer. Ankle sprains are treated by rest, ice, compression, elevation, casting, or surgical intervention, depending on the severity of the sprain.

Tendinitis

Tendinitis of the Achilles tendon, the flexor hallucis longus, and the peroneal tendons is very common among all classical ballet, modern, and "show-biz" dancers. This is undoubtedly due to the fact that a great deal of plantar flexion and dorsiflexion and other movements of the ankle are required in all of these dance forms. Tendinitis is best treated by rest, physical therapy, and oral anti-inflammatory medications. Should the tendinitis of the medial tendons become a chronic problem, surgical intervention for release of the flexor hallucis longus from a stenosed tunnel or correction of other problems in the area may be necessary.[4]

The Knee and Foreleg

Contusions about the Knee

Modern dancers, because they do a great deal of kneeling on the dance surface, may suffer trauma to the anterior aspect of the knee. Because of certain activities that are done lying on the side, they may experience trauma to the lateral aspect of the knee. These abrasions, bruises, or contusions are treated as appropriate. Any maneuver requiring twisting of the femur on the tibia done by a dancer in any dance form may result in tearing of the meniscus. I have encountered one case of a male modern dancer who performed a rotation of the body to his left while bearing weight entirely upon the right lower extremity. This required shifting the femur while the foreleg and foot were stationary. He developed a tear of the medial meniscus and partial tearing of the medial collateral ligament, requiring surgery.

The Snapping Hip

The snapping hip, seen in all types of dancers, has been variously described as being caused by the movement of various tendons over bony prominences of the lateral and medial aspects of the hip joint. In most cases, this condition can be treated conservatively with warm-up exercises and/or strengthening of the anterolateral musculature in the hip joint. Surgical intervention for release of the iliopsoas tendon has been described, but is rarely necessary.[7]

Spine and Upper Extremities

We have not observed any significant difference in injury patterns between various dance forms in spine and upper extremity problems. Dancers in all of the various disciplines, particularly male dancers who perform lifts, develop pulled muscles in the back, osteoarthritic changes of the spine, and herniation of lumbar disks. Tendinitis about the shoulder may be seen in dancers who engage in a great deal of *port de bras* work. Badnin has described an increased incidence of osteoarthritis of the cervical spine in Russian female classical ballet dancers.[2] He attributes this to the increased amount of more elaborate cervical spine movements required of the classical Russian ballerina as compared to the male dancer. Degenerative arthritis in general is thought to occur earlier in dancers than in nondancers because dancers subject their musculoskeletal systems to more "wear and tear."

Summary

The major differences in the occurrence of soft tissue and musculoskeletal injuries between the modern jazz and "show-biz" dancers and classical ballet dancers appear to be in the lower extremities. In the modern dancer, the absence of protective shoe covering and the absence of tights covering the feet produce certain problems. Modern dance movements requiring sitting, kneeling, and lying on the floor are also a contributing factor in producing lower extremity problems. Problems of the cervical, thoracic, and lumbar spine and of the upper extremities are probably equal in most of the major dance forms.

References

1. Washington EL. Musculoskeletal injuries in theatrical dancers: site, frequency and severity. Am J Sports Med 1978; 6,2:75-98.
2. Badnin I, Nironova ZS. Injuries and diseases of the locomotor apparatus in ballet dancers. 1st ed. Moscow: Central Institute for Traumatology and Orthopaedics, 1976.
3. Sammarco GJ, Miller EH. Forefoot conditions in dancers, part 1 and part 2. Foot Ankle 1982; 3:85-98.
4. Hamilton WG. Stenosing tenosynovitis of the flexor hallucis longus tendon and posterior impingement upon the os trigonum in ballet dancers. Foot Ankle 1982; 3:74.
5. Kleiger B. Anterior tibial talar impingement syndrome in dancers. Foot Ankle 1982; 3:69.
6. Hardaker WT Jr, Margello S, Goldner JL. Foot and ankle injuries in theatrical dancers. Foot Ankle 1985; 6:59-69.
7. Schaberg JE, Harper MC, Allan WC. The snapping hip syndrome. Am J Sports Med1984; 12:361-365.

16

A MEDICAL AND SOCIOLOGICAL CONSIDERATION OF BREAK DANCERS AND POP-LOCKERS

Ernest L. Washington, M.D.

Introduction

THE TERM *BREAK DANCING* has been used in the news media and medical literature to refer to both true break dancing and the related, but different, form of street dancing known as pop-locking. There are significant differences between the types and styles of movement in these two forms of street dance. Recognition of these differences will subsequently be shown to be important from a medical standpoint.

Break dancing is characterized by elaborate acrobatic, gymnastlike movements with leaps into the air and spins on the crown of the head and on the back. "Floor work" or "foot work" with the body in a semihorizontal position and supported on one or the other arms is also characteristic of break dancing (figure 16-1).

Pop-lockers, on the other hand, rarely, if ever, allow the body or upper extremities to touch the dancing surface. The dance movement in this form of street dance consists of robotlike movements of the spine, arms, and legs (figures 16-2-A, 16-2-B, 16-2-C). The fact that the pop-lockers rarely, if ever, touch the dancing surface with the body or upper extremities is a very significant difference between these two forms of street dance from a medical standpoint. This and other differences apparently have not been recognized previously in the medical literature.

Break dancing emerged 15 years ago in the South Bronx, a section of New York City, as a less destructive, nonviolent form of confrontation between urban youth gangs. Pop-locking, on the other hand, had its origins in the black urban areas of Los Angeles. Both "breaking" and "popping" have become

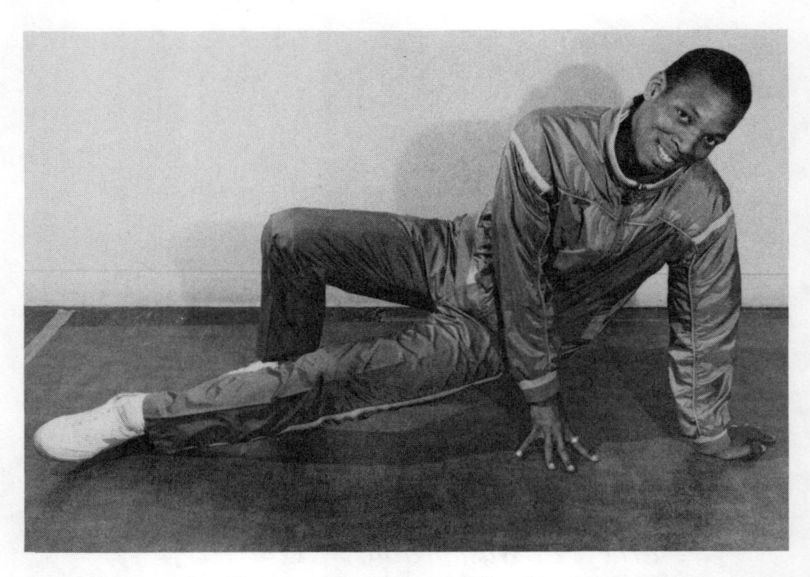

Figure 16-1. The "foot work" characteristic of break dancing is accomplished with the body in a semihorizontal position supported on one upper extremity or the other. Note that the wrist of the supporting upper extremity is in extreme dorsiflexion with weight bearing through the wrist.

popular as a means of nonviolent confrontation between rival groups and groups with different ethnic origins. Law enforcement agencies in many areas have noted a decrease in criminal activity among youths, and have attributed the decrease to the redirection of destructive energy into break dance and pop-locking. In a survey of 48 break dancers, Smith found that 73% of those surveyed showed no lowering of school grades as a result of engaging in this activity.[1] It appears that the overall social impact of the two forms of dance on urban youth has been a positive one.

Review of Medical Literature

Norman and Grodin have described their experience with break dance-related medical problems at the Boston City Hospital.[2] They describe what they called the "break dance back syndrome" seen in eight male break dancers in a 3-month period of 1984. The patients, ranging in age from 11 to 18 years, each presented with symptoms of lower back pain and difficulty in bending over after a day of break dancing. They found no neuromuscular deficits, and the patients were treated with rest, heat, and analgesia as well as instruction in proper safety and training for break dancing. They also describe an adolescent male with back pain following break dancing who was diagnosed as having a fracture of the spinuous process of the third thoracic vertebra. They also report break dance injuries involving the elbow, wrist, knee, ankle, and foot as well as

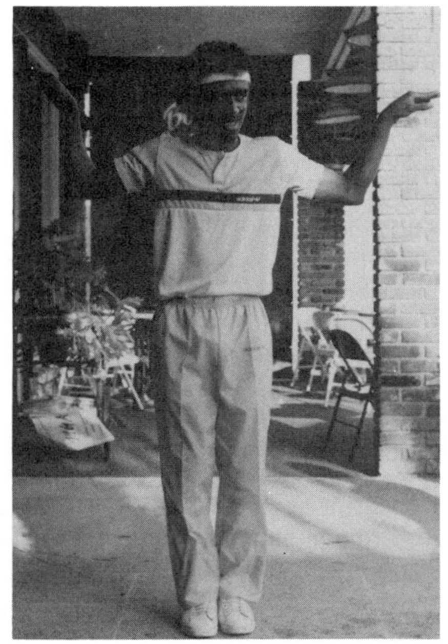

A

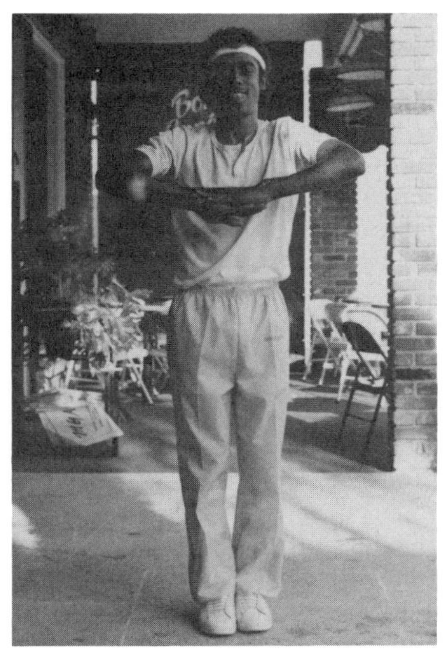

B

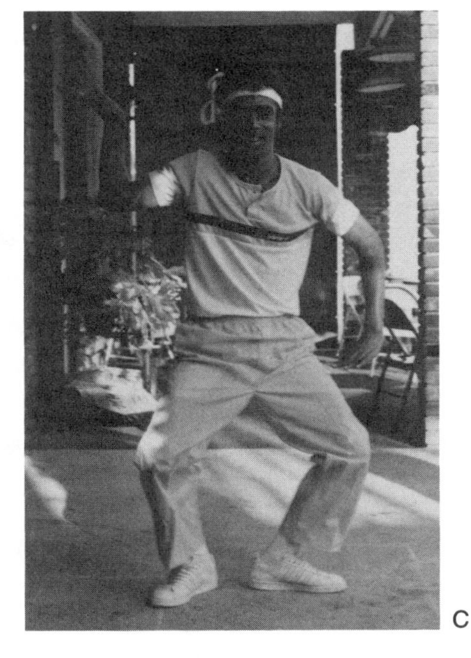

C

Figure 16-2-A, 16-2-B, 16-2-C. This dancer specializes in pop-locking and has an amazing variety of movements consisting of percussive snapping and popping of the cervical, thoracic, and lumbar spines as well as the upper and lower extremities. Notice that the arms, hands and upper part of the body never touch the dancing surface.

three fractures of both the radius and ulna. These authors believe that the incidence of injury in break dancing is similar to that in other unsupervised athletic activities. The authors recommend that break dancers practice on mats that are 4 in. thick, and express their belief that a "sprung" wood floor is the best surface for practice or performance because it decreases the incidence of stress fractures. They also suggest that adequate warm-up prior to dancing and cool-down after dancing are extremely important. They point out that many problems can be prevented by careful screening, instruction, supervision, and training.

Goscienski and Luevanos describe three cases presenting with a firm swelling and pain in the mid- and lower back area in boys who had been engaging in break dancing with repeated "spins" on the thoracolumbar area with the thoracolumbar spine flexed[3] (figure 16-3). The swellings, found to be in the area of the lower thoracic and upper lumbar spine, measured about 6- to 9 cm. They noted minimal hyperpigmentation of the overlying skin, but no ecchymosis or tenderness. They also found that the swelling was considerably more prominent when the patient bent forward from the waist. X-rays showed no fractures of the spinous processes or calcification within the swellings. Treatment consisted of advising the patient to discontinue back spins. No further treatment was necessary if the patient followed this instruction. In consulting with other physicians in the San Diego area, the authors learned of other injuries related to break dancing. These included two fractures of the radius, two fractures of the clavicle, an atlantoaxial dislocation, a torn medialcollateral ligament of the knee, neck strain with torticollis, and severe sprains of the ankle and thumb. They indicate that although most problems seen in break dancers

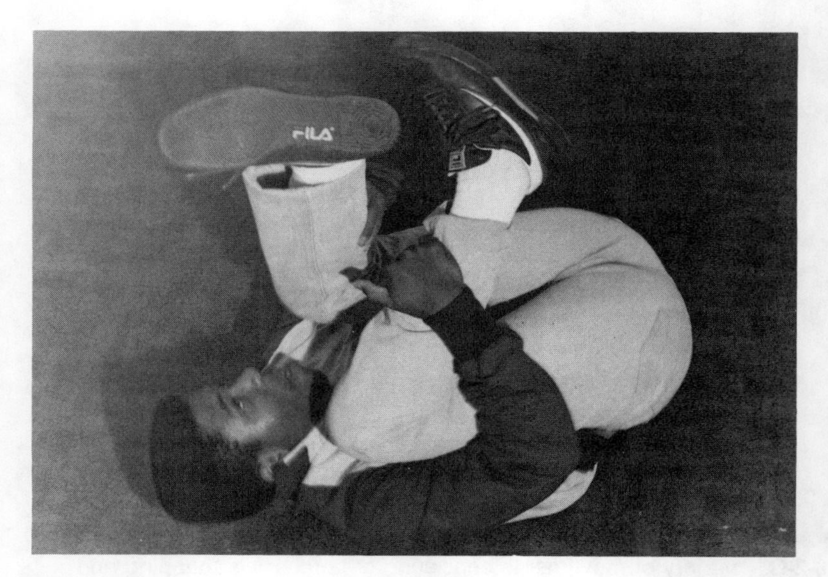

Figure 16-3. Spins on the thoracolumbar spine with the thoracolumbar spine and hips flexed may cause soft tissue masses on the thoracolumbar area associated with lower back pain.

have been minor, the potential for severe life-threatening injuries is great. They caution physicians to inquire more thoroughly into the nature of activity that results in both common and uncommon injuries. Copperman describes two cases of alopecia that he attributed to the "head spins" commonly seen in break dancing.[4] The author suggested that this condition be named "alopecia breakdancia." In a short letter to the editor of the *New York State Journal of Medicine,* Leung reports cervical cord injury as a result of break dancing.[5] He indicates that other kinds of injuries may result from break dancing such as muscular strains, tendinitis, stress fractures, spondylolysis, dislocations of the elbow, and ankle capsulitis. He stresses the importance of public education regarding the potential hazards of break dancing.

McBride and Lehman of the New York University-Bellevue Hospital Center in New York City describe three cases of cervical spine injury resulting from break dancing.[6] These authors point out that the acrobatic dance movements seen in break dancing carry considerable risk, as evidenced by three cervical spine injuries, one of which resulted in permanent quadriplegia. This severe injury was sustained by a 25-year-old professional dancer who attempted a flip, but landed on the top of his head instead of on the shoulder. He was rendered immediately quadriplegic, and x-rays showed a compression fracture and subluxation of the fifth cervical vertebra. He was placed in halo cervical traction and underwent C-4 to C-6 laminectomy and fusion. The patient had not, at the time the article was written, recovered neurologic function, and somatosensory-evoked potentials remained absent.

A second case reported by these authors was that of a 13-year-old boy who developed severe neck and right arm pain after falling on his head while attempting to do a flip. X-rays revealed a fracture of the spinous process of C-7 and loss of the normal lordotic curvature of the cervical spine. He was treated with a soft cervical collar, and his pain lessened over the following 3 weeks. The third patient was a 15-year-old boy who sustained neck injury while doing a head spin when the cardboard mat on which he was spinning slipped on the pavement. He sustained a flexion injury of the cervical spine and felt shooting pain down the spine to the lower back. Numbness in the left arm and hand was also reported. Decreased deep pain sensation over the C-6 and C-7 dermatomes to the left upper extremity were noted, but he was otherwise neurologically intact. Cervical spine x-rays revealed straightening and slight prevertebral soft tissue swelling. No bone injuries were noted, and the patient's symptomatology resolved over a 7-day period.

An unusual spiral fracture of the distal midshaft of the fifth metatarsal as a result of break dancing is reported by Dieden.[7] This fracture may occur either from inversion of the supporting foot during the crossover step or improper planting of the crossover foot during the crossover step (figures 16-4-A, 16-4-B, 16-4-C). The author notes that break dancing can be expected to produce uncommon injuries, including fractures in unusual locations.

Smith describes the types of injuries he found in a study of 48 break dancers.[1] In this rather extensive review of the social and medical aspects of break dancing, the author, who at the time was a fourth-year medical student at the University of San Diego School of Medicine, reports that this study showed back injuries that were apparently related to hyperextension of the

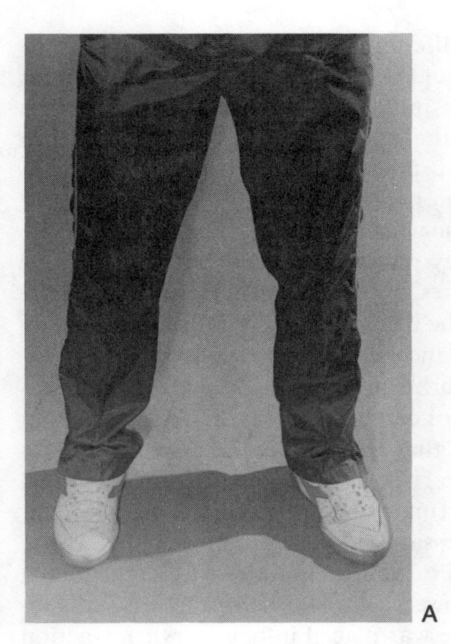

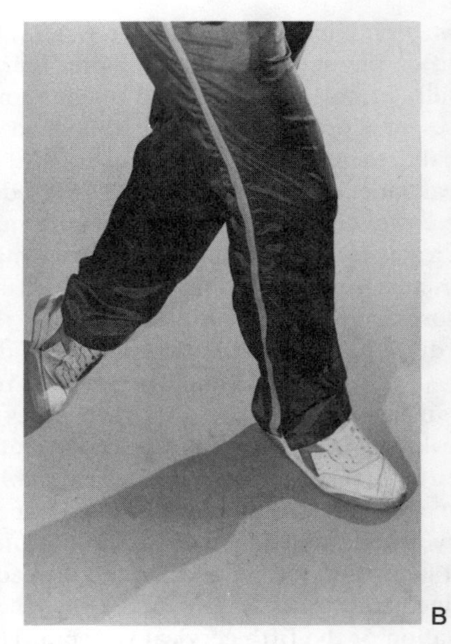

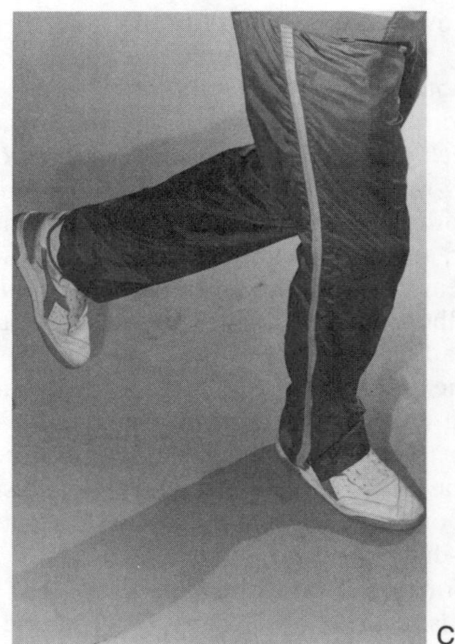

Figure 16-4 A, B, C. (A) The cross step is begun with both feet planted on the dancing surface. (B) One foot then crosses over the other foot. If the foot is not in proper position at this time, or if it is prematurely planted with the foot in some inversion, a fracture of the fifth metatarsal may occur. (C) The final position of the crossover step with the crossing over foot firmly planted on the dancing surface. If this final step is performed properly, fracture of the fifth metatarsal may be avoided.

spine. He also describes swellings in the thoracolumbar spine area that were associated with back spins and finger fractures and sprains that were usually related to "floor moves" or "foot work." ("Foot work" is a break dance movement where the dancer supports his weight on his hands while he uses his feet to "run" around the body and occasionally kick, alternately shifting weight from one hand to the other [figure 16-5].) The fingers are vulnerable in many other moves as well, most notably the "windmill" and "hand spins." Fractures of the forearms are described as occurring during "head spins" and "hand glides," where the entire body is balanced on the weight of one arm with the wrist in extreme dorsiflexion. The "cricket," in which the dancer squats with his legs twisted around his arms, has also reportedly been the cause of forearm fractures. Smith also describes groin injuries where the ligaments are overstretched when the legs get caught on the dance surface during scissoring movement such as that done during the "windmill." He also describes testicular injuries that may occur during the "worm," in which a dancer flips and rolls on his chest, pelvis, forearms, and thighs. Alopecia was also reported in this study.

Broome and Heppenstall have described "break dancer's bursitis."[8] The lesion they describe is essentially the same as that described by other investigators reporting patients presenting with a swelling in the midback area associated with a hypertrophic reaction to back spins and windmills. They state that there was no discoloration or trauma to the overlying skin. In one of the three

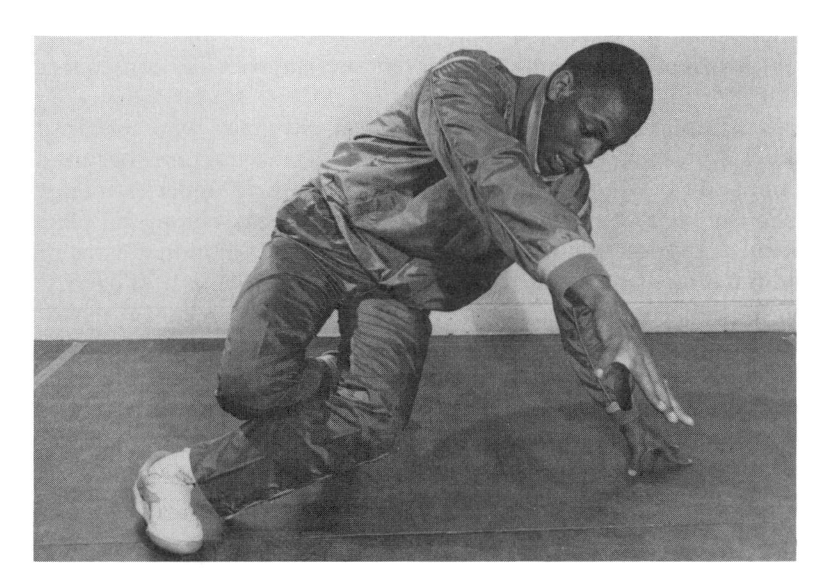

Figure 16-5. As "foot work" progresses, rapid scissoring movements of the legs occur as the body rotates around the supporting upper extremity. Note that weight bearing is now occurring through the tips of the fingers of the hand of the supporting upper extremity. This position of the hand is said to predispose the dancer to fractures and sprains of the fingers and thumb.

cases reported, the mass was surgically removed. Histology showed a preponderance of dense, reactive, fibrous tissue with an increased amount of vascularity. They felt that this histological picture was most consistent with a reactive fibrosis and adventitial bursitis secondary to repetitive, chronic trauma such as "housemaid's knee" (a great deal of kneeling), and "policeman's heel" (extensive walking, with impact being mainly on the heel).

Bithoney has reported three additional cases of lower back pain in children associated with a mass in the thoracolumbar area.[9] All three children had been break dancing extensively. The author points out that complaints of back pain are unusual in a child, but that many elements of break dancing apply stress to the back and put the dancer at considerable risk for soft tissue and muscle damage compatible with a mechanical derangement of the lower back. He reports that the injury seems self-limiting and reversible, but whether it predisposes the individual to a more serious back condition later in life is unknown. Treatment consists of discontinuing break dancing, applying moist heat locally, rest on a firm sleeping surface, and symptomatic use of analgesics as well as follow-up to document resolution of the mass in the midback area.

Moses and Shannon have reported the development of osteomyelitis in a fracture of the spinous process of a thoracic vertebra in a 9-year-old male break dancer.[10] They postulate that break dancing had somehow altered the mucous makeup of the nasal passage, allowing the entrance of *Staphylococcus aureus* into the blood stream. The combination of *S. aureus* septicemia superimposed upon a nondisplaced fracture of the spinous process allowed the development of osteomyelitis at the fracture site in the spinous process of the vertebra. The authors conclude that this is but one example of break dance injuries and that appropriate supervision and training may prevent such injuries and consequent complications.

Hansen has reported the cases of two 14-year-old males who sustained fractures (Salter type 1) of the proximal humerus.[11] These fractures occurred while the entire body weight was supported upon the injured upper extremity. The author states that a shearing force on a relatively weak epiphyseal plate was the probable cause of fracture. He also predicts that additional cases of this uncommon fracture will result from break dancing, particularly in dancers younger than 18. In his opinion, youngsters under 18 should not engage in maneuvers in which the full body weight is borne on one arm.

Surpure et al describe generalized aches and pains in a 9-year-old male break dancer.[12] The patient also had a stiff neck and a mass in the scapular area. The history of break dancing was not elicited until the examination was almost over. The authors suggest that the medical community should, in young people presenting with generalized aches and pains, lumps and masses, and complaints of pain in the low back area, consider the possibility that break dancing is a causative factor. They observe that break dancing can cause a wide range of injuries, the most serious of which so far appears to be a slipped capital femoral epiphysis. Wrist and finger fractures and soft tissue injuries also occurred. They also point out that muscle and joint sprains accompany slips and spins and that break dancing applies stress and strain to the soft tissue, placing the dancer at considerable risk for muscle and ligament damage. According to these authors, the damage seems to be self-limiting, but whether this could predispose to a more chronic condition is unknown.

Gerber et al have described "break dancer's wrist."[13] This is the first report of a growth plate abnormality caused by chronic, repetitive trauma in break dancing. X-rays of the 14-year-old patient's painful wrist revealed widening and displacement of the distal ulna physis with metaphyseal irregularity. This resulted from the patient's having supported the weight of the entire body on one arm with the wrist in maximal dorsiflexion. This apparently was an important part of this patient's routine, and the authors concluded that the chronic trauma from the maneuver produced the epiphyseal changes in the distal ulna. The patient was immobilized in a short arm cast for 6 weeks, with resultant resolution of his symptoms and radiographic evidence of healing of the distal ulna.

It is obvious from the literature that a wide range of injuries can result from break dancing. Not one of the articles reviewed distinguished between break dancing and pop-locking. Our experience with break dancers in the Los Angeles area indicates that there are significant differences and the medical problems with which the dancers present differ to some extent.

Medical Problems: The Los Angeles Experience

The following section is based on the author's experience with the 120-member Los Angeles Breakers Break Dance Company, other break dance companies in the Los Angeles area, and individual break dance patients. The author became company physician to the Los Angeles Breakers Break Dance Company in early 1984. The dancers range in age from 4 to 25 years; some consider themselves professional dancers, while others engage in the activity on a recreational basis.

Injuries I have encountered have been principally muscle sprains, contusions, and abrasions. A number of thumb sprains have been reported, and one dancer who was not seen by me was hospitalized for a thumb fracture that eventually was placed in a cast but did not require surgery. In discussion of finger and hand injuries, many of the dancers stated that injuries of the thumb are very common, one declaring that "the broken thumb is the trademark of the break dancer." The dancers also report that the "windmill" appears to be the most consistent cause of abrasions and contusions as well as other trauma to the musculoskeletal system. The windmill is done on the floor in the supine position, with the hips widely abducted and the lower spine, midspine, shoulders, and cervical spine alternately coming in contact with the dancing surface. The body "spins like a top" during the maneuver. The elbows also come into contact with the dancing surface in a repetitive, consistent pattern. In observing them in action, we noted that the dancers had themselves devised makeshift padding to protect bony prominences such as the illiac crest and the spinous processes of the spine (particularly the seventh cervical spinous process) from trauma. Knee pads, elbow pads, and gloves were commonly worn by the break dancers but not by the exclusive pop-lockers because the pop-lockers do not engage in movement requiring arms, hands or upper body to touch the dancing surface. These precautions had not been recommended by me or by any other medical personnel.

Of particular interest to me were the problems reported by the exclusive pop-lockers in the company. The mother of one 9-year-old dancer reported that he frequently complained of headaches after pop-locking for several hours. The mother reported that the child engaged in the activity almost constantly. She stated that the headache pain seemed to be self-limiting if the child refrained from the repeated snapping of the cervical spine called for in pop-locking. Other pop-lockers in the company indicated that they would develop pain after "hitting too hard," referring to the percussive snapping of the cervical spine and upper extremities during pop-locking. They stated that if the snapping was "softened," they did not develop headache. The mechanism of injury and etiology of the headache is probably very similar to that of the whiplash injury sustained in automobile accidents when the vehicle is struck from the rear. The percussive snapping forward and back of the cervical spine in this type of accident produces muscle spasm and subsequent referred headache. It is therefore worthwhile when presented with headache of apparent undetermined etiology in a child or adolescent to ask whether the patient engages in pop-locking.

Membership of the Los Angeles Breakers has dropped from 120 in 1984 to a nucleus of approximately 10 to 15 dancers at this writing, indicating an apparent decline in interest and participation in break dancing and pop-locking. A combination break dancing and pop-locker patient 26 years of age presented information that could help explain the decreased participation and popularity. He said that many of his friends had stopped because they were "hurting all over." He said he had discontinued head spins because he had developed significant neck pain and an x-ray had shown a loss of the normal lordotic curvature of the cervical spine. He stated that a number of his friends had discontinued head spins because of pain in the cervical spine. After discontinuation of head spins, the pain and discomfort in the cervical spine reportedly subsided.

Other patients have pointed out that the position of the hands during the floor work or foot work while break dancing may be important in preventing finger and thumb fractures. The best position to prevent finger injury is with the wrist in maximal dorsiflexion and with the palm flat on the dancing surface. Other positions, such as with the metacarpophalangeal joint in dorsiflexion or the fingertips supporting the weight of the body, are more likely to produce fractures and injuries to the fingers and thumb.

Injury Surveys of Dancers, Physicians, and Teachers

In June 1984, about 50 break dancers were asked to complete a questionnaire concerning their experience with injuries associated with break dancing or pop-locking. A total of 69 injuries were reported by 22 out of 30 respondents; 8 reported no injuries. All respondents were male. The age range was 13-23 years, with a mean age of 17.35 years and a median age of 18 years. The results are displayed in table 16-1. Injuries to the hand were most frequently reported, followed by pulled thigh muscles and problems affecting the hip.

Another survey form was sent to 210 physicians in the Los Angeles area. The form, which asked the respondent to describe any injuries seen that were related to break dancing or pop-locking, went primarily to orthopedic sur-

Table 16-1. Sites of Injury, in Order of Anatomic Frequency, in 69 Break Dance and Pop-Lock Injuries

Site of Injury	No. Injuries	% of Total
1. Hand	16	23
Thumb	10	
Fingers	3	
2. Thigh	9	13
Pulled muscles	8	
3. Hip	8	11.8
Bruised	6	
Swelling	2	
4. Ankle	6	8.7
Sprained	6	
Shoulder	6	
Sprained	1	
Bruised	5	
5. Wrist	5	7.5
Sprained	3	
Knee	5	7.5
Sprained	1	
Pulled muscles	3	
Back	5	7.5
Bruised	3	
Swelling	2	
6. Neck	4	5.75
Pulled muscles	3	
Bruised	1	
7. Foot	3	4.5
Bruised	2	
Broken	1	
8. Head	2	3
Bruised	1	
Cuts	1	

geons, but some pediatricians and general practitioners were also included. Of the 16 responses received, only 3 physicians stated that they had seen injuries resulting from break dancing or pop-locking. The first physician described a "lump on the back" as a result of break dance activity. The second described a fracture of the radius in a 14-year-old male break dancer, and the third told of three ligamentous injuries of the thumb he had seen. Two of these injuries required surgical repair of the ulnar collateral ligament and the other required casting only. We concluded from the low response to the survey that most of the recipients had not seen injuries resulting from break dancing. This reinforced our impression that the incidence of serious injury in break dancers is probably very low. It should be remembered, however, that the few injuries that do occur can be quite serious, and the medical community must must be prepared to evaluate and deal with them.

Emergency room physicians at a 400-bed hospital were sent a form requesting information on injuries or problems related to break dancing. Respondents indicted that they had seen no such injuries, but noted that they had not specifically inquired if an injury had resulted from the activity. Very often the patients would say, "I was playing." It is therefore important for the physician when confronted with a problem that may be related to break dancing to specifically question the patient about possible break dancing or pop-locking.

Break dancing and pop-locking often come under the supervision of a classically trained dance teacher. Communication with one such teacher[14] with rather extensive experience with break dancers revealed the following problems: (1) loss of hair as a result of head spins, (2) complaints of mid- and lower back pain, (3) skin bruises, (4) shoulder and elbow injuries from performing windmills, and (5) many wrist complaints. This teacher stated that the wrist problems seemed to occur when weight bearing on one upper extremity is required with the wrist in maximal dorsiflexion. She also has noted a significant decline in break dancing because many of the dancers were having pain in the arms, legs, and back.

Summary and Conclusions

A review of the medical literature and the author's experience with break dancers and pop-lockers in the Los Angeles area indicates that the incidence of serious injury to participants is probably very low. The literature revealed that each investigator reporting problems seen in this group had no more than 8 to 10 cases to report, in many instances only 2 or 3 cases. These numbers are very low considering the large numbers of patients who participate in break dancing and pop-locking and the significant number of patients seen at the medical centers from which many of the reports came. When it does occur however, injury can be very serious.

According to the literature, the most common significant problem appears to be back pain associated with a mass in the thoracolumbar area. Because low back pain is an unusual complaint in pediatric or adolescent age groups, it may be an indication that the patient is engaging extensively in break dance activity; if so, back pain and a lump or mass on the back do not necessarily require an extensive (and expensive) workup to identify other causes of the symptoms.

Fractures about the growth centers of immature bones may also be a significant factor in young dancers who attempt full-body weight bearing on one upper extremity. Of particular interest are reports of testicular torsion or groin pain after engaging in break dancing and the loss of hair due to head spins. It should be noted that most of these problems are unlikely to occur in the pop-lockers because, unlike break dancers, these dancers do not do extensive floor work in the semihorizontal position or other gymnast-like movements. The rapid crossing over and scissoring of the legs on floor work is thought to be an etiologic factor in the testicular torsion reported in the literature. The literature repeatedly stresses (and this author agrees) that supervision, adequate warm-up and cool-down, and use of protective padding are very important factors in preventing injuries in these dancers.

The two forms of dance discussed in this chapter apparently have had positive social impacts. Decrease in criminal activity among urban youth participants in these activities and improved scholastic performance in some cases have been reported. Although the popularity and number of participants in break dancing and pop-locking have significantly decreased from peaks in the early 1980s, it seems likely that the activities will continue to be enjoyed by children and adolescents all over the country for some time to come. It is therefore particularly important that the general medical community, and certainly those members of the medical community who treat dancers, maintain a high index of suspicion for the particular and peculiar types of medical problems that have been described in break dancers and pop-lockers.

References

1. Smith CE. Break dance injuries. Dance Med-Health Newsletter Winter 1984-Spring 1985; 2-10.
2. Norman RA, Grodin M A. Injuries from break dancing. Am Fam Phys 1984; 30(4): 109-12.
3. Goscienski PJ., Luevanos L. Injury caused by break dancing. JAMA 1984; 252(24):3367.
4. Copperman SM, Two new cases of alopecia (letter). JAMA 1984; 252(24):3367.
5. Leung AKC. Hazards of break dancing. N.Y. State Med 1984; 85(12): 592.
6. McBride DQ, Lehman LP, Mangiardi JR. Break-dancing neck. New Engl J Medicine 1985; 312(3):186.
7. Dieden JD. Break dancer's fracture of the fifth metatarsal (letter). West J Med 1985; 142(1):101.
8. Broome HE, Heppenstall RB. Break dancer's bursitis. JAMA 1985; 253(6):777.
9. Bithoney WG. Breaker's back (letter). Pediatrics 1985; 75(3):616.
10. Moses J, Shannon M. Back pain, vomiting after break dance mishap. Hosp Pract (off) Mar 15, 1985; 20(3): 100K-100L, 100P.
11. Hansen GR. Breaks and other bad breaks for breakers. JAMA 1985; 253(14):2047.
12. Surpure JS, Reeves J, Coussons H. Breaking pains and arthralgias! (letter). Am J Dis Child 1985; 139(11):1072-3.
13. Gerber SD, Griffin P P, Simmons B P. Break dancer's wrist. Pediatr Orthop 1986; 6(1): 98-9.
14. Lawrence BEM. Personal communication June 1986, Los Angeles, CA.

17

AEROBIC DANCE INJURIES AND THEIR PREVENTION

James G. Garrick, M.D.

SOME MAY CONSIDER A chapter on aerobic dance out of place in a book dealing with various dance forms because they regard aerobic "dance" as merely exercise to music. This may be true, but the activity can hardly be ignored in view of the fact that there are currently some 23 million participants, many of whom find the activity appealing because they consider it dancing.

Aerobic dance currently exists in many forms. Some programs have been heavily influenced by the instructor's jazz or ballet background; others are more purely athletic, with some even employing weight-lifting activities or movements. Some of the recent nonimpact aerobic programs have their origins in the martial arts.

Unlike many other dance forms requiring a formal studio setting, aerobic dance is performed in a variety of environments. Although classes appear to have the greatest appeal, the availability of many videotapes provides the opportunity to participate in the home at one's convenience.

The popularity of the activity, along with the quest for variety—and sometimes safety—has spawned numerous aerobic offshoots, including non- and low-impact aerobics, stretch aerobics, programs using wrist and ankle weights, water aerobics, aerobics during pregnancy, and even aerobics for the elderly. Although many of these activities have strayed from the dance orientation seen in the original programs, they are nonetheless considered part of aerobic dancing.

Most aerobic dance classes follow a similar pattern. The session starts with a warm-up period consisting of exercises that gradually become more strenuous, increasing the heart rate to a "training" level. These exercises often include stretching the major muscle groups to be employed later in the aerobic portion of the class. The second section of the class is the "aerobic" portion, lasting 20-30 min. and designed to maintain a heart rate of 65-80% of an age-corrected maximum (figure 17-1). The final activities allow a gradual decrease in heart rate and include antigravity floor exercises as well as a more extensive series of stretching exercises.

Aerobic Dance Participants

Participants can be divided into three groups according to their general activity levels. The most sedentary of these groups makes up 40-50% of the aerobic dance population. These participants are usually women 30-50 years old. Except for the activities of daily living, aerobic dance is their only effort toward fitness enhancement or athletics. If they engage in other activities, such as tennis, golf, skiing, or cycling, it is usually intermittent and desultory. This group merits medical consideration because its members are—often for the first time—attempting to become "more fit," but are the least prepared for these new activities.

The second group is roughly the same size as the first. This group consists of individuals who have added aerobic dance to a menu that already contains a variety of sport and recreational activities. Activities and activity levels vary widely within this group. Running, tennis, cycling, skiing, and swimming are among the other activities most frequently pursued in the group. The time committed to these activities can vary from 5 to 30 hr. per week. Although still in a distinct minority, male participants are more common in this group.

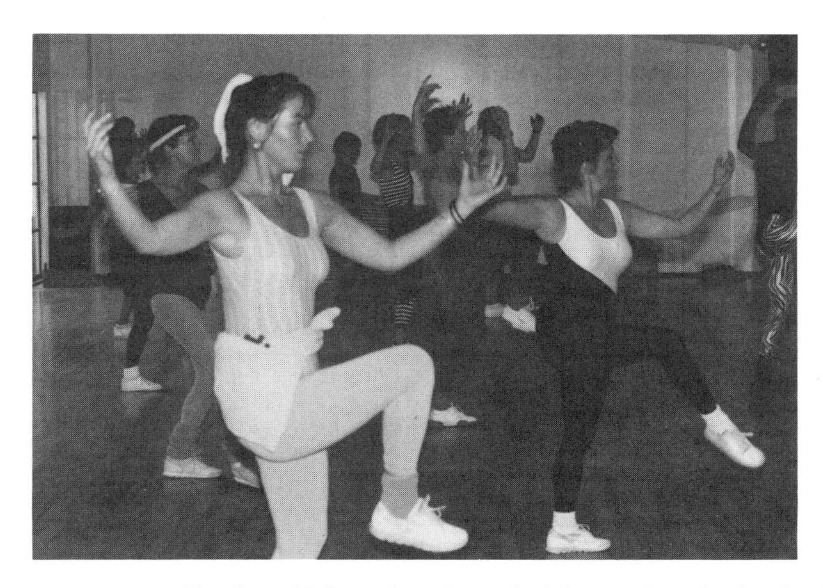

Figure 17-1. The "aerobic" portion of a typical dance class, lasting for 20 to 30 minutes, is designed to maintain a heart rate of 65-80% of an age-corrected maximum.

The third group is made up of aerobic dance instructors. Unlike instructors or coaches in other athletic activities, these teachers are actually demonstrators; thus, the hours spent teaching are, at the same time, hours of intense participation. Although most instructors are remarkably fit, they come from a diversity of backgrounds—from physical education to professional dance.

Injury Studies

Little scientific information dealing with the medical problems associated with aerobic dance is available. Before publication of the study to be reported here, accounts of aerobic dance injuries were either anecdotal or the result of retrospective surveys. Although there was no lack of a willingness to express the usually negative opinions on the "dangers" of aerobic dance, such reports were based either on limited personal experience or on theory. Criticism was based not on the fact that aerobic dance had been shown to be dangerous, but rather that it was developed and taught by those unschooled in exercise physiology, kinesiology, and medicine.

Francis et al in 1985 reported the results of a questionnaire given to instructors attending a workshop dealing with aerobic dance safety.[1] Based on the responses of 135 instructors, the authors characterized the injuries seen in both aerobic dance instructors and students.

They emphasized the fact that 76.3% (103–135) of the instructors had sustained or aggravated one or more injuries as a result of aerobic dancing, going on to indict "impact shock" as a major causative factor. They presented the frequency with which various anatomic sites were involved (table 17-1). No definition of an "injury" was provided, thus one must assume that exactly what constituted an injury was left up to the respondents.

The instructors involved in this survey were relatively experienced; more than 60% had taught aerobic dance for more than 2 years. On average, they

Table 17-1. Sites and Frequency of Injuries (%) Among Aerobic Dance Students and Instructors—Reported in 4 Studies

	Study				
	Ritchie	Francis	Garrick	Garrick et al	
Injury site		(a)	(b)	Students	Instructors
Upper extremity	4.1	—	4.5	2.8	3.6
Spine	14.0	13.2	11.0	11.9	7.2
Hip	2.9	5.5	8.7	4.5	3.6
Thigh	2.8	—	4.8	—	—
Knee	8.9	11.8	32.6	14.7	13.3
Leg/calf/Achilles	38.2	34.5	16.4	28.7	24.1
Ankle	7.1	10.9	6.9	22.9	24.1
Foot	13.5	17.7	13.9	22.9	24.1
Other	8.5	17.7	—	1.2	—

a. Cases included only instructors.
b. All cases required formal medical care.

taught 1.7 classes per day for 4.2 days per week (7.14 classes/week per instructor). No attempt was made to establish relationships between the likelihood of sustaining an injury and length of experience, hours taught, background education, or the age or sex of the instructors.

Using the data presented in the report, one can arrive at a rough estimate of exposure and, hence, injury rates. Assuming 7.14 classes per week, classes lasting 1 hr., and the average instructor (in this group) teaching for 2 years, one arrives at 100,246 hr. of exposure, which produced 220 injuries. The injury rate for these instructors would be 0.22 injuries per 100 hr. of exposure (table 17-2).

Richie and associates also reported the results of a survey of aerobic dance participants.[2] Questionnaires were given to students and instructors at 28 aerobic dance facilities in Sacramento and Long Beach, CA. They noted that the 1,233 respondents represented a "more than 50%" response rate.

Defining an injury as "any condition causing significant pain and/or limiting participation", 534 participants reported 1,075 injuries (43.3% of the students and 75.9% of the instructors). One hundred (9.3%) of the injuries were reported to instructors. Anatomic sites of injuries for both groups were tabulated (table 17-1).

Like the Francis group, the authors emphasized the importance of the role played by footwear and flooring, additionally suggesting that "foot stability is of major importance (figure 17-2)." They examined the relationship between flooring types and the percentage of participants (participating on a particular floor) who reported injuries. The highest proportion of injuries (50%) occurred on a concrete floor covered with carpet, followed by wood-over-airspace floor covered with padded carpet (47%), wood-over airspace floor (38%), and concrete floor "heavily padded and covered with carpet" (36%).

These authors reported an increased likelihood of sustaining an injury with frequency of participation as well as increased length of time as a participant. Whether these findings were merely the result of increased exposure was not reported.

Rough estimates of exposure and injury rates can be calculated from the data presented in the report. Assuming 1-hr. classes, the students logged a total of 106,112 hr. of participation (3.31 classes × 26 weeks × 1,233 students), resulting in an injury rate of 1.01 injuries per 100 hr. of participation. The (similarly calculated) rate for instructors as 0.32 per 100 hr. of participation (table 17-2).

In a paper discussing the patient population of a sports medicine clinic, Garrick presented data dealing with 681 aerobic dance injuries seen during a 5-

Table 17-2. Number of Injuries per 100 Hours of Aerobic Dance

Study		No. Injuries/100 hr.
Francis	(instructors)	0.22
Richie	(students and instructors)	1.01
Garrick	(students)	1.16
	(instructors)	0.96

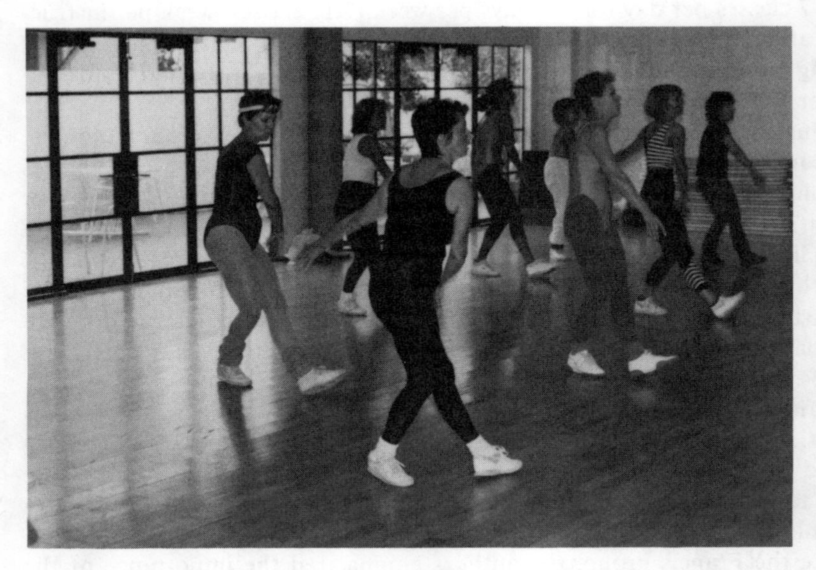

Figure 17-2. Studies of aerobic dancing injuries have emphasized the importance of proper footwear and flooring, additionally suggesting that foot stability is of major importance in minimizing injuries.

year period[1] (table 17-1). In addition, the injuries were characterized by type (table 17-3) and ages of those injured (table 17-4).

Injuries in this report were defined as musculoskeletal problems arising from aerobic dance activities that required the services of a physician. Injury rates could not be ascertained because there was no practical means of establishing the population at risk. Inherent in the definition of injury was a measure of severity, as all of the injuries necessitated a physician visit—"severe" injuries if for no more than economic reasons.

In 1986, Garrick et al reported the results of the first prospective, epidemiologic study of aerobic dance injuries.[4] In a 16-week study, they followed 411 participants with weekly phone calls, documenting the time actually spent engaged in aerobic dance activities as well as the incidence of any musculoskeletal problems. The "injuries" were classified by severity. Grade 1 problems were those producing discomfort but no disability; grade 2 problems resulted in the temporary avoidance or alteration of aerobic dance activities; grade 3 problems resulted in an alteration of the activities of daily living; and grade 4 injuries required formal medical care.

Table 17-3. Severity of 681 Aerobic Dance Injuries over a 5-year period

Severity of injury	Students	Instructors
Grade 1	74.6	72.3
Grade 2	18.4	21.7
Grade 3	4.5	4.8
Grade 4	2.5	1.2

Table 17-4. Age of Patient (% of total) (681 patients)

Age	%
0–12	0.1
13–18	0.6
19–25	14.7
26–39	70.9
40 +	13.2

The study encompassed both students (N = 351) and instructors (N = 60) who amassed 29,924 hr. of collective aerobic dance activity, for an average of 59.8 hr. per student and 148.7 hr. per instructor. Among the students, 155 reported 244 complaints; 45 instructors reported 83 problems. Injury rates for students were 1.16 per 100 hr. of activity and 0.96 per 100 hr. of activity for instructors (table 17-2). The sites of the injuries in both students and instructors are presented in table 17-1.

Nearly three-fourths of the problems were of the grade 1 variety, resulting in no disability (table 17-5). The severity of the injuries differed little between students and instructors. In-depth analysis of the data failed to reveal statistically significant relationships between injury rates and brand of shoe, type of flooring, or age or sex of the participants. Participants with a history of previous orthopedic problems and students who had no other fitness activity appeared to be more likely to sustain an injury.

Discussion and Comment

The main reason for undertaking studies such as those presented here is to attempt to identify potentially alterable variables associated with an increased likelihood of sustaining an injury while participating in aerobic dance activities. Examining an activity from this epidemiologic perspective, however, requires that one know as much about the uninjured (controls) as about those who sustained injuries. Perhaps more important, one must also be able to measure exposure or time at risk (of injury). Finally, the information should be gathered within reasonable proximity to the time the injuries occurred in order to minimize the vagaries and biases of long-term recall.

Careful examination of some of the "conclusions" drawn from these studies helps place the information in the proper epidemiologic perspective. Both Richie and Francis indicted "improper floors" and "inappropriate

Table 17-5. Injury Severity

Student injuries (%)	Injury gradient	Instructor injuries (%)
74.6	I	72.3
18.4	II	21.7
4.5	III	4.8
2.5	IV	1.2

shoes" as major contributors to aerobic dance injuries. With either of these variable, the only attempt made to compare exposure was presented by Richie when he noted "injury frequencies" on various surfaces. This was accomplished by compiling the percentage injured on various types of floors. Even in the unlikely event that exposure was comparable on the various flooring surfaces, the injury frequencies varied little, and his conclusion that "a hard, nonresilient floor surface will definitely increase injury frequency. . ." is not supported by the data.

It appears that these authors have, a priori, associated the high percentage of knee, leg, ankle, and foot injuries with the "conventional wisdom" of the running world and have thus indicated the shoes and the surface on which the activity is performed. They fail to note that there is no epidemiologic support for this contention either in their data or the "running literature."[5] It is also difficult to make a case for a potential causative role played by shoes or floors when one considers that the average student was involved in but 3.7 hr. of aerobic dancing per week, at least half of which involved warming up, cooling down, and stretching—activities that would seem to involve minimal weight bearing.[4]

Although examination of the patterns of anatomic injury sites yields little hard data regarding the biomechanical causes of injuries, it does provide some information regarding the relative importance of various medical problems. The studies of aerobic dancers all indicate that complaints associated with the leg, ankle, and knee are of some appreciable importance, inasmuch as these anatomic regions loom large in the constellation of injuries. In a medical sense, however, knee injuries appear to be a much greater problem; they appear at least twice as frequently as leg, ankle, or foot injuries among patients seen in a formal medical setting (table 17-1).

Nearly all of the knee injuries seen in the sports medicine facility were of the overuse variety—usually some form of patellofemoral dysfunction. Although some might suggest that most of these problems are associated with improper foot biomechanics, few factual data support this thesis. Additionally, these knee problems are similar to the overuse injuries seen in other athletic and fitness activities, many of which (ballet, skiing, gymnastics, etc.) employ the foot in a far different manner. This suggests that the problems, those involving the knee at the very least, may be associated with some variable inherent in many athletic activities. In the author's estimation, this variable is **overuse** or **inappropriate use.**

The overuse thesis also seems consistent with other findings supported by hard data, namely the high frequency of injuries seen in (1) those with prior orthopedic problems, (2) those for whom aerobic dance was their only fitness activity, and (3) those who participated infrequently in aerobic dance. Thus, a program aimed at safety enhancement might more appropriately encompass issues such as a gradual but consistent involvement in the activity, education regarding the recognition and management of overuse injuries, and the presence of an instructor or supervisor who can provide medically appropriate advice on physical complaints.

It is admirable that the field of aerobic dance questions its practices and safety record. Even though aerobic dance appears less hazardous than most of the "fitness alternatives" such as running and tennis, it obviously can be made even safer. It is difficult to understand, however, why aerobic dance participants have so readily embraced the self-flagellation common within the group. It should be apparent that the heaviest criticism comes from those offering "solutions" for the problems they have described (or perhaps created). Those blaming footwear come forth with a new shoe design. Those decrying the educational credentials of instructors offer "certification" courses and tests. Those blaming "bad floors" become consultants to flooring manufacturers. Those who use injury statistics inappropriately to describe the activity as being too hazardous "solve" the problem with an aerobic program of their own design.

When viewed from a purely medical perspective, aerobic dance appears to offer well-documented fitness enhancement with a minimum of risk. Perhaps even more important, it has appealed to a large group of women previously uninvolved in any fitness activity. it would be unfortunate if the efforts of the highly vocal detractors serve only to discourage participation by those who are both the most impressionable and most in need of such a program.

References

1. Francis LL, Francis PR, Welshens-Smith K. Aerobic dance injuries: a survey of instructors. Phys Sportsmed 1985; 13:105-11.
2. Richie DH, Kelso SF, Belluci PA. Aerobic dance injuries: a retrospective study of instructors and participants. Phys Sportsmed 1985; 13:130-40.
3. Garrick JG. Characterization of the patient population in a sports medicine facility. Phys Sportsmed 1985; 13:73-76.
4. Garrick JG. Gillien DM, Whiteside P. The epidemiology of aerobic dance injuries. Am J Sports Med 1986; 14:67-72.
5. Powell KE, Kohl HW, Caspersen CJ, Blair SN. An epidemiological perspective on the causes of running injuries. Phys Sportsmed 1986; 14:100-14.

18

REHABILITATION OF THE INJURED DANCER

Marika E. Molnar, M.A., R.P.T.

PHYSICAL THERAPY FOR DANCERS with disorders of the musculoskeletal system is based on the results of a systematic, thorough evaluation preceded by subjective and objective history-taking. In most cases, the findings of this examination will lead to the selection of the correct treatment modality, proper aftercare treatment, education in injury prevention, and guidance during the return to previous artistic endeavors.

The objectives of treatment are multifold:

- Pain relief
- Restoration of full range of motion
- Stability of the joint
- Normal muscular strength, endurance, control and coordination
- Proper proprioceptive responses
- Restoration of confidence in dancing ability
- Education about (1) the musculoskeletal system, (2) immediate first-aid care, and (3) prevention of future injuries

Life-Style as a Cause of Injuries

Essential to the rehabilitative process is the physical therapist's understanding of the professional dancer's life-style. Dancing is not a 9 to 5 job; it is full time, all the time. With class every morning, rehearsals throughout the afternoon, and performances in the evening, professional dancers push their bodies to the limit.

Their bodies allow them to become the creative expression of the choreographer, the visual component to the music, and an ephemeral entity for the audience. Yet, the sheer physicality of dancing is also what sets the limitation on the dancer's artistic life and career.

The roots of all American dance forms can be traced to classical ballet's disciplined technique and formalized language. Not only professional ballet dancers study ballet, but most modern, jazz, and theatrical dancers take ballet classes as part of their daily routine to keep themselves fit. Besides the many obvious differences in movement qualities, differences in the use of space and choreographic demands exist between modern dance and ballet. Therefore, it is important to know the type of dancing to which the injured dancer will be returning.

A comprehensive history of a dancer's career is a vital component in determining the guidelines for full return to preinjury level of activity. In addition, a detailed account of previous injuries, their precipitating factors, and the actual mechanisms of the injury itself is essential. It is during the interviews held for assembling this information that the therapist and dancer develop the rapport that will enable them to work together confidently and cooperatively.

In my capacity as physical therapist for the New York City Ballet, I have responsibilities to the dancers and to the administration. My philosophy is that the dancer is more essential than the dancing. If there is risk of reinjury or predisposition to serious injury, the dancer involved and I make the decision to speak to the ballet mistress in charge. We then decide on a course of action that gives the most importance to the best interests of the dancer. This policy has prevented some of the younger dancers from sustaining more serious injuries and also has assured that they are rehabilitated so that they can get back into peak condition as soon as possible. The communication between therapist, dancer, and administration is vital to the health and nurturing of the dancers, especially new members of the company.

Most dancers join the company at the age of 17 as members of the corps de ballet. Within 1 or 2 seasons, they will inevitably be disabled for a time by a traumatic injury. Most of these accidents are to the foot and ankle: metatarsal stress fractures, first- or second-degree lateral ankle sprains, or flexor hallicus longus or Achilles tendinitis.

Unfortunately, the reasons for these injuries are obvious. As students, dancers work perhaps 3-4 hr. daily without the stress of performing at night. As company members, they increase their daily work load to 6-8 hrs. Their daily routine is changed from being solely in the classroom to being in the classroom for 1½ hr.; in the rehearsal studio for up to 6 hr., some of which is standing around, waiting, or repeating certain steps over and over again; and then to performing on stage during the season. This increase in training can be the cause of overuse injuries. An eagerness to dance and the quest for perfection are other precipitating factors that contribute to injuries traceable to fatigue. Most of the more serious injuries occur at the end of a long rehearsal period or after a difficult class, when the dancer attempts that difficult step one more time.

To discourage these events from being perpetuated, a neuromusculoskeletal screening is performed prior to the season. The results of this evaluation are taken into consideration when assigning the dancers to the various new corps roles. The entire repertoire for the season is balanced as much as possible to allow for a gradual induction into professional life.

The dancers have access to my office at the theater on a daily basis to work out their problems, whether they be a painful blister, the need for a back evaluation, foot and ankle exercises, or a checkup for a recent returnee to the stage. I have the opportunity to watch class and rehearsals and thus can spot possible problems before they become real problems.

When time off from performing is the only alternative, the dancers keep in shape by such activities as swimming, weight training, floor barre, yoga, etc. The usual daily routine is doing whatever exercises they can do without aggravating the injury and attending a physical therapy session. Maintaining proper nutrition and a positive attitude are helpful adjuncts.

Other Causative Factors

Choreographic Demands

As the dancer's body becomes more finely tuned and capable of performing more difficult feats, the choreographer may increase creative demands without recognizing the limitations of the human body. When an injury of any severity does occur to a company member, usually another dancer is waiting to substitute. The fear of losing a part or being considered undependable or injury prone often deters young dancers from acknowledging their injuries.

Frequently, what the choreographer asks of the dancers artistically is not in their repertory of movement training, i.e., taking a ballet class in the morning does not prepare the body to move with the loose torso and turned-in legs required in modern-dance choreography. Therefore, it is advisable for the dancers to supplement their daily class with a routine of exercises that will condition their bodies to respond to the demands placed on them. An individualized exercise program should be developed by the physical therapist with the dancer's physique in mind. The dancer thus can take the responsibility for preparing the body to move as called upon. Specifically, home exercises should correct any muscle imbalances, improve the aerobic capacity, and maintain proper alignment of all the body parts.

Incorrect or Faulty Technique

Bad habits or patterns of movement are difficult to relinquish without hard work and good coaching. The lack of external rotation (turn-out) at the hip joint is often compensated for at the knee or ankle, causing excessive shear forces across the joint surfaces and resulting in a breakdown of tissue. Once an acute episode subsides, it is essential to eliminate the pathomechanics.

Along with retraining technique, balancing the muscles around the pelvic girdle and mobilizing the hip joints to work more efficiently are a priority. If tight hip flexors and weak hip extensors are not corrected, the lumbar spine will be overused, resulting in lower back dysfunction. The hip flexors must be stretched appropriately, and the hip extensors must be strengthened to allow normal range of motion to be produced at the hip joint before the paravertebrals fire. Therefore, any step requiring hip extension must be verbally and manually corrected so that the improper pattern is not repeated. In performing a *relevé* (rising up on the ball of the foot), everyone strives to rise as high as possible. To accomplish this, many young dancers place weight onto the lateral borders of their feet (sickling), placing increased strain on the lateral collateral ligaments of the ankle. Along with being given exercises to strengthen the peroneals and surrounding musculature, these dancers must be retrained to place the weight more between the first and second toe to assure that the movement is synchronous and correct. Proprioceptive training (position sense) should also be instituted to reestablish kinesthetic awareness. (See figures 18-1 through 18-20.)

Correction of Faulty Technique

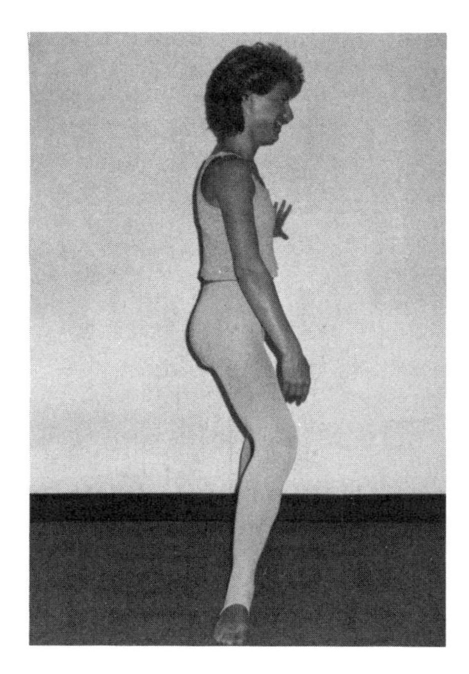

Figure 18-1. Lack of turn-out at hip—foot turned out 180° placing excess stress on knee joint.

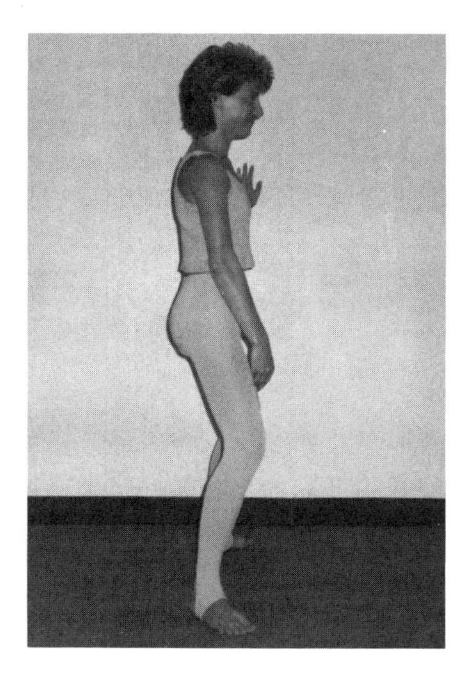

Figure 18-2. Proper placement of feet for available turnout.

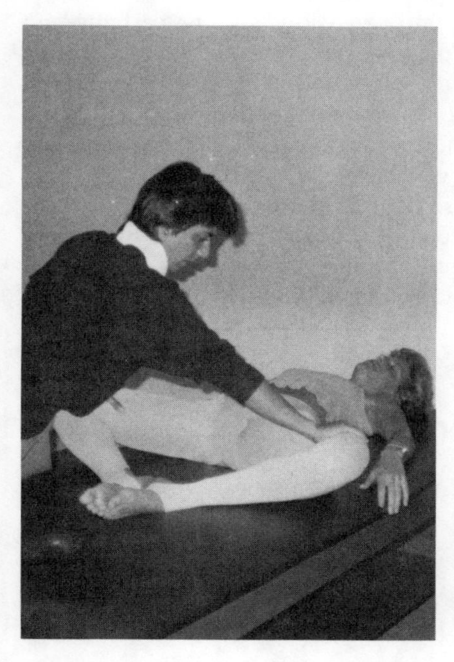

Figure 18-3. Therapist stretching hip capsule.

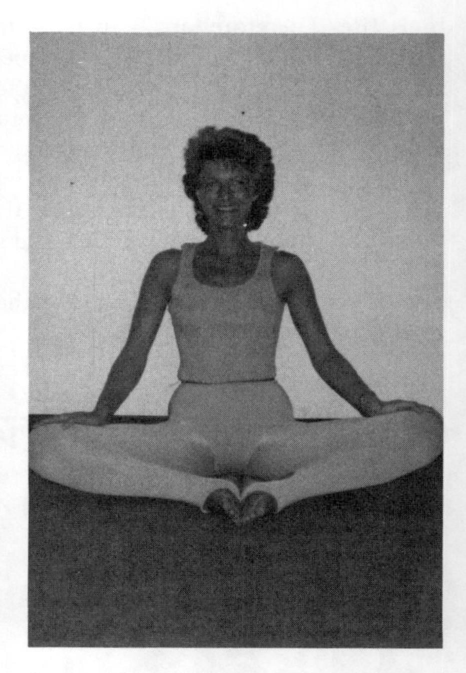

Figure 18-4. Self-stretching against wall.

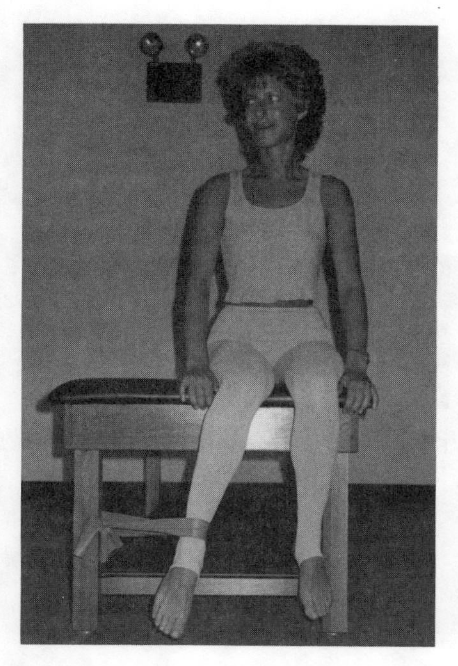

Figure 18-5-A. Strengthening external rotators: starting position.

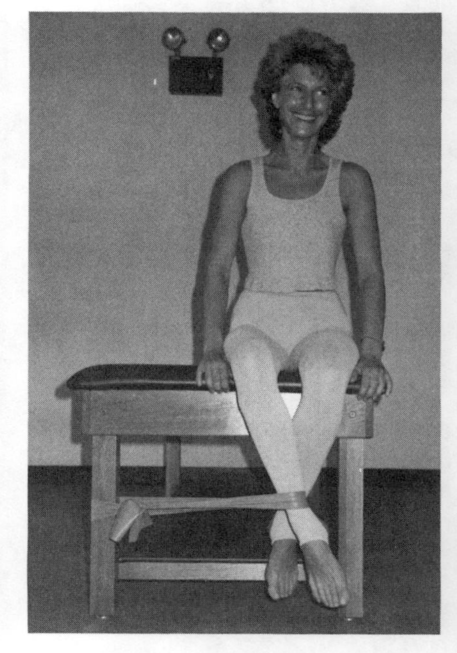

Figure 18-5-B. Strengthening external rotators: ending position.

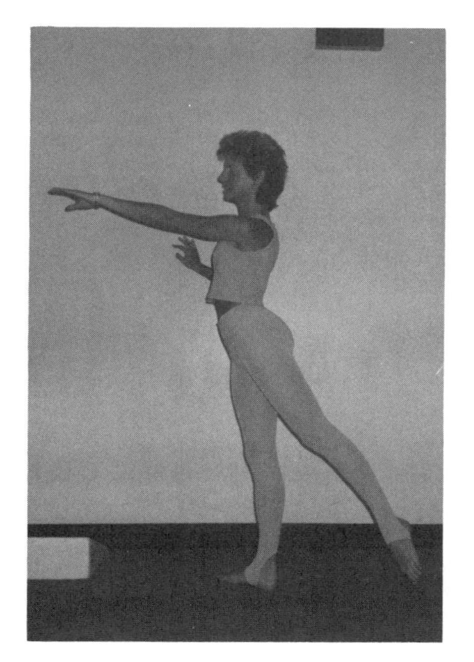

Figure 18-6. Incorrect *tendu* to the back using lumbar spine too early.

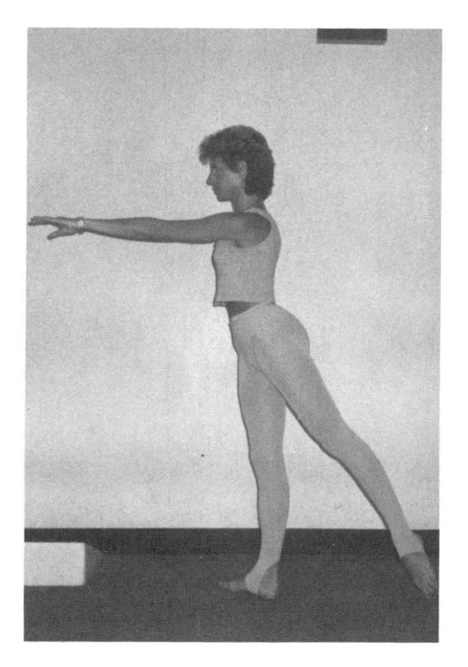

Figure 18-7. Proper use of hip extension.

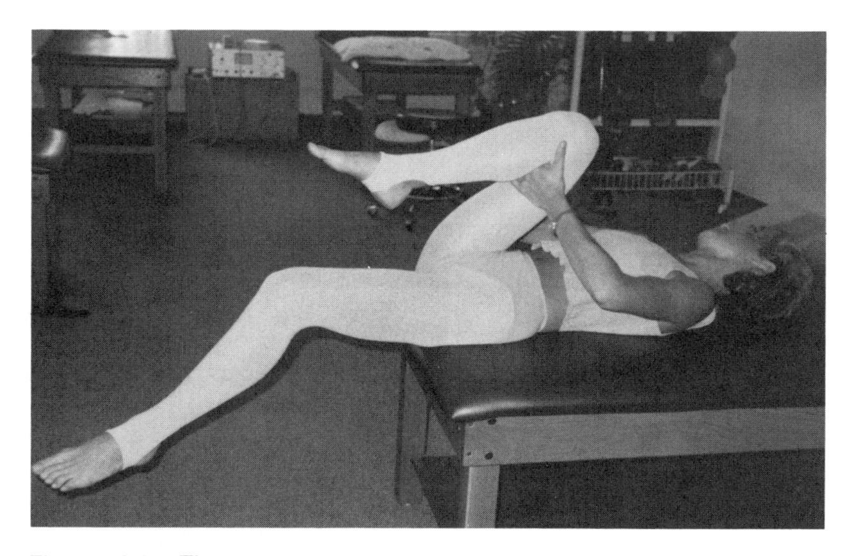

Figure 18-8. Thomas test for hip flexors showing tightness.

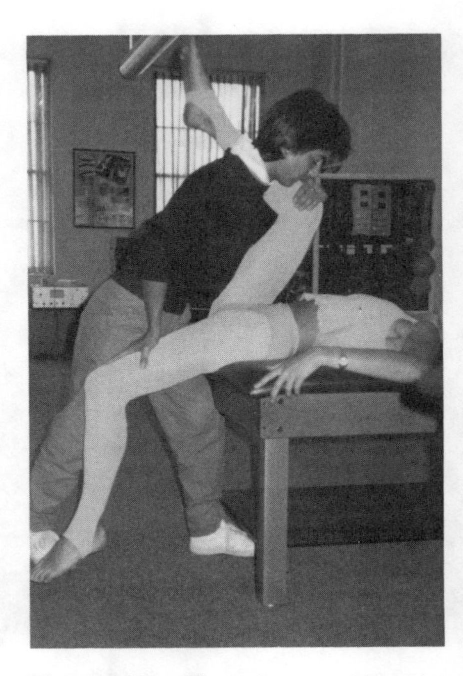

Figure 18-9. Therapist stretching hip flexors—muscle energy technique.

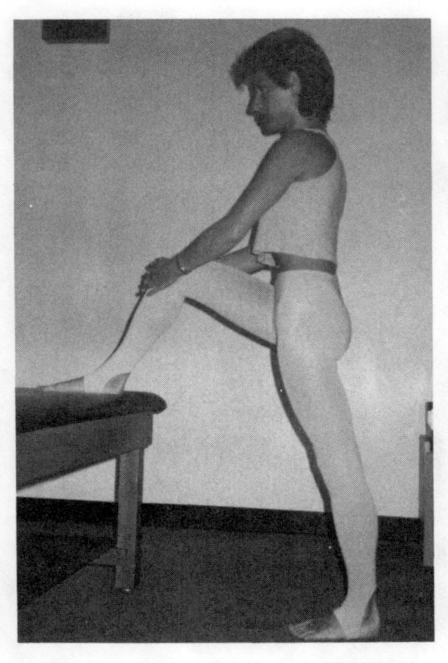

Figure 18-10-A. Starting position for self-stretch of hip flexors and gastrocnemius.

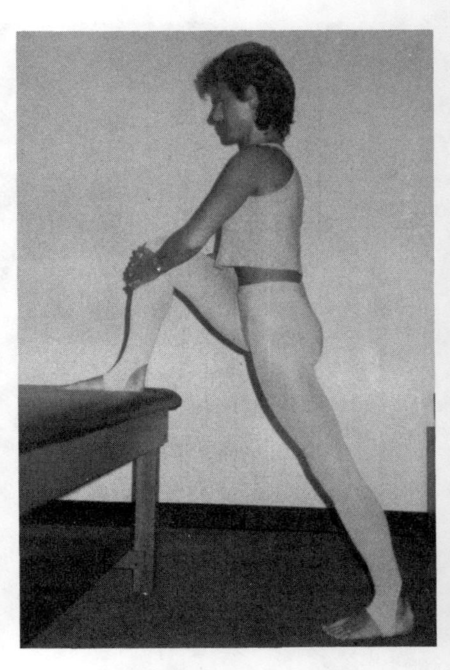

Figure 18-10-B. Ending position—hip flexor stretch.

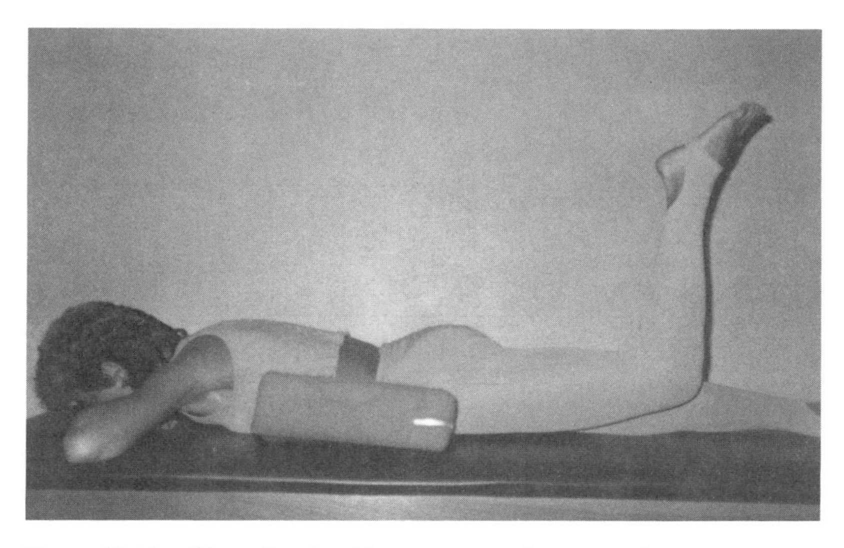

Figure 18-11. Strengthening hip extensor—gluteus maximus.

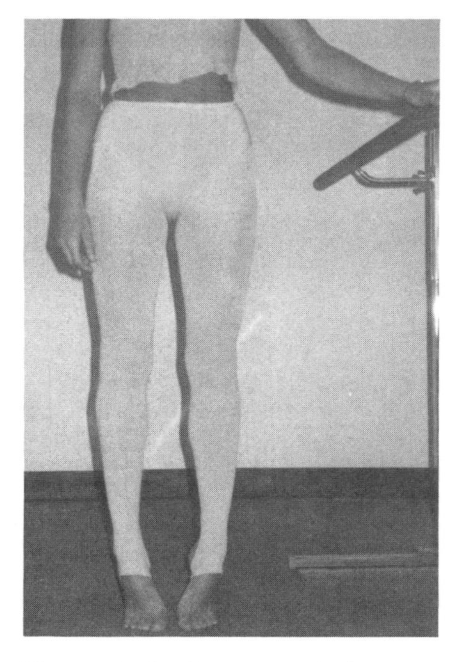

Figure 18-12. Incorrect *relevé.*

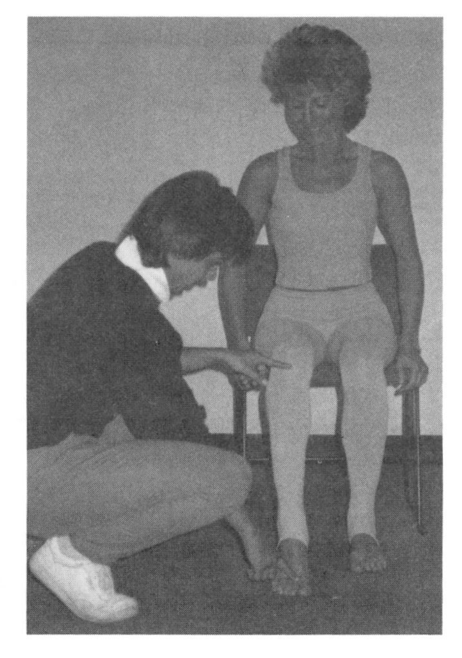

Figure 18-13. Therapist instruction in proper placement of feet.

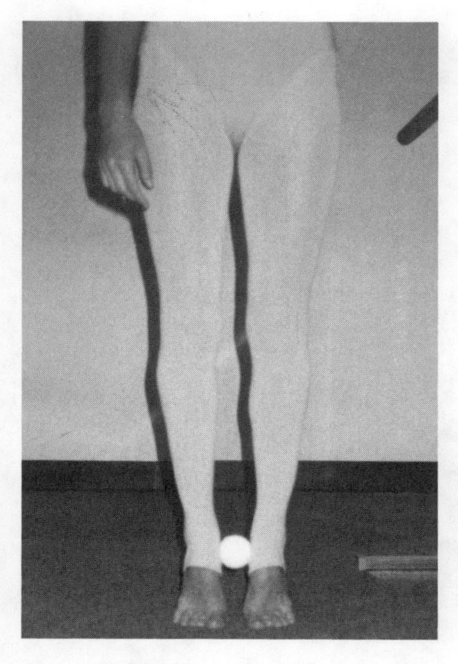

Figure 18-14. Proprioceptive retraining with tennis ball for proper alignment.

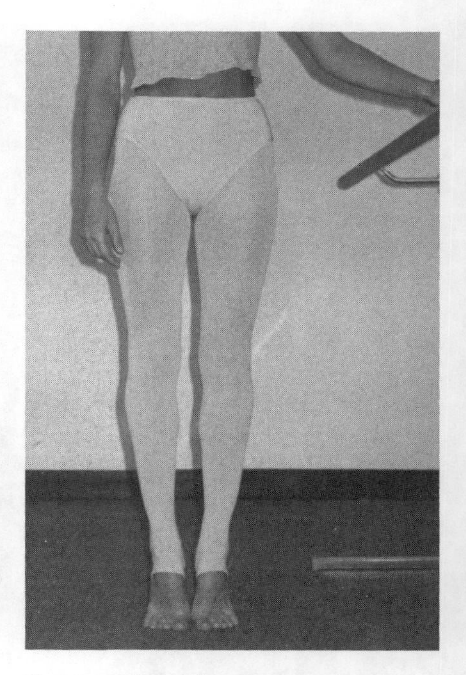

Figure 18-15. Correct *relevé.*

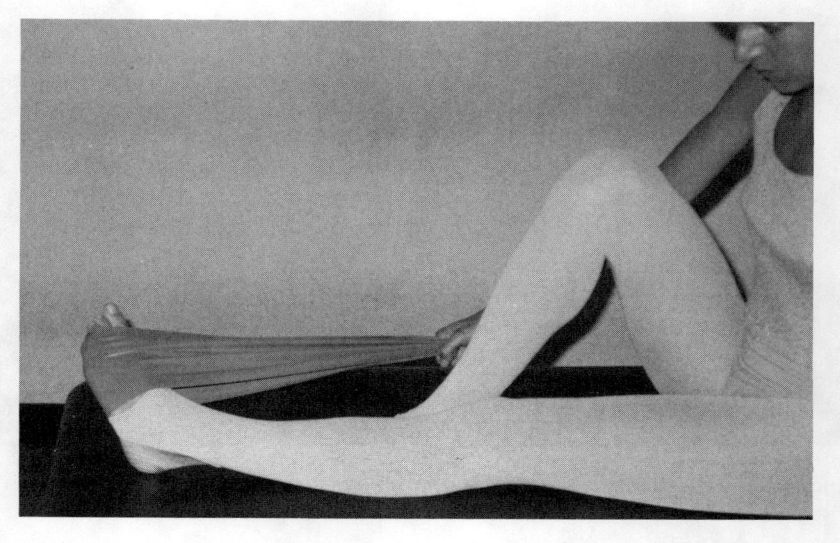

Figure 18-16-A. Theraband exercises for peroneals: starting position.

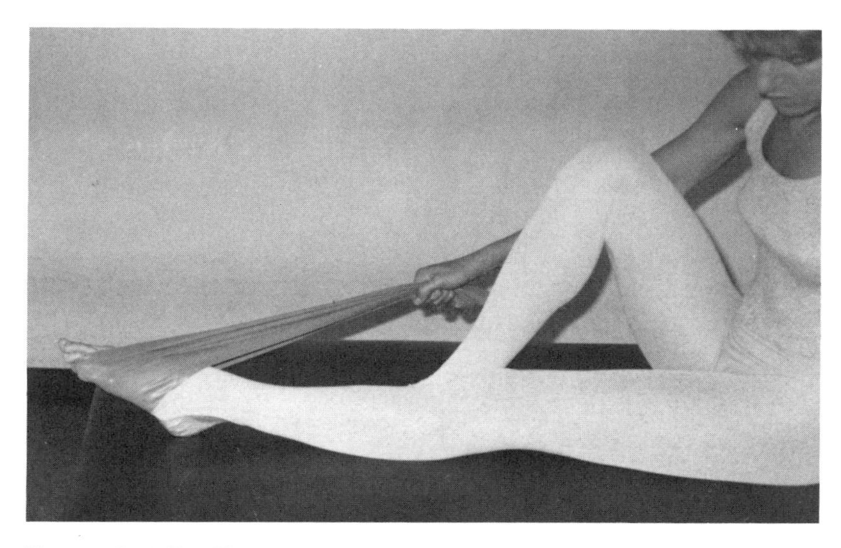

Figure 18-16-B. Theraband exercises for peroneals: ending position.

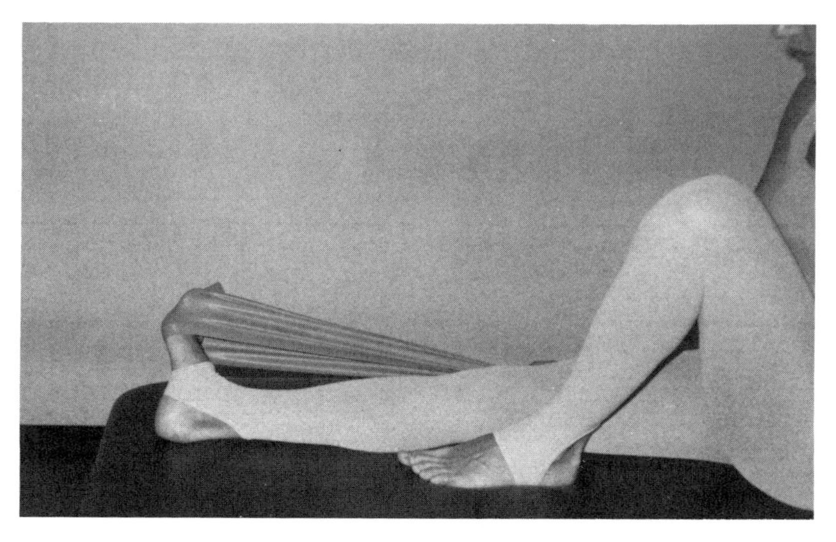

Figure 18-17-A. Theraband exercises for posterior tibialis muscle: starting position.

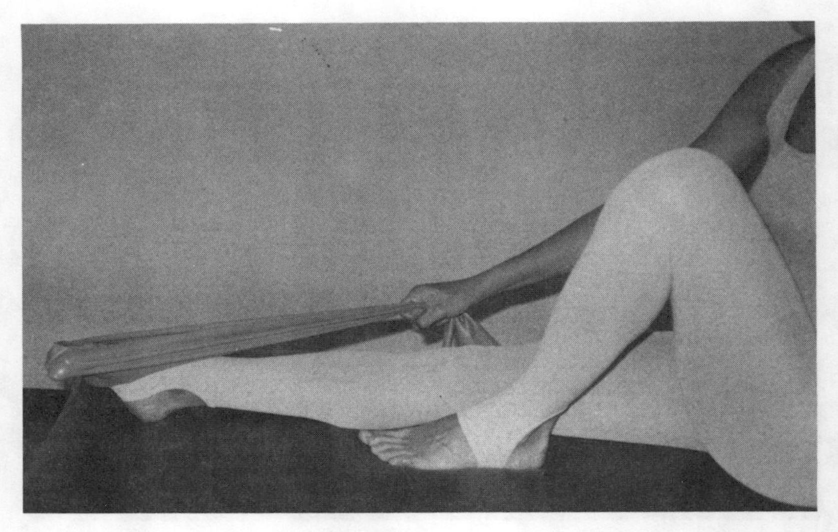

Figure 18-17-B. Theraband exercises for posterior tibialis muscle: ending position.

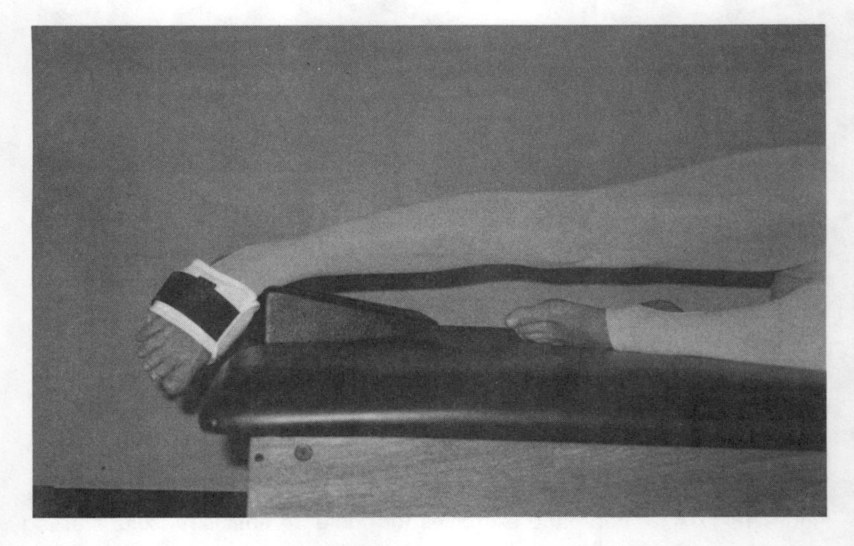

Figure 18-18-A. Weight training for peroneals: starting position.

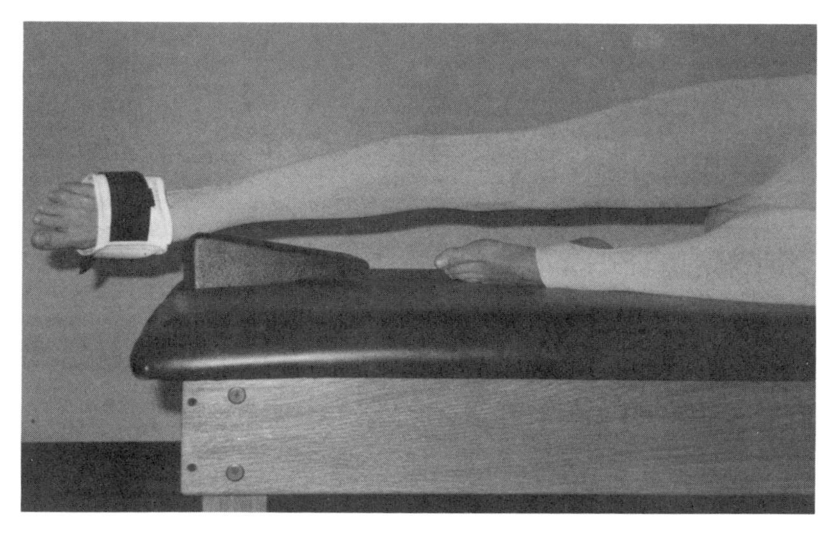

Figure 18-18-B. Weight training for peroneals: ending position.

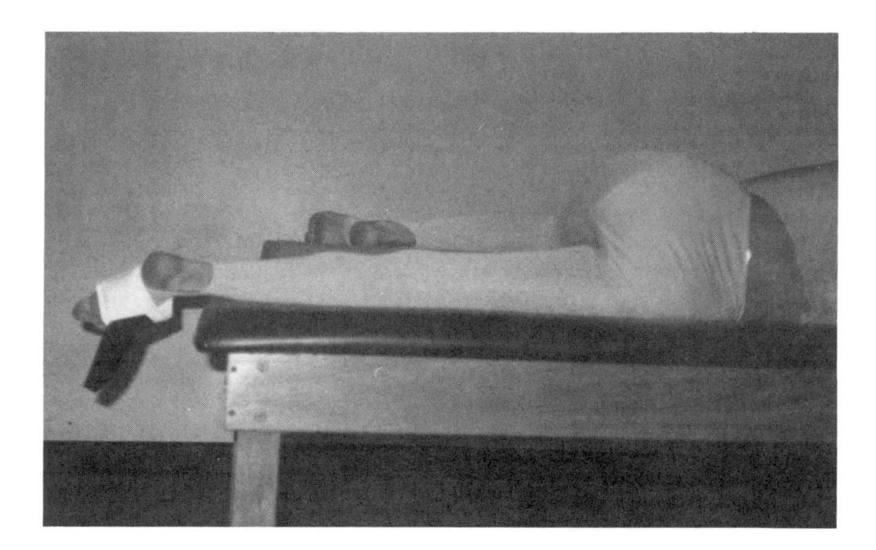

Figure 18-19-A. Weight training—posterior tibial: starting position.

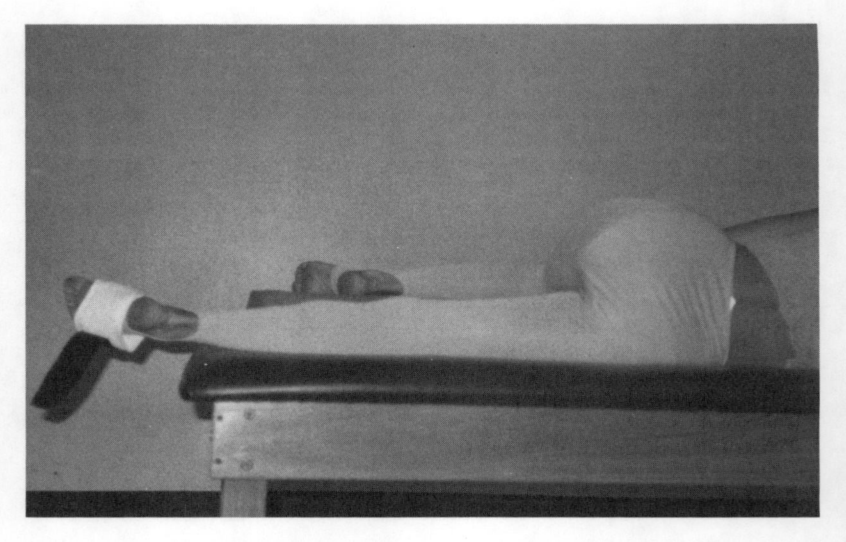

Figure 18-19-B. Weight training—posterior tibial: ending position.

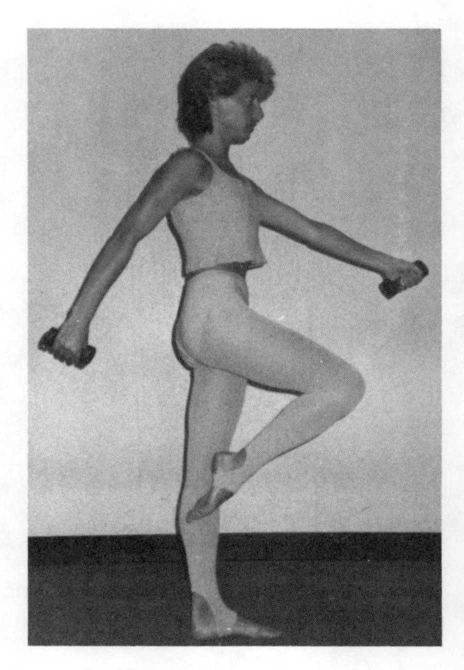

Figure 18-20. Proprioceptive reconditioning of ankles.

Improper Footwear, Clumsy Costumes and Sets, Bad Stages

It is particularly useful to have the dancer bring in shoes used in dancing. Very often, the shoe is no longer the correct size for the dancer's foot. The foot has grown, but the dancer is still ordering the same size as before. In a ballet slipper, the dancer must be able to stand with the feet parallel and the toes straight and not curled. If the toes are curled or crunched in the shoe, they cannot be used effectively, and undue stress is placed upon the metatarsal heads and the tendons to the toes. Blisters, corns, and callouses also result, all of which can lead to infections.

Most larger theaters in the United States have stage floors suitable for dancing or can install portable floors made especially for dancing. Unfortunately, many of the stages in Europe are old, raked, and hard, with little or no wing space. This environmental factor needs to be reevaluated by the theater management so that it will not be detrimental to the dancers' health.

Anatomical Abnormalities

Structural malalignment and accessory bones often can cause injuries that come on insidiously. A perfect example of this is the inability to point one foot as much as the other due to an os trigonum (posterolateral tubercle of the talus), which becomes impacted between the calcaneus and tibia during extremes of plantarflexion. This supernumerary bone occurs in the general population, but does not cause problems unless extreme ranges of plantarflexion are needed. It often takes years of serious training before pain or inflammation forces the dancer to seek help. The dancer will readily acknowledge that one foot always pointed more than the other, but had not caused pain until now. Often, a traumatic foot or ankle injury that left one ankle weak will be reported in the past history. Surgical removal is the best method of relieving pain and increasing range of motion, especially for the dancer who must work on *pointe.*

Treatments alternative to surgery that have helped dancers include:

- Stretching the dorsal structures of the foot slowly and carefully to eliminate myofascial restrictions to plantarflexion
- Stretching the gastroc-soleus complex.
- Strengthening the weak muscles around the foot and ankle, especially the intrinsics, peroneals, and posterior tibialis.
- Reeducating the proprioceptive feedback system using weight-bearing positions
- Ice to decrease inflammation after exercises
- Joint mobilization of the inferior tibiofibular, talocrural, subtalar, and midtarsal joints.

The above rehabilitation process can often alleviate the need for surgery if the injury is not yet chronic. Retraining to eliminate past bad habits due to compensation is essential, whether or not surgery is performed. (See figures 18-21 through 18-27-B.)

Overcoming Anatomical Abnormalities

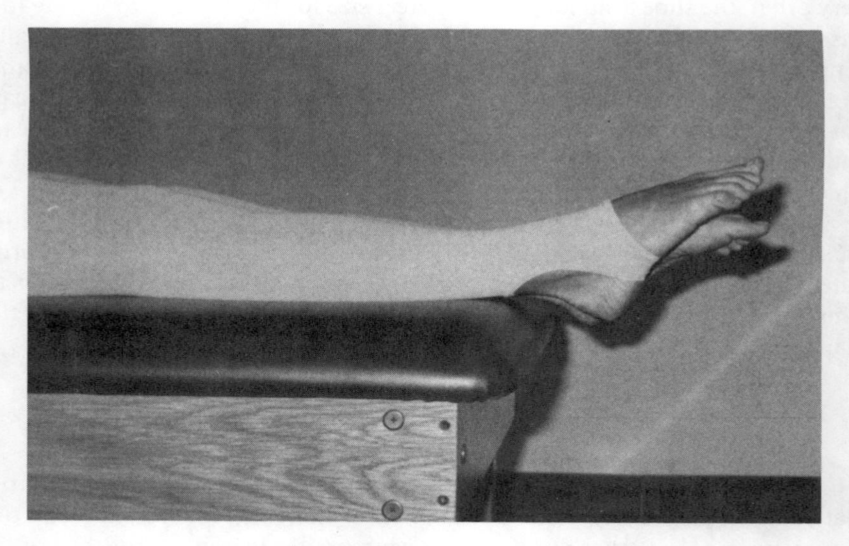

Figure 18-21. Decreased range of motion in one foot.

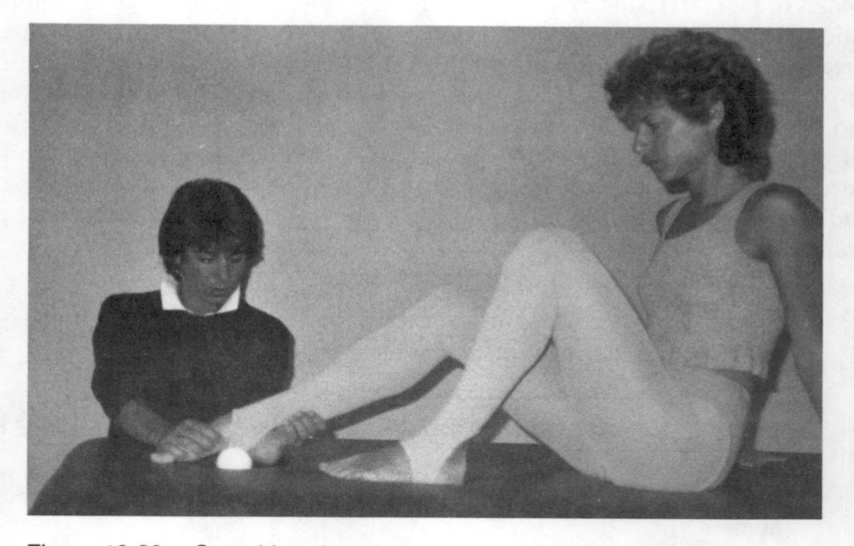

Figure 18-22. Stretching dorsal structures of foot by therapist.

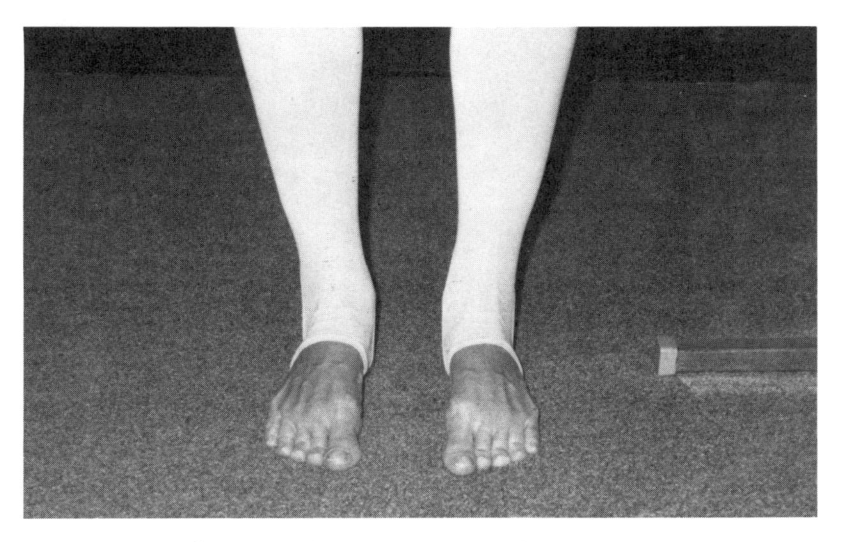

Figure 18-23. Strengthening intrinsics—doming.

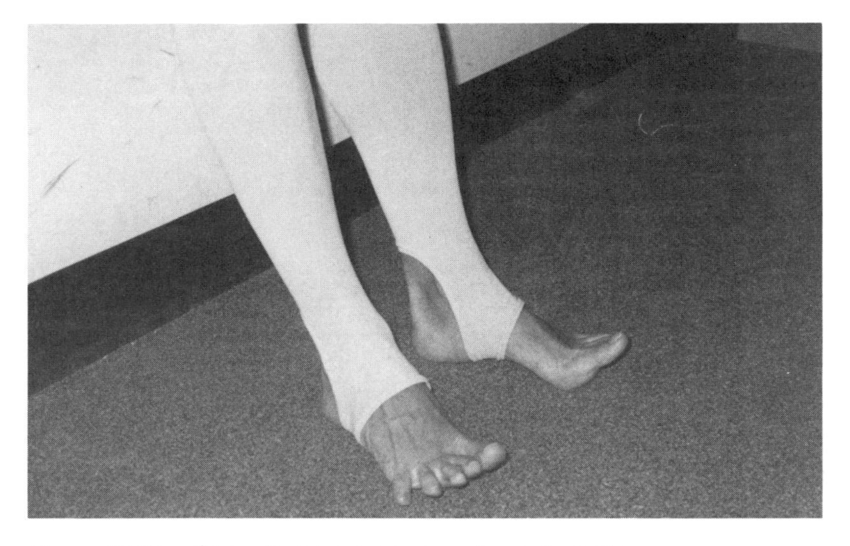

Figure 18-24. Strengthening intrinsics—toe extensors.

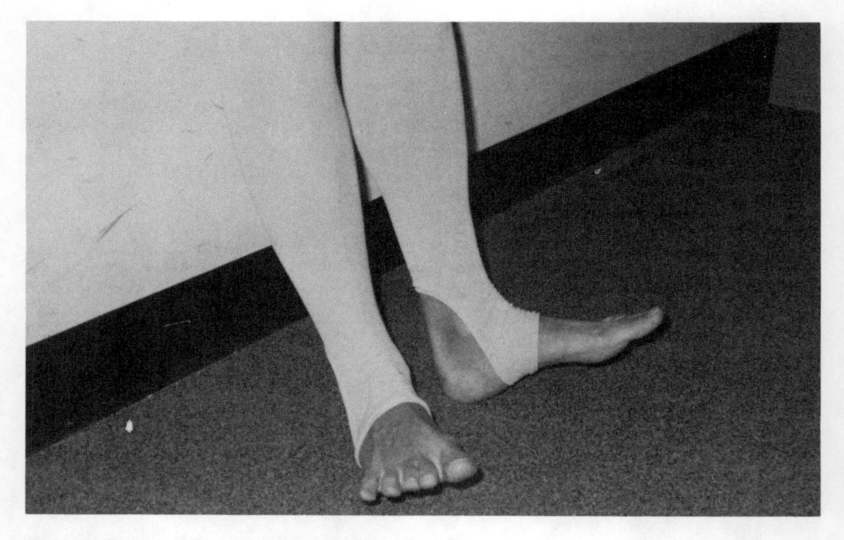

Figure 18-25. Strengthening dorsiflexors.

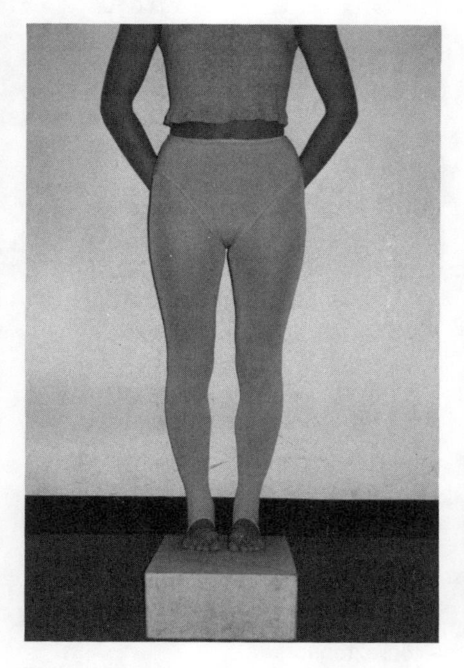

Figure 18-26-A. Stretching triceps surae group: gastrocnemius.

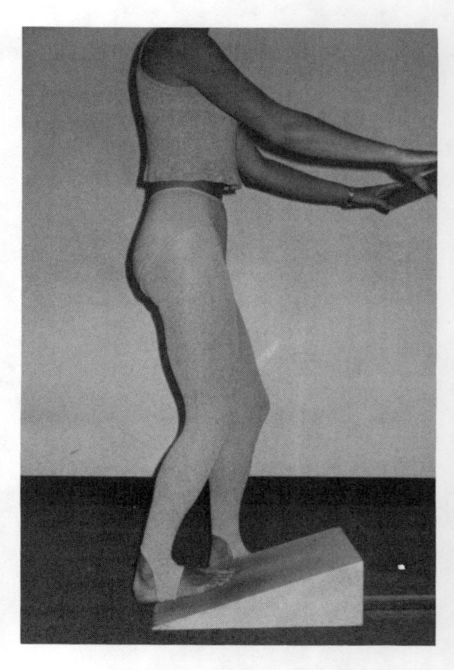

Figure 18-26-B. Stretching triceps surae group: soleus.

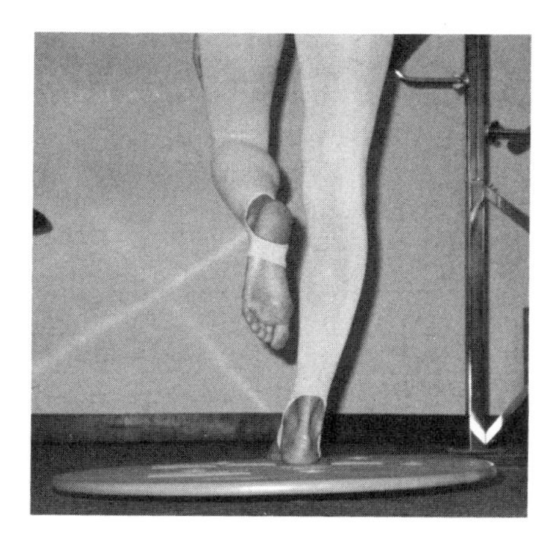

Figure 18-27-A. Proprioceptive reconditioning: BAPS board (Biomechanical Ankle Platform System).

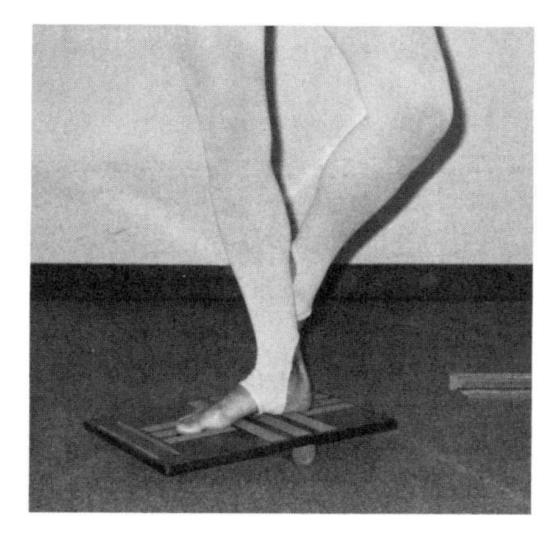

Figure 18-27-B. Proprioceptive reconditioning: tilt board.

Identifying Causes of Pain or Movement Limitations

Normal functioning of the musculoskeletal system requires (1) full and pain-free range of motion of the joints, (2) stability of the joints at the extremes of the range of motion, (3) adequate muscular control of joint motion, (4) well-conditioned proprioceptive sense, and (5) proper muscle length, strength, and endurance. If these requirements are not met, examination of the dancer may reveal the following signs or symptoms:

1. Pain (local or referred)
2. Limited range of motion due to:
   - bony restriction
   - adaptive shortening of capsule and ligaments of the joint
   - adaptive shortening of muscle
   - fast or slow muscle guarding
   - empty end feel
   - internal derangement—springy block
3. Excessive range of motion (hypermobility)
   - with pain caused by:
     —continued postural imbalance
     —coordination/proprioceptive abnormalities
     —delayed stretch pain from overstretching tendons
   - without pain
   - complete instability
     (Local [segmental hypermobility] is usually compensatory for a hypomobile segment above or below it; general constitutional hypermobility is usually acquired among dancers and gymnasts.)
4. Weakness of musculature controlling the joint (The weak muscle is often antagonist to a shortened muscle.)

Normal values for dancers are difficult to determine. Joints and muscles are examined bilaterally and compared to each other for each individual. Once the total body picture (neuromusculoskeletal profile) has been evaluated for normal function, the specific structure involved must be evaluated. Pain and joint muscle dysfunction often occur simultaneously. It is a difficult task at best to determine the underlying pathomechanics of the injury, but with proper information and knowledge of the dancer and the dancer's work/training schedule, a treatment philosophy can be developed that will be a safe guide back to artistic endeavors.

It is the dancer's responsibility to follow through with the advice and rehabilitation exercises given by the therapist; it is the therapist's responsibility to become more familiar with the dancer's world—vocabulary, movements, style, etc.

The therapist and dancer must take into consideration the following time factors:

- Length of rehabilitation time (weeks, months) to ensure full healing and recovery
- Dancers' readiness to recognize faults and correct them
- Length of time before an important performance
- Time involved in progressing from class to rehearsal to actual performance
- Chronological age and the needs of younger dancers within their musculoskeletal development
- Chronic versus acute injuries

The physical therapist must be highly motivated, creative, and sensitive to the dancer's life. The dancer must have confidence in the therapist's skills and knowledge. Together, with mutual trust and respect, the rehabilitation process will be a beneficial, enjoyable experience.

Bibliography

1. Chaitow L. Neuromuscular technique. Wellingborough, Northamptonshire: Thorsons Publishers, 1980.
2. Evjenth O, Hamberg J. Muscle stretching in manual therapy, vol 1. Alfta Rehab, 1984.
3. Gustavsen R. Training therapy. Thieme, 1985.
4. IFOMT. Proc 5th Intl Conf. Gillaine F, Sweeting L, eds. Whakatane NZ: IFOMT.
5. Janda V. Muscle function testing. London: Butterworths, 1983.
6. Kessler RM, Hertling D. Management of common musculoskeletal disorders. New York: Harper and Row, 1983.
7. Kopandji IA. The physiology of joints, vols 1-3. New York: Churchill, Livingstone, 1974.
8. Paris SV. The spine: etiology and treatment of dysfunction (course notes), 1979.
9. Root M, Orien W, Weed J. Normal and abnormal function of the foot, vol 2. Los Angeles: Clinical Biomechanics Corp, 1977.
10. Travell J, Simons D. Myofascial pain and dysfunction—the trigger point manual. Baltimore: Williams & Wilkens, 1983.
11. Upledger E, Vredevoogd JD. Craniosacral therapy. Seattle: Eastland Press, 1983.
12. Walther D. Applied kinesiology, vol 1. Pueblo, CO: Systems DC.

19

DANCE SURFACES

Jay Seals

DANCE PROFESSIONALS PAY CLOSE attention to the quality and characteristics of dance surfaces because they regard the dance floor as one of the most important variables (second to physical conditioning) affecting performance. Unfortunately, when dance surfaces are installed in a new or remodeled dance facility, the professional dancer is rarely consulted. The specifying decision often lies with construction professionals, who may or may not be concerned with how a dance surface affects a dancer's performance and health.

Although styles and techniques in dance range dramatically from the highly trained ballet professional to the dance exercise enthusiast, there is a shared concern for and growing recognition of the value of working out on a proper and safe dance surface. Liken the dance surface to other, far less intricate kinds of professional performing surfaces, and dancers have a right to demand more attention to their needs.

Comfort, protection, and overall suitability of a dance surface are often overlooked or compromised when a floor is installed. As institutional and commercial expansion of dance facilities continues, more emphasis is being given to addressing the needs of the performer, instructor, and recreational participant during the floor specifying process.

Through evaluating the experiences and subjective floor surface assessments of diverse members of the dance community and tapping the flooring industries' existing research and more recent case histories on the performance of various recreational flooring systems, general consensus can be reached regarding the appropriate qualities of dance floor systems. Numerous designs are available that incorporate qualities that enhance performance, user comfort, and injury reduction. Compounding any overwhelming consensus are varying opinions of the ideal floor system among dancers, even among those trained in the same style; however, a core of evidence suggests that the dance community is not far off in defining the very specific flooring needs of its industry. More extensive and collaborative research and—even more important—building technical knowledge of recreational flooring systems among the architects, designers, and engineers who create dance facilities are among the greatest challenges facing the dance industry.

Dancer on Dance Floor: A Dynamic System

Dancing is a complex interaction between two dynamic systems—the dancer and the floor. The layman may not consider the floor as a dynamic system, but the dancer knows that the floor can dramatically affect performance, stamina, and health.

The dynamics of the dancer are apparent even to the most casual observer. Grace, athleticism, precision, and style are discernible components of a dancer's "dynamics" (figures 19-1, 19-2). Dance floors also have dynamic components that are more structural in nature, but are every bit as evident in a given floor's "performance." Two of the most important characteristics of a dance floor are resiliency and shock absorption. Dance floors must have shock-absorbing properties, but at the same time, they must return a certain amount of energy to the dancer. Without this resiliency, various movements in dance would require considerably more physical effort. An extreme example of a highly shock-absorbent surface with virtually no resiliency is a sand beach.

The surface of a dance floor must be firm in order to provide resistance to the force exerted by the dancers' feet as they push off for leaps. However, if the surface is too firm, with little or no "give"—as with concrete or asphalt—the musculoskeletal system of the lower extremities absorbs most of the shock, likely leading to early muscular fatigue. If the musculoskeletal system fails to attenuate adequately the shock of the foot strike, afflictions of the feet and legs such as shin splints, painful arches, stress fractures, and sore joints may develop.[1]

The optimum resilience of dance surfaces varies with the style of dance and the conditioning of individual participants. A floor with high resiliency is equally appreciated, however, by highly conditioned and less-conditioned dance athletes alike. To the experienced dance professional, a dance floor system designed to provide the ideal qualities of resilience and shock absorption is readily distinguishable from an average or substandard dance floor.

Shock Absorbency and Resiliency

Resiliency and shock absorption are two of the three major criteria for judging a dance floor (the third, surface friction, will be discussed later in this chapter).

For a flooring system to be resilient and shock absorbent, it must have certain properties and/or perform certain functions for the user:

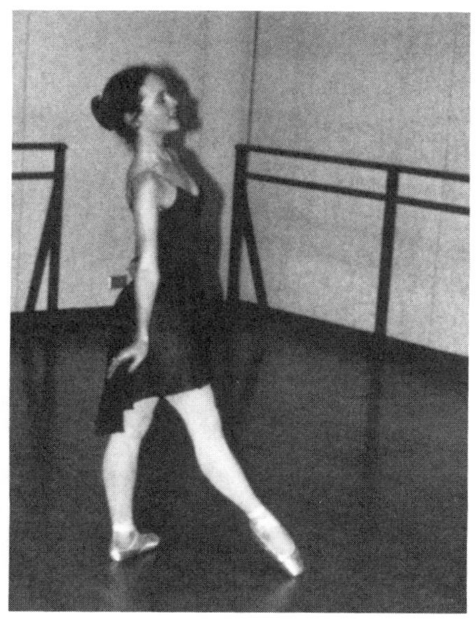

19-1

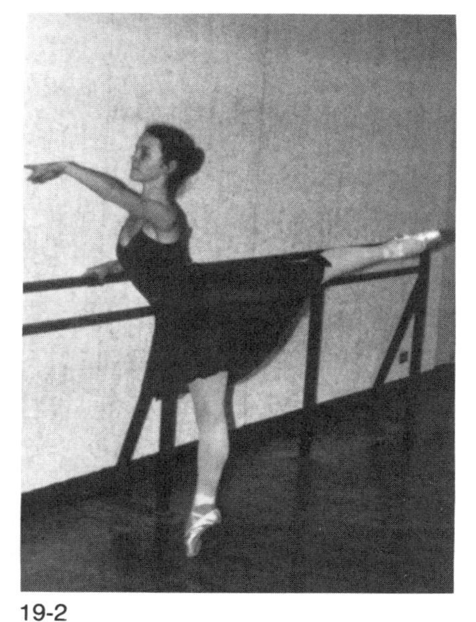

19-2

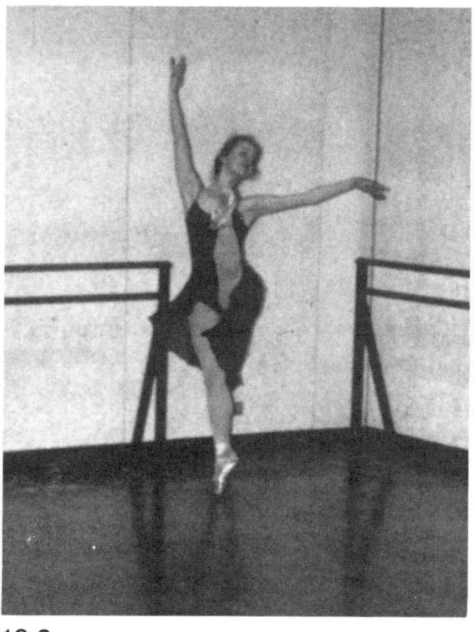

19-3

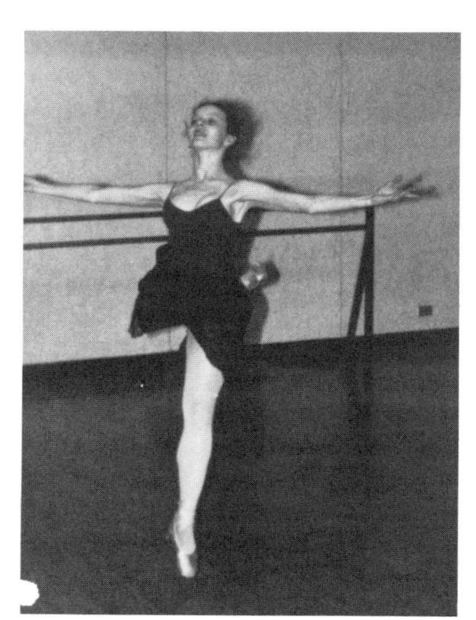

19-4

Figures 19-1, 19-2, 19-3, 19-4. The above figures show the interaction of the ballet artist, movement performed and the dance surface. During the various movements the dance surface provides the delicate balance between slide and traction. As the foot of the dancer impacts with the surface, different ground reaction forces are created. Suspended systems absorb the low and high energy of impact and return part of that energy back to the dancer—reducing potential for injury and discomfort during rehearsal or performance.

- It should have shock-absorbing qualities.
- It should "give" under impact to some degree and absorb some of the impact energy in the process.
- It should not deform permanently or dent under the pressures or impacts of normal usage.
- It should not be so springy that it acts as a trampoline.
- It should not be absolutely rigid or hard and should not give the impression of so being.[2]

By definition, an ideally resilient floor system would have to return as much energy as a trampoline, but do so while deflecting or compressing as little as concrete and have a surface as soft as sand.[3] Although it would be impossible to design such a system because some of the requirements of the ideal state are contradictory,[3] many floor systems today have at least some of the ideal qualities listed.

Because the art of the dance does vary in style and technique, a floor system can be designed to meet the requirements of the style of dance for which it is intended. For example, modern dance programs may enlist techniques that create low-frequency shocks on a floor surface, whereas classical ballet may, at times, include high-impact movements that result in high-frequency impact with the floor surface. In each case, the floor system's dynamic response must be sensitive to the degree of impact energy delivered into the floor system by the dancer, attenuating shock and returning a sufficient amount of energy to the dancer. Thus, the ideal floor enhances performance and minimizes fatigue and possible injury.

Proper body alignment, technique, and conditioning all play important parts in injury-free dancing (figures 19-3, 19-4). Over a long period, a forgiving floor system can aid in compensating when proper technique and body alignment during moves are not practiced. The ideal stage or studio floor is a built-up floor system commonly referred to as a "floating floor," or a suspended floor system. Dancers working on a suspended wood floor tend to suffer fewer and less severe injuries than do those using a nonsuspended floor.[4] A suspended dance floor designed with a hardwood or vinyl surface provides dancers the opportunity to perform full-out movement during performance or rehearsals relatively free of injury and physical risk.[5]

Practice Versus Performance

The ideal rehearsal studio floor may be at variance with the ideal performance floor, for dancers may spend many hours a week in the studio perfecting their art and tuning their bodies. Intensity, duration, and frequency of rehearsals mandate the need for a compliant, forgiving floor system. Also, a resilient and shock-absorbent floor system with the proper traction or surface friction is especially helpful to the beginning dance student. The floor helps the beginner learn to move, jump, and work as a dancer with confidence and less risk of impact-related injuries.[6] Similarly, teachers instructing several classes a day on a properly specified floor will not experience the fatigue or throbbing in the lower back and legs usually encountered when teaching on rigid surfaces.[7]

When they dance on hard surfaces such as concrete, tile, and thin floor coverings, dancers compensate internally within the body to offset the stress and trauma that develops on hard surfaces during the course of a session. In many cases, shin splints and stress fractures result from extended dancing on noncompliant, unsympathetic floor surfaces. These surfaces typically occur on tour, where appropriate facilities are not always available.[8]

Unfortunately, performances in many areas of the United States are held in facilities with stages that are very rigid and inflexible. Although the time spent performing is minimal compared to rehearsal hours, the frequency is enough to present problems for dancers. Fortunately, many of the new stages being constructed recognize the needs of the dancers, providing user comfort through controlled compression, deflection, and recovery of the floor system under impact of the various moves during performance. However, because many of these stages must also allow for various stage props, bleachers, and even walking elephants, most ballet and professional dance companies tour with portable floors that provide a familiar uniform surface on which to perform. However, these floors do not have sufficient mass or thickness to mask a rigid stage floor. Portable synthetic floors do, however, provide superior levels of traction and surface friction. Because existing stage floors are generally in less-than-ideal condition, covering the existing stage floor with sheet vinyl helps to eliminate uneven surface traction. Resilient northern hard maple, widely preferred by traditionalists in the dance community, is used extensively as a dance surface in studios and rehearsal halls. This wood is desirable because of its light color and its durability, hardness and tight grain, qualities that provide splinter resistance.[9] In addition, a properly prepared maple floor provides better glide than vinyl surfaces, creating less friction (and less heat buildup) with the dancer's foot. Painful blisters can result from excessive friction and heat.

The following are time-tested systems that provide the important properties of dance floor construction:

- Resilient rubber-padded sleeper floating floor systems (figures 19-5, 19-6)
- Multi-layered basket weave sleeper or joist construction (figures 19-7, 19-8)
- Spring Coil flooring systems (figures 19-9, 19-10, 19-11, 19-12)
- SpringAire or spring leaf systems (figures 19-13, 19-14)
- Resilient low-profile foam underlayment systems of varying densities (figure 19-15)

The most popular floor systems for ballet and classical dance over the years have been the basket weave, spring leaf, and spring coil systems. The characteristics of these systems provide the dancer and instructor the ability to rehearse for long periods without the strain and trauma experienced on less-forgiving floor systems.[6]

Studies in Floor Resiliency

The benefits of the sleeper and spring leaf systems under impact were detailed in 1966 in a study funded by the Maple Flooring Manufacturers Association.[10] Twelve flooring systems, including tile, wood direct to concrete, and additional designs of suspended systems were all compared to concrete under impact. Snell Laboratories constructed a special testing apparatus to measure the resiliency characteristics of various flooring systems. The design premise for the testing was that its action should simulate the stress condition affecting a gymnasium floor when an athlete or athletes landed from a vertical jump such as might occur in a rebound play in basketball. Such impacts would approximate one or two men (400–500 foot-pounds) landing simultaneously in a close area.[11] The testing design allowed for the following variables to be measured:

- Transmitted vibrations
- Instantaneous deflection (in inches) of the flooring surface
- Permanent deflection (in inches) of the flooring surface
- Height of rebound of the weight after striking the test surface (in inches)
- Compression of the spring coil flooring structure system during impact (in inches)
- Time of compression (in seconds) of the spring flooring structure system during impact
- Time of return of the spring flooring system on rebound (in seconds)
- Time of rebound of the weight to maximum height (in seconds)

Using the above information, the compression, deflection, and rate of recovery of each floor system were compared to the values of concrete[12] (figure 19-16).

The report indicated that additional research would be required to evaluate the contributions to foot/body comfort and fatigue of shock absorption (deflection and rate), rebound height, and rate of energy transferred. The results of the test clearly indicated the benefits of suspended systems. Additionally, subjective assessments by users of the various dance floor types further reinforced the clinical importance of appropriately designed dance surfaces. It is important to note that the science of relating injury to impact is still in its embryonic stages.

The bionegative effect of impact forces in connection with pain and injuries is widely accepted, but a clearer understanding of this set of questions needs further research. Externally measured impact forces are not identical to internal impact forces in the joints, ligaments, and/or tendons.[13] However, it would be apparent from surveys of dance professionals and other athletes that

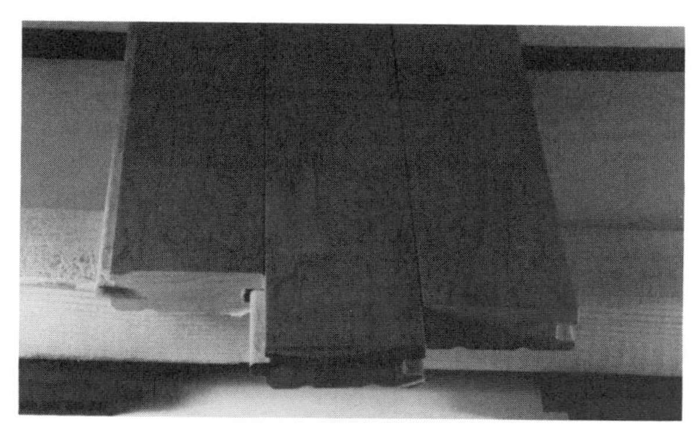

Figure 19-5. A resilient rubber-padded sleeper floating floor system.

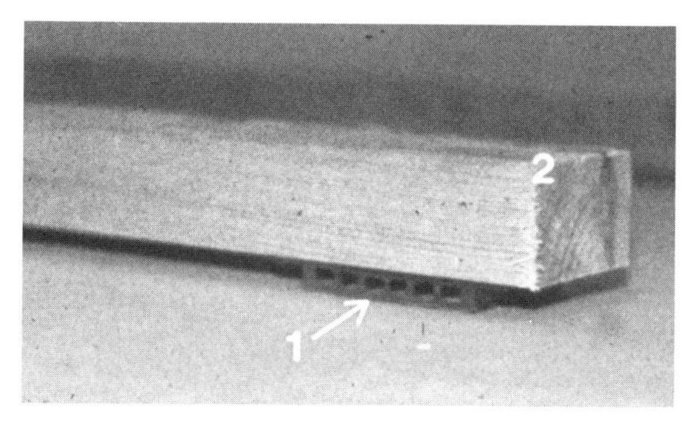

Figure 19-6. Sleeper construction, with resilient 3/8-in. rubber pads (1) placed underneath 2 × 3-in. sleepers (2) placed 9, 12, or 16-in. on center to provide varying degrees of shock absorption and resiliency.

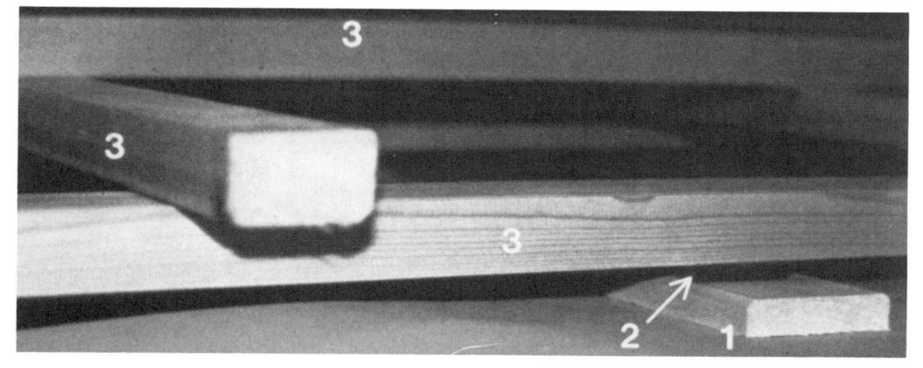

Figure 19-7. Multi-layered basket weave sleeper or joist construction (Robbins). Stacked layers of 1 × 4-in. or 2 × 3-in. (3) are cushioned with permacushion pads (2), alternating perpendicular to one another (that is, alternated 24-in. on center, creating a resilient undercarriage). Spacing of sleepers can be decreased to provide less dampening characteristics.

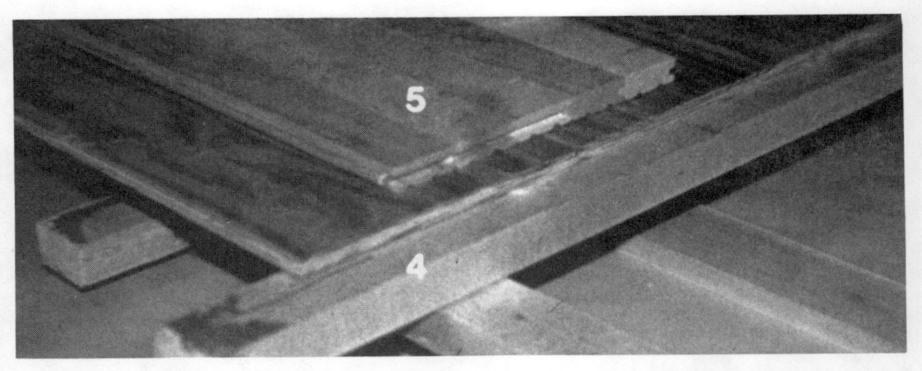

Figure 19-8. Over the top of the tongue and grooved northern hard maple suspension system (4), a plywood and maple flooring surface is installed (5). Vinyl or northern maple may be used for the surface.

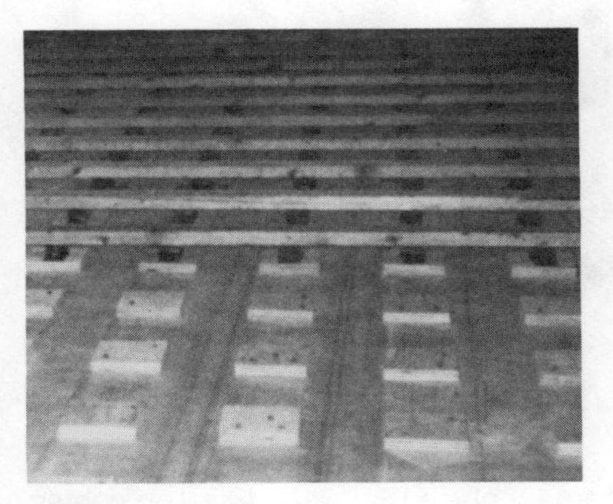

Figure 19-9. Installation of Spring Coil ballet floor system at Towson State University.

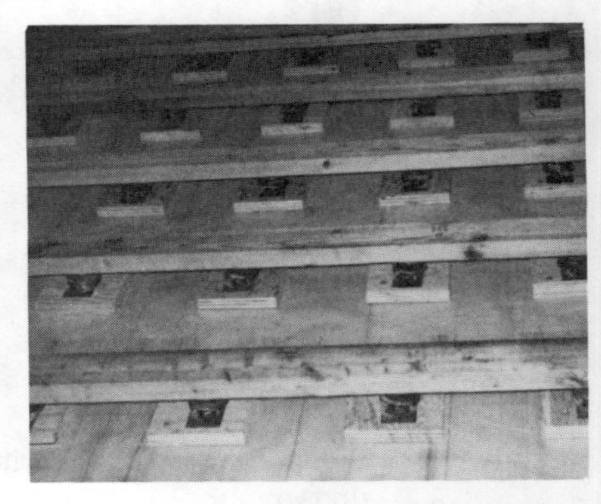

Figure 19-10. Closeup of leveling blocks, special spring coils attached 12-in. on center to 2 × 4-in. sleepers spaced 16-in. on center across short dimension of floor area.

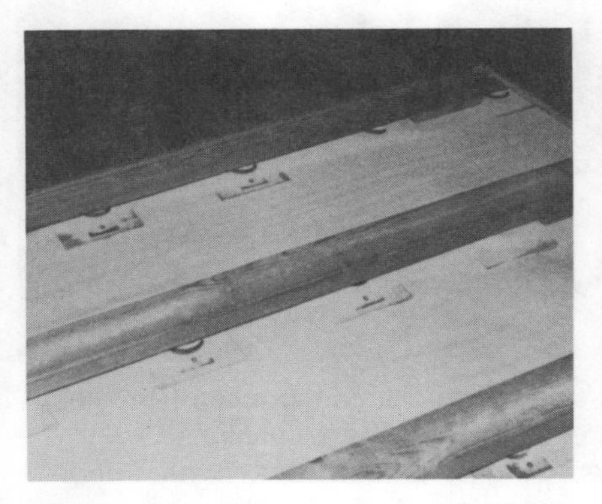

Figure 19-11. Sound deadening placed in and between springs and sleepers, and $^1/_2$-in. plywood nailed to sleepers.

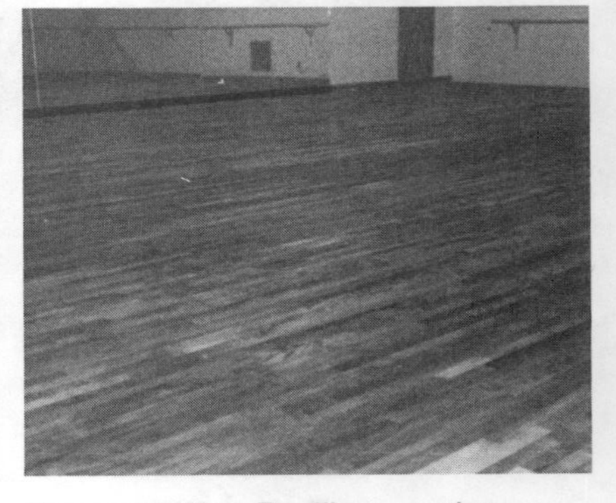

Figure 19-12. Resilient northern strip maple installed over plywood sleeper spring system.

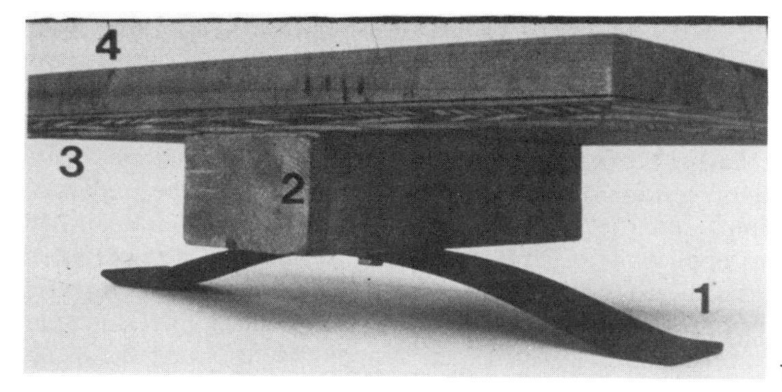

19-13

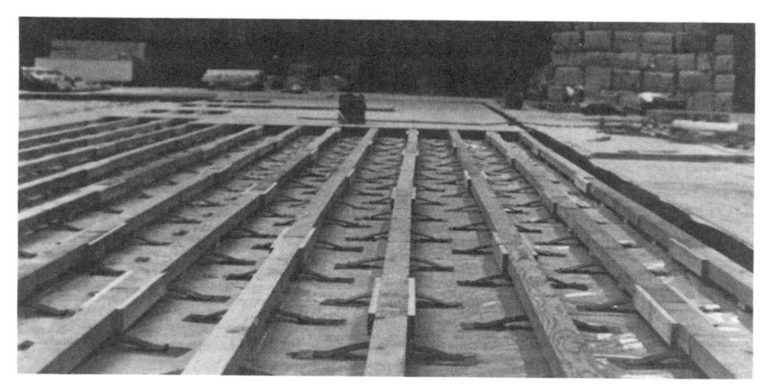

19-14

Figures 19-13, 19-14. SpringAire floor system, comprised of spring leaf (1) attached to 3 × 4-in. sleepers (2) placed 16-in. on center. Spring leaves are attached 32-in. on center at the underside of 3 × 4-in. joists. Springs provide ideal compression, deflection and recovery for dance with plywood (3) and northern maple (4) installed over the top of the suspended substructure.

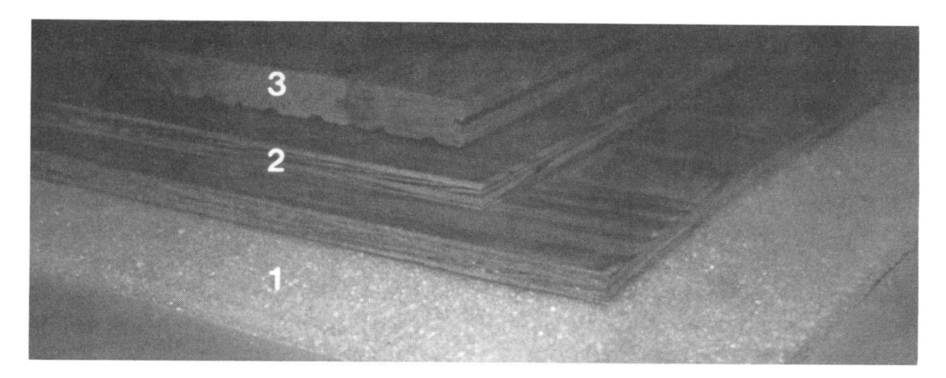

Figure 19-15. Low-profile system resilient foam underlayment sheets (1) of varying thicknesses and densities deaden sound and absorb shock. Plywood subflooring (2) is laid over the top of foam and tongue and grooved hard maple (3) nailed to plywood as the dance surface.

impact-related injuries are reduced by the installation of suspended wood floor systems.[14]

Because there are currently no established test methods to evaluate shock absorption of hard playing surfaces, the flooring industry and the author adopted the ASTM F355-78 Standard Test Method for Shock-Absorbing Properties of Playing Surface Systems and Materials.[15] This method covers the measurement of certain shock-absorbing characteristics, the impact force/time relationship, and the rebound properties of playing surface systems. This method is applicable to natural and artificial playing surface systems and to components thereof. This test method was very helpful in evaluating the dynamic response characteristics of 3/16- to 1/2-in. sheet vinyl urethane and rubber in comparison with suspended system designs using the same material placed over the top. Hardwood flooring over these systems was also evaluated.

In performing the test, a standard object is dropped from a given height (6 to 24-in.) and its velocity is measured at the baseline (surface sample). An accelerator then measures the deceleration of the object as it travels into the sample surface until it comes to an instantaneous halt. This represents the G-max. The object acceleration is then measured as the sample surface pushes the object back on the rebound. The rebound velocity is measured as the object passes back through the baseline. The oscilloscope trace shows time versus acceleration. The G-max is measured as the maximum deceleration the object received. In terms of injury potential, the lower the G-max, the better.[16] The factors derived from this test method will give some indication of how different materials react under the conditions of the test. Impulsive testing is by far the most rapid technique that can be applied to the study of a complex structure such as dance floors.[17] Dance floor systems absorb energy by deflection; if the impact energy created by a dance floor is not enough to deflect the dance floor or if there is too much energy (i.e., the impact energy of the foot bottoms out straight through the material), the system is not effective as a shock absorber.[16] In comparison, the suspended systems under impact developed lower G-max than 1/4-in. synthetic sheeting.

The essential benefit in a floor system responding dynamically in this manner is the ability of the floor system to provide user comfort during performance and at the same time return sufficient energy to the dancer to enhance performance and reduce fatigue. In the case of a concrete surface, an instantaneous jolt is delivered to the lower extremities upon impact due to the failure of the concrete to yield. Concrete covered with a thin mat material that consolidates under contact bottoms out as the deceleration forces increase rapidly back to the legs. The previous conditions are avoided with suspended systems in that during performance, the body is not forced to absorb the instantaneous jolt that can be created upon contact. As the floor system deflects or yields, the energy of impact from the foot is absorbed into the floor system and stored in its component's molecular structure. As the floor system recovers, much of this energy is lost to internal friction and heat of the flooring components. Depending on the design of the system, a percentage of the energy is returned back to the foot in the form of kinetic energy of elastic recovery. A floor system that yields on contact provides delaying action, thus applying lower external impact forces to the lower body.

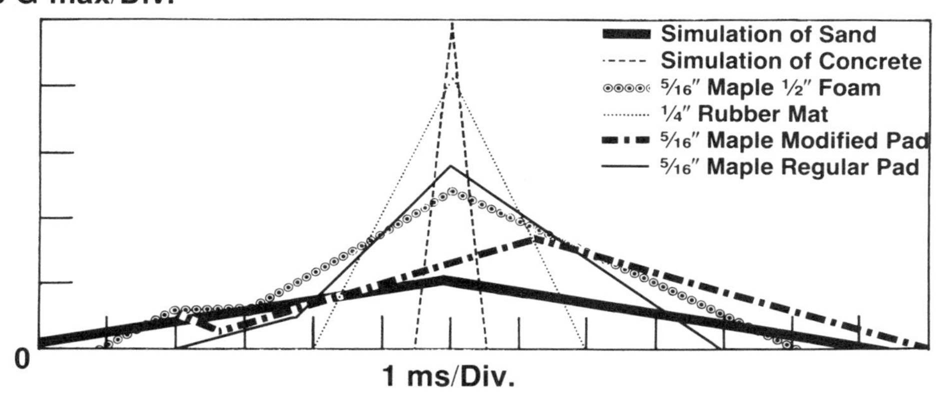

Figure 19-16. The above graph illustrates the shock attenuation characteristics of various floor systems under dynamic testing. The vertical axis illustrates maximum force in units of 50 Gs and the horizontal axis illustrates time of impact in 1 millisecond division. The graph thus illustrates a force time relationship of the various floor systems under the same test method F-355-F8 drop test 18-in. drop height.

1. The highest G forces under impact would be generated with concrete. The above illustration is a simulation of concrete, since physical damage to the testing equipment would occur during higher impact forces.
2. A 1/4-in. rubber mat impacted yielded a G max of 200. The time to G max or maximum force was approximately 3 milliseconds.
3. The third spike from the top illustrates a maple suspended flooring system incorporating 3/8-in. rubber pads underneath the system yielding a G max of 130 and a time to G max of 4 milliseconds.
4. The fourth spike from the top illustrates a maple suspended flooring system encorporating 5/8-in. rubber pads underneath the system yielding of G max of 113 and a time to G max of 5 milliseconds.
5. The fifth spike from the top illustrates the same maple flooring system with 1/2-in. crosslinked polyethylene foam pad underneath the maple suspended flooring system yielding a G max of 85 and a time to G max of 7 milliseconds.
6. The last spike from the top is a simulation of sand showing very low G forces under impact. Dance floor systems are designed with dynamic characteristics that fall inbetween the characteristics of concrete and sand. A compromise is made after careful consideration and evaluation of the dance programs surfacing needs.

Surface Friction

The surface, or traction, of a dance floor is very important when static and dynamic movements of the foot interface with the flooring surface. There is a very delicate balance between the needed slide and traction during performance and rehearsal. In order to provide freedom of movement without slippage, the surface preparation and maintenance of natural wood surfaces must be carefully done. Proper evaluation of the sanding and finishing process during installation will contribute substantially to the failure or success of the surface as it is used. Unfortunately, dance programs in many facilities share the same area. Often, the surfaces suffer from improper maintenance and buildup of rosin, body oils, and traction treatments. In many cases, these contaminants contribute to the creation of an uneven surface that can lead to slippage problems during rehearsal and performance.

During the planning stages of a dance studio, careful consideration should be given to the finishing process. It is important to have dance professionals decide on the proper finish application that will meet performers' needs. This can be accomplished by their dancing at other facilities with the same program and collecting information about materials used, properties, and trade names. The chemical composition of the finishing materials can spell disaster or success. If this information is not available, the flooring contractor's specialist can provide sample panels to the dance department for evaluation. At that time, maintenance requirements should be explained to those who will be responsible for this function after the studio is in operation. Whatever maintenance program is decided upon—and this will vary with the surface and dance program—a test should be applied to the panels and the dancers allowed to test the surface again.

The objective of this evaluation is to determine if the original finish surface will maintain a constant surface friction under the maintenance program selected. Generally, dance floors for classical ballet are sanded and sealed with penetrating sealers that seal the pores of the wood and leave very little (if any) film on the wood surface. Correctly applied, the coating will provide the proper traction for the artist.

Summary

Participation in classical ballet, modern, and jazz dancing continues to grow; along with interest in dance as a sport and recreational activity. Coupled with this growth is the need to evaluate the dancer, dance style, and dance surface as they interact dynamically with one another. The bionegative and biopositive loading of impact forces on the muscloskeletal system during participation needs to be further researched.

The lower incidence of impact injuries when suspended dance floor systems are used is widely accepted; but further research is needed into the significance of impact loading externally and internally on the dancer. Although dynamic drop tests provide indications of a dance system's resilient nature, they are not necessarily reflective of the actual ground reaction forces created between the surface and the dancer while in motion. Subject tests run on various systems installed over force platforms would provide comparative information to evaluate between drop tests and subject tests. The determination of external and internal forces acting on the dancer's body and how these loading forces affect the internal structure of the locomotor system would help to clarify the etiology of dance injuries. [18]

References

1. Morehouse C. Comparison of resiliencies of synthetic athletic surfaces: a final report. University Park, PA: Pennsylvania State Univ, 1981.
2. Snell F D Inc. Snell report on resilient factors of different flooring constructions to maple flooring manufacturers association. New York: F D Snell, 1966.
3. Snell F D Inc., op. cit.
4. Teitz C M D. Sports medicine concerns in dance and gymnastics. Clin Sports Med Nov 1983.
5. Roe R. Communication on SpringAire dance floor system.
6. Fox P. Communication on Spring Coil dance system.
7. Durr D. Communication on SpringAire dance floor system.
8. Quirk R. Ballet injuries: the Australian experience. Clin Sports Med Nov 1983.
9. Stoehr J. An examination of life cycle costs of three sports surface options, advantages, disadvantages of surface types. Wood May 1982.
10. Snell F D op. cit.
11. Snell F D op. cit.
12. Snell F D op. cit.
13. Nigg B M. External force measurements with sports shoes and playing surfaces, conclusions biomechanical aspects of sports shoes and playing surfaces. Calgary: Univ of Calgary, 1983.
14. Teitz C. Sports medicine concerns in dance and gymnastics. Clin Sports Med. Nov 1983.
15. American Society For Testing and Materials. Standard test method for shock absorbing properties of playing surface systems and materials. Philadelphia: ASTM, 1978.
16. Waterman N. Research report sport surfaces (description of test method used to test Robbins experimental floating gym floor and jogging track system). Lawrence MA: Voltek, 1983.
17. Jayarmaman G. Dynamic response characteristics of floor structural systems used for indoor sports: a research proposal. Michigan Technological University 4, Dynamic response characteristics of floor systems, 1985.
18. Nigg BM. The assessment of loads acting on the locomotor system in running and other activities; measuring techniques for load assessment. Calgary: Univ of Calgary, 1986.

20

PSYCHOLOGICAL ISSUES IN A DANCER'S CAREER

Jerome M. Schnitt, M.D., and Diana Schnitt, M.F.A., C.M.A.

IN THE UNITED STATES, dance study is a part of the lives of several million students at any given time. It has been informally estimated that as many children study dance as participate in athletics. If the term "dance study" is additionally broadened to include "aerobic" classes (usually considered to be exercise rather than dance by the fine arts community), this number swells considerably.

What are these dancers seeking? Why do they enter dance study, who leaves it (early or late), who stays, and what happens to all these students? This chapter looks at typical career paths of dancers from descriptive, developmental and conjectural points of view and reviews relevant scientific literature on dance.

Much of what is "known" about the psychology of dance is anecdotal; teaching is typically based on the apprenticeship model and is therefore experiential. It is not surprising that the psychological life of the dancer is not as well understood as the biological; this parallels the situation in medicine in general, where the biological sciences are further developed than the psychological. Some scientific studies have been made of some aspects of the psychology of dance, however. This literature includes such topics as body image, eating disorders, locus of control, and perception. Review of this body of work can be useful to the clinician attempting to work with dancers. Additionally, as has been found in sports medicine in general, understanding the attitudes and experiences of dance students may make it much easier for health personnel at all levels to communicate with dance students, and thus to gain the trust and compliance with treatment so essential to health maintenance and recovery.

A large popular literature on dance will not be directly addressed here. This literature, while often fascinating, usually is based on retrospective (often stylized) biographies and autobiographies of major figures in the field. The public is naturally curious about the lives of successful people, and well-known dancers are no exception.

It has become fashionable of late to "tell all," as Kirkland has done in her recent book relating her perspectives on some of the realities of the life of the adolescent dancer.[1] This type of account can vividly convey the intensity of some of the challenges dancers encounter. However, no matter how honestly such a work is constructed, it still must be recognized as a subjective recounting of an individual's experiences, which complements but does not replace scientific study.

The popular literature focuses on the few dancers who make it to the top. This chapter looks instead at issues common to most dancers during their career development.

Mind–Body Issues

To understand and work with dancers, physicians must understand that the dance world makes some assumptions about the relationship between the mind and the body that are fundamentally different from those of traditional medicine. Much of the skill needed in medicine is cognitive, based on scientific learning as applied to clinical situations in a logical way. As a group, physicians are not often called on to consider their own emotional states, and even more rarely must consider their postural alignment, their movement patterns, or the sensations in their muscles as they move. There are some exceptions; surgeons must consciously develop certain physical coordinations; psychiatrists must consciously focus on their own emotional states to conduct psychotherapy. Typically, however, medicine can be viewed as a cognitive science.

Dance training is very different; dancers are not encouraged to isolate cognition from emotion or perceptual and movement skills; they must be able to convey to an audience a wide range of feelings through their movements. They are not simply playing the role of an actor, convincing the audience to believe in an artifice; rather, performance is a reflection of the dancer's world view and life-style.

Contrasting Images within the Dance World

Ballet, modern, and jazz dance are the core techniques in American dance training. Each has a very different inner structure and conveys a unique image to the audience and to prospective students. Although it is possible to be trained in only one of these forms, most dance students are at least briefly exposed to all three, usually choosing a distinct favorite from among them.

Ballet

The classical image of ballet is a stage of purity, of innocence, of beauty and light, of elegance and grace. Movement often appears effortless; gravity seems readily defied. Even the villains are graceful. When well executed, it is a high art form, one of the most moving artistic experiences constructed by Western culture. From this perspective, it is a world that feels artistic, safe and secure; we readily send our small children, of preschool and primary school ages, to study ballet.

The underpinnings of this carefully constructed subculture are striking. It is a prepubertal world of structure and obedience, of conformity and pattern. Traditionally, in the ballet school, all students dress the same way, and there is only one correct way to perform each movement. In traditional settings, the ballet teacher conducts class with a definite style of authority, with a clear expectation of obedience and full respect. Displays of emotion are the prerogative of the teacher; students are not expected to respond with feelings, even if, in the extremes of the moment, the teacher expresses strong emotion directed at one or several students.

It is an asexual world; here are men and women, boys and girls, dressed in skin-tight clothing, genitals and breasts concealed by thin layers of stretch cloth. They move in ways that display their bodies, they touch and hold each other, sometimes in pseudocaresses, and yet sexuality seems entirely out of place. Paradoxically, although the perception is general that there is an unusually large proportion of homosexual men among ballet students, this perception is entirely anecdotal and not based on research.

The world of ballet has changed very little over several hundred years. The clarity of roles; the expectation that learning should be by rote; the authority of the teacher, who may be feared as much as respected; the lack of conscious recognition of sexuality (even in the face of sexually explicit stimuli)—all these would fit in a nineteenth-century European school, and many would fit in the eighteenth and even seventeenth centuries.

The products of this tradition, the top-notch ballet dancers, require 10-15 years of training from an early age to refine the requisite movement skills. These skills are only part of the picture; from a social system perspective, other skills are just as necessary. For example, the ability to work within the subculture also requires particular attitudes, high motivation, and a willingness to sacrifice nondance activities and relationships that might compete.

Modern Dance

Early modern dance conveyed a different image: Modern had an earthier, grounded style, which originally capitalized on "natural" movement and gesture. Modern dance allows motions not inherently attractive, such as angular movement, contractions, and a broad range of expressed feelings and impulses (including a symbolic sexual quality). In modern dance, except within individual companies' technical styles, there is often no "one right way" to execute a movement; any human movement can be acceptable in the right circumstances.

There was no required style of clothing for classes (although some schools chose a standard, such as black leotards and tights). They dance without shoes, originally as an expression of rebellion against the image of ballet. There is broader tolerance for body type and size than in ballet. The performers and the choreography may be quite abstract and cerebral, or may be demonstrative of feeling states. Dancers may not necessarily appear to be playing to an audience.

The underpinnings of modern dance are equally contrasting to ballet. Born out of dissatisfaction with the classicism of ballet, modern dance was a rebellion against an earlier era of dance and often against the prevailing social system outside of dance.[2] Humphrey's now-classic work on choreography opens the first chapter with a critique of ballet: "The dance has been, until recently, entirely ingenue, a sweet obedient child brought up in the theater and the court, and told to be young, pretty and amusing."[3]

In contrast, early modern dance attempted to rediscover natural movement. According to Humphrey, the "essential purpose [of modern dance] is to reveal something about people, to communicate to each individual some emotional state, idea or situation which he can identify with his own experience.... If one word were to be used to characterize the whole trend, the word would be 'subjective'.... Dancers found that they were people first, with new attitudes and feelings about life, in a world with vast sociological, psychological and historic change."[4]

As a structure, then, modern dance traditionally attracted persons who were less likely to support the prevailing social structures in dance and outside the dance world. It follows that those with special-interest issues might feel more at home within such an "antiestablishment" structure; this may in part explain the presence of homosexual males and the purported larger representation of feminists and lesbians in modern than in ballet or jazz.

Students *may* successfully begin modern dance training at a later age than ballet training. Classes are not necessarily less formal or more casual than ballet classes, but the teaching model commonly uses less fear; it is not really a democratic world of equality between student and teacher, but it can feel to be a more relaxed setting than ballet.

From its inception, modern dance attempted to integrate choreography with technique. This was in contrast to ballet, which separated these functions. In modern dance, in order to be able both to create and execute, being both a performer *and* choreographer was the ideal.

Jazz Dance

In jazz dance, assertion, aggression, and sex are often the central drives and themes displayed. What is forbidden in ballet and alluded to in modern is often much more explicit in jazz. Women are active, assertive, often adult sexual beings, often equal partners with men in the types of roles they play. There is an open quality to the notion of being on stage and exhibitionistic; at times there is purposeful eye contact with the audience; facial expressions may include flirtations—even seductive—looks or open smiles.

The pelvis and shoulders move in a more demonstrative, at times openly exaggerated sexual or flirtatious way; hip and shoulder isolations occur more frequently than in modern or ballet. Typically, the jazz dancer must express a type of assertive sexuality absent from both modern and ballet. Students have traditionally come to jazz through tap and character lessons and sometimes through more popular dance forms.

The underpinnings of jazz also focus on sexual and assertive drives. There is an overt sexuality in costuming and behavior; in class, language can be sexually provocative, often in an exaggerated way that communicates an awareness that the dancers have the potential to be adult male and female sexual beings and that the dance can communicate this to an audience in a stylish and entertaining fashion.

Developmental Stages in a Dancer's Career

The following section proposes an outline of several psychological and sociocultural issues typically encountered at different points in a dance student's career. These stages are hypothetical and may overlap considerably, varying according to type of dance and individual development. This outline attempts to integrate material from several perspectives, including psychodynamic, developmental, sociological, and historical.

Stage 1: Parental Choices

Most 3- to 4-year-olds love to move; they hop and run with great abandon, trying out their increasing sense of mastery over their limbs. Parents, observing this investment of energy, may try to encourage dancing as a constructive, even refined channel for their children's seemingly endless supply of energy. Although dance may provide a constructive outlet for this type of energy, some parents may mistake this love of movement as evidence of unusual talent and develop unrealistic expectations for their child.

Children this age also may have a sense that dancing makes them special in some way. Putting on leotards and tights and performing can be an extremely gratifying experience for a young child. Many mothers may enter their children in a dance class at age 4-6. The decision to be made here is whether to choose a ballet class, a jazz class, or a less structured "movement" class. The choice is often based on sociocultural variables such as social class, ethnic background, and evaluation of the fine arts or popular dance forms.

Parents must encourage the process, purchase clothing, arrange for transportation, and pay for lessons, usually in a supportive way. In ballet, if there is little parental support at this point, there is little chance of a child's becoming a successful company member for several reasons. First, by the time the child is able to make independent choices about what to study (at age 12-15), crucial bony structure changes are no longer possible. For example, many professional company schools screen students for bone structure. Second, mastery of technique to a professional level takes at least 10 years, and there is an early entry age for major companies.

Even if the child shows little interest in pursuing dance, the mother may encourage the child, at times strongly, to remain in class. At this level, classes are taught in the broadest array of settings, ranging from neighborhood dance schools to formal settings. The relationship with the dance teacher is secondary to those with school teachers and parents.

Stage 2: Early Dedication

This stage is marked by a shift from parental interest in lessons to increasing interest and commitment on the part of the student to the dance, usually somewhere after age 7, often ending with puberty. The amount of time devoted to dance increases though this period, often gradually, from one class per week to as much as 2-3 hr. per day after school plus much of Saturday (and, at times, part of Sunday). This shifting schedule requires increasing sacrifices of normal activities in the service of the dance experience.

In ballet, by this point, some students who have been encouraged by teachers, parents, or inner commitment are enrolled in regional schools some distance from home; transportation can become a major issue. Students also become highly invested in the identity of "dancer"; they begin to feel like dancers, taking on the characteristics of others they admire in the school. The relationship with the teacher can become highly important, with much time spent trying to please the teacher with increasing levels of skill and grace—that is, with "good" behavior (as defined by the teacher).In ballet as traditionally taught, "bad," unacceptable behaviors and attitudes (such as not concentrating on the work, not trying as hard as possible, not dressing neatly, not obeying politely and fully, putting on too much weight, being out of preferred alignment) may be punished by public admonishment from the teacher, with subsequent loss of face or by nonacceptance in the form of cliquish exclusion by successful students.

Nationwide, modern dance classes for this age group are not as numerous as ballet and jazz classes. In local modern dance settings, classes may take on the characteristics of a helping family, appearing to support the improvement of all members; external punishments are less apparent. In the average modern setting, "bad" behaviors are confronted by the teacher in a more supportive way, resulting in less overt loss of face. However, because of the preadolescent's powerful need to please the teacher, the student still faces the internal feeling of nonacceptance, which can be equally significant.

In order to earn and keep the teacher's respect, students who remain invested in the process begin to make increasing demands on themselves for discipline and self-denial. This can become a self-reinforcing system, because other relationships may take on lesser importance. The teacher may become the central figure in the student's life, spending more hours of the day with the student and at times directing the student more forcefully than the parents.

The relationship thus takes on a distinctly parental flavor; if this new "parent" plays the classical role, he or she is a demanding but caring judgmental influence, reinforcing the development of the student's desire to master his or her body and to channel impulses and feelings into the movements of the dance, rewarding good behavior, and, directly or indirectly, punishing bad. As the students identify with the teacher, they often idealize the teacher as having the appropriate life-style for a dancer; this is the person they want to please, and this is the person they want to be like. Thus, other peers and adults can seem less important than the idealized teacher. This can increase the gulf between the student and other nondancing cohorts as well as parents.

Clearly, this type of discipline is not for everyone. Although the reasons for leaving the dance world in childhood are many, conflicts between dance training and other models of behavior and attitude must certainly cause some students to lose interest and withdraw.

So far, this picture of the rigors of dance training may seem at odds with the literature: several studies of children, college students, and adults have shown that dance classes raise self-esteem, lower anxiety and depression, and promote a sense of well-being.[5-7] This literature supports the initial sense of self-satisfaction experienced by most who enter dance. However, these reports are all short-term studies of persons who had not already self-selected into dance, two factors that may render them irrelevant in looking at long-term issues in dance.

Stage 3: Maximal Conflict

As the child reaches puberty and moves into midadolescence, a number of issues arise that force responses. First, the effect of the sex hormones leaves little doubt that sexuality must be addressed in some fashion. Puberty is a time of conflicting feelings, of having a body that changes faster than one's capacity to adapt psychologically. In the case of the dance student, several forces seem important. First, except in jazz, the nature of the relationship with the teacher ordinarily has been one in which sexuality is ignored. In order to keep the system intact, the student must avoid awareness of these feelings, recognizing only respect and caring for the teacher. This may result in overidentification with and overidealization of a same-sexed teacher or a "crush" on an opposite-sexed teacher.

Second, with low body weight often an issue in dancers, many girls have late onset menarche, with low levels of sex hormones and minimal development of secondary sex characteristics. Although puberty is thus delayed, psychic and biological complications may develop, such as the sense that it is possible and desirable to retain the preference for presexual behavior and to prevent disruption of the prepubertal identity. Low body weight becomes an important issue, in that a sylphlike thinness is typically preferred, especially in ballet. Maintenance of low body weight in the face of adolescent growth spurts may be literally impossible without severe restrictions of diet or extreme exercise/purgative regimens.[8]

The dance student's changing body also changes alignment. The growth of the long bones, increased muscle mass (and breast development in girls) all shift posture and alignment. Ironically, it is at this most physically awkward stage of life that the dance student is faced with the inner demand (and the teacher's requirements) to remain the same: coordinated, slim, graceful.

The teenage years are also a time of testing of authority, of experimenting with new styles of behavior, appearance, and attitude. To remain faithful to dance and the teacher is often to postpone or avoid these tasks.

The chance to work through the complexities of adolescence typically is postponed because of lack of time and because the important relationships and skills seem to be within the dance world, not outside it. Thus, too, academic interests may fade; even if academics are valued by the student or supported by the parents, it is difficult to complete homework after a day of school followed by a trip to the dance class, several hours of dance, and then the trip back home. In contrast to student athletes, whose sports seasons usually last only several months, dancers often take classes throughout the school year.

Clinically, we are unaware of any formal reports of the incidence of clinical psychopathology in dancers. Anecdotally, one begins to see occasional students with depression marked by a joyless commitment to work and discipline. They may have an overbearing conscience and a brittle, idealized sense of self-esteem highly identified with the degree of perceived mastery of dance and the resulting reinforcement/rejection from the teacher and peers. One also may see eating disorders emerging, although it can be difficult to diagnose an eating disorder in a dancer because so many of the hallmark symptoms must be taken in the context of the dance setting.[9]

Decisions are often made between ages 12 to 14 about whether to continue with the increasing, and sometimes total, commitment to dance. Successful ballet students are faced with the decision whether to enter high school and attend a regional dance school after hours, or to leave high school and audition for a national school. In some larger metropolitan areas, a further option is application to a high school for performing arts. Because considerable amounts of energy, time, and finances have been invested to this point, the dance student may experience many internal and external pressures to continue (or to stop, if parents, student, or both have had enough).

Students who have developed strong identities as dancers, and who not only have body types conducive to their chosen dance form but also effectively identify with a growth-oriented teacher in a setting that promises later rewards, may appear not to suffer through this transition; at this point, the choices may seem easy. For some, the role may be reminiscent of that of the favorite child: Others in the class may receive less approval or may even leave dance altogether, but the favored student may have a self-image of being on the way to stardom. In addition, positive memories of the sense of being special when dancing may reinforce the desire to keep going in dance.

This situation helps lead to self-selection of those who can and will work harder at the task rather than refuse or crumble. Those who stay are likely to be precisely the type of students ballet-masters have typically preferred: talented pupils who are hard-working, devoted, and willing to please and to follow unquestioningly.

With rare exception, modern and jazz dance students at this age do not have the choice of year-round national schools; rather, they may opt to attend a national summer dance festival. But for those in ballet who enter professional company schools, the immersion is total. Several articles describe in detail the life of the ballet student at these schools.[10-12] In brief, and painted in the extreme, contact with those outside of ballet is minimal, and the demands of the ballet-master become the important external cues. Internally, one tries to master one's body, to make it do what is asked of it. Preoccupations with body shape, weight, and successful execution of movement combinations become paramount. The influence of the group is important, especially with respect to competition. Success no longer comes naturally; competition for a few coveted roles is intense, as is competition for the approval of the ballet-master, who emerges as a powerful parental figure surrounded by adolescent and post-adolescent students striving for a relationship that is essentially prepubertal.

Clearly, most dance students have chosen (or have *been* chosen) not to enter this intense world. Of the several million taking beginning classes and the tens of thousands of applicants to nationally prominent schools, only several thousand are accepted by these schools (and less than a hundred will have principal roles with major companies). However, the fantasies of those who have not entered these schools may not necessarily have vanished. A high school senior who has done well in a local dance studio may still harbor fantasies of a professional ballet performance career in thinking about the future.

Stage 4: The Major Commitment

For those who show promise of a successful ballet career, by now the decision has been made whether or not to study full time at a regional or national school. This is a crucial point in any ballet career. If the student is not in line to be a company member by age 14-16, a major performance career is highly unlikely. For those admitted to a national school, attendance is clearly a statement of commitment to a career in ballet. Those who prefer less intensive ballet may maintain an active presence in ballet in after-school and weekend study. Before this point is reached, the serious dance student has often made an implicit (and sometime explicit) bargain with parents and/or teachers: If the student gives full commitment to dance, this will lead inevitably to success and fulfillment (often including fame and fortune). In ballet, the student may still be working on this principle despite the odds against a performance career at this late stage.

Those who focus on modern dance or jazz in the mid- to late teens typically are still enrolled in local or regional studios or local companies and attend summer festivals. Although they are not working at a national company level, the best of these students may still have opportunities for performance careers in dance.

Some students first enter dance in high school or college, sometimes skipping over earlier stages of career development. Some of these students, because of talent and commitment, achieve success in nonballet dance forms. Because of the smaller numbers of younger male dance students, late entry into dance is less restrictive for them; a late adolescent male of moderate talent may be strongly encouraged to continue.

Stage 5: (A) Working in Ballet—Pinnacle Versus Precipice

Careers in classical ballet begin at an earlier age than those in modern and jazz. For this reason, this discussion of the fifth stage of a dance student's is divided into two parts. Those who enter national ballet schools and who become professional performers in ballet companies typically do so by their late teens or, occasionally, early 20s. Rather than being able to relax with a feeling of having made it to the top, company dancers face the dual challenges of holding onto their positions despite the pressures of competition from below (from the company school) and of emerging from the corps (chorus). One study of the culture of a dance company reports this phenomenon running in parallel with a sense of teamlike cooperation.[13]

Thus, the old pressures remain high: to be thin, to be healthy, and trying always to please the master and/or choreographer. Friendships with other dancers are important, but any dancer may become a direct competitor. Failure may mean more than a period of disfavor in the back of the classroom; it may literally spell the end of employment (and possibly of career).

For some, the knowledge that they have made it to the top reinforces their memories and sense of being special and rekindles the often-cherished belief that all good will now finally come to them. Although there is audience applause, and there can be some satisfaction in feeling superior to those who haven't made it to the top, disappointment may occur in finding that some of the sought-after rewards are not there. Fame may come and, rarely, fortune; happiness can be achieved if it is based on the satisfaction of accomplishment. But happiness cannot be based on fulfillment of a childhood fantasy of being the most favored, the most beloved, nor can it be based on having gained the teacher's ultimate approval. Even if the latter is achievable, it does not last. Serious disillusionment is possible at this point.

Stage 5: (B) Modern and Jazz—Choice Points

In the later high school years, dancers interested in careers in modern and jazz must choose from several basic settings for further training. Students who have chosen the style they wish to pursue may enroll in the appropriate company school or major studio, first as students, then perhaps as part-time teachers in the school and/or as company members. In modern, company schools are the most direct route to performance careers (although not necessarily for performer-choreographer careers). In jazz, the parallel choices also include study with a nationally recognized teacher and auditioning for theatrical or other professional work.

Within modern, those who have not identified with a particular style choose between conservatory and college or university settings. Conservatories usually train students in dance-related subjects such as technique, composition, music, etc., over a 2- 4-year period. Two-year graduates may then enter college; 4-year graduates often enter their choice of company schools.

University dance departments often are large enough to provide a wide variety of dance specializations, not only ballet, jazz, and modern, but also majors in dance studies such as criticism, movement analysis, and teaching. Most college dance programs are small, specializing in modern dance, the style most adaptable to postcollege performance careers.

Whereas most students in company schools continue their major emphases on improving their technique in order to become a company member, college and conservatory settings usually attempt to expand their students' talents to include choreographic skills, with a goal of training future company leaders. This is not a simple task. The marriage of technique and choreography is one of opposites complementing each other; the requisite skills and mind-set are quite different. The importance of this divergence in training requires an understanding of the working principles inherent in technique and choregraphy.

Through a student's training, mastery of technique typically is by rote, repetition, and discipline. The student develops a set of behavioral skills to adapt to this mode of learning; students learn to accept, to obey, to fit in. There is a higher authority who defines what to do; teachers are unambiguous about what is to be learned.

For technique to succeed on stage, another set of skills is also needed, These skills, usually acquired later in a performer's career, involve mastery of transitions, phrasing, musicality, the ability to "play" with an audience, and timing. These skills, which allow a shift from executing the movements to "dancing" in a way that visually and emotionally moves an audience, may be described as expressivity.

Expressivity is very different from what is required in the choreographic process. Choreography requires the capacity to cross boundaries, to suspend judgments, to associate freely, to find metaphor and simile in movement forms, to find order out of disorder, to dismantle order to find new order.[14] These tasks require a type of autonomous functioning absent from (and potentially at odds with) standard technical training, especially in traditional ballet.

The identity change from obedient pupil to independent thinker and director of others is profound. Humphrey reported the truism that the performing arts have a hundred interpreters for every creator and that only rarely do performer-choreographers emerge.[3] Many students do not adapt to the different characteristics required of the choreographer, preferring to remain in the performer role. College departments usually have as one primary goal the training of dancers to become choreographer-performers. How and whether this goal is achieved will help determine the student's future in dance, whether as performer, choreographer or both, or whether the student decides to deemphasize dance as a career choice.

In modern, if the student's identity shifts from that of performer to choreographer-performer, the ideal of success is slowly redefined. Rather than fame and fortune, the choreographer-performer may also find fulfillment in the role of the creative artist-performer and in the *process* of the creative act.

Dancers who enter companies directly, bypassing college, still learn choreography indirectly by being the subjects of choreography within the company. Performers with innate talent and interest may arise as budding choreographers within the company. These dancers usually bypass or postpone college.

Stage 6: The Mature Dancer

In ballet, many company dancers have relatively brief careers as performers. By the mid- to late 20s, many performance careers are over. Injuries take their toll and competition for space in the corps from younger company school members is keen. Also, the growing realization that most of the company's dancers will never rise above the corps can force some to reconsider their careers. Those who leave ballet at this time often retrain for second careers, leaving the dance world. In modern dance, careers are also often short; it has been said that there are no mature company members, but only mature choreographers. Of course, there are exceptions to this generality. Some successful ballet performers continue dancing into their mid- to late 30s, and some modern dancers are still performing in their 40s. However, most performers stop at earlier ages. Theoretically, some dancers may reach the point of being what might be called the mature company member: This is someone who has accepted the limitations of being a professional dancer but still finds enjoyment in the process.

Is the dance ever over? At this level, dance is a way of life. Some adult dancers report difficulty coming to grips with the limitations of their aging bodies. For some, it becomes a preoccupation, a staving off of the eventual deterioration that ultimately will lead to death. This might be viewed as a continuation of the earlier issue of control and mastery over one's body.

Information on former company members is only anecdotal. Reports of high rates of alcoholism and drug abuse remain to be substantiated. One might expect the desire to be on stage would remain a force in some dancers' lives, whether remaining on the performance stage long past their physical prime or seeking to be the center of attention in their personal or professional lives. Adaptations are possible, even onstage; some senior choreographer-performers create physically less demanding theatrical roles for themselves onstage, thus maintaining a viable performing presence.

At a physical level, those who suffer multiple injuries in their dancing days are likely to experience the long-term complications of these, such as post-traumatic arthritis. Psychologically, one could expect significant difficulties for the dancer forced to adjust to a body that no longer does what is consciously asked, a body becoming less graceful and less beautiful. These transitions apparently have not been formally studied in dancers.

Correlations with Scientific Literature

We have presented a descriptive picture of dance training as having profound effects on its students, of steering them on a particular course through the developmental issues of youth, adolescence, and adult life. Each of the three dance forms presented carries its own most prominent issues and dynamics. Given the potential for initial interest and parental (and peer) steering into one dance form or another, one can readily imagine self-selection into ballet, modern, or jazz to be another potent force. Students would be more likely to prefer the form that fits their body type, interests, and issues. It is not clear why students choose one or the other of these dance forms. However, one is tempted to assume a correlation with the developmental psychic issues and temperament of the individual. There is virtually no research into this area beyond the descriptive.[10,12,15]

The psychological dance literature in total comprises fewer than 100 scholarly articles, typically focusing on specific issues relating to dancers. These may be classified into several categories, some of which are briefly reviewed below.

Eating Disorders

In American culture at this time, dancers are thin.[16] Ballet dancers are expected to be especially thin. Does being thin in a dancer correlate with abnormal eating attitudes, abnormal eating behaviors, and with presence of eating disorders such as anorexia nervosa and bulimia?

The eating disorders literature has looked at student ballerinas, expecting them to have disordered eating.[11,17,18] Several studies have reported a higher incidence of true anorexia nervosa and abnormal eating attitudes in a student ballerina population,[11,19] whereas others have found a lesser problem with this population[20] and with modern dancers.[21] Diagnosis can be difficult because of the presence of low body weight and food faddism throughout the populations of dancers studied.[7,9] One study reported that ballet students differed from anorexia nervosa patients in that whereas both groups have a heightened drive to achieve, anorectics have an avoidant, negative fear of failure style, and ballet students have an achievement-oriented positive fear of failure drive.[22] Another concluded that the advanced and professional ballerinas maintained their thin states by voluntary but not compulsive self-deprivation of food together with the use of diuretics and self-induced vomiting to satisfy their directors and meet contract weights.[11]

Body Imagery

Given the nature of dance study, where students are placed in mirror-lined classrooms 5–6 hr. per day, 5–7 days per week for years and where these same students are expected to look and act certain ways and are applauded for thinness and carriage, it is no wonder that their images of themselves are affected by their study.

The most intensive work on body imagery has been done in relationship to anorexia nervosa, where emaciation may coexist with a self-image of being overweight.[18,23] One intensive review of ballet students revealed that no matter how thin, all subjects wanted to be thinner and felt better if the teachers commented on their thinness; the researchers were concerned about the degree of distortion of body imagery.[10] In contrast to these effects of years of dance study on body image, seven weeks of intensive study in dance for nondancers had no effect on body image.[24]

A recent review of body imagery suggests that how one perceives others is a crucial part of body imagery, and that anyone's body image is actually a composite of multiple images of self and others.[25] Given this perspective, the psychological literature on perception is also pertinent.

Dancers' visual and depth perception does not differ from that of athletes and nonathelete, nondancer college students.[26] In contrast, on tests of motor response to rhythm, dancers and athletes are better than nonathletes. One study reported that dancers do not improve their perceptual abilities with later training.[27]

Locus of Control

Given the hypothetical student who is trying to master his or her body and who is simultaneously submissive to a powerful dance teacher, one would expect that dance students should have a strong sense of control over their bodies but not much control over the world around them. A method of testing for these beliefs has been developed and applied in a limited way to student dancers.

The original locus of control scale[28] differentiates a sense of inner control over one's life from a sense of being subject to outside controls (Am I "master of my fate" or is my life largely influenced by the dictates of situations and other people?). Subsequent locus of control scales subdivide belief in external control into control by chance, by random events, or by powerful people.[29,30]

One study of 36 college students taking dance classes, some of whom were serious dance students, found that the group had a high internal control belief system and low beliefs in chance or powerful other controls.[31] A more directly relevant project studied modern dancers; on the original locus of control scale, subjects had very high belief in external controls over their lives.[32] This same group was given a scale measuring health locus of control, which ascertains beliefs that good health (1) is a product of external forces such as chance and luck, (2) comes from following the advice of powerful others such as doctors and nutritionists, or (3) is determined internally by personal attitudes or behaviors.[33] Subjects had very high belief in internal controls over health and low belief in the two external measures. This result appears to support the idea that serious dance students see their bodies as being under their own control but their lives being controlled by outside forces. Further work done on ballet students, jazz students, and a replication with modern dance students would be helpful.

Future Research

The dancer's career is profoundly affected by the type of dance studied, its culture and values, and by the individual teacher and approach used. This is in addition to the personality, body build, talent, and outside support the individual brings to the setting. But as may be seen from this chapter, much remains to be determined; at this point, studied speculation is all that is available. A recent review of the dance literature attempts to help the interested clinician or researcher define areas of interest for future work.[34] Basic questions include asking to what degree the type of dance one chooses is a reflection of personality and to what degree the setting and culture of dance alter personality. The differentiation of psychopathology from normal response to a specialized setting (growing up in the dance culture) is worked out only in a preliminary way. The current chapter proposes that dance study significantly affects its students, and that the several subcultures present in different dance styles may act differently.

Other areas of interest exist at the interfaces with related disciplines. Dance therapy and sports psychology have literatures and journals of their own. The eating disorders literature touches on dance; one recent review of eating disorders in dancers suggests further areas for study, including the need to determine the efficacy of educational models versus clinical case-finding methods to deal with abnormal eating attitudes and eating disorders in dance training settings.[9] Also advocated are concrete research projects to further determine the "normal" psychological attributes of dance students studying specific forms of dance.

Little is known about the psychology of male dancers as a group beyond the public assumption that many are probably homosexual. Many males have traditionally entered dance long after females have begun. Recent changes in societal attitudes about dance have allowed males to enter the dance field in larger numbers and at an earlier age. How much this will affect dance, and the public perception of sex roles, is unclear.

Given the finding that gymnasts and dancers have a number of physical and setting-specific issues in common, further study of this relationship might be worthwhile.[35]

In conclusion, the study of dance psychology is a relatively new field that has not been well represented in the past. The recent emergence of performance medicine, along with the popularization of sports medicine and sports psychology, should help focus more attention on the issues common to dance students and help develop a sounder understanding of the effects of different settings on dancers. The dancer's career is not typically that of a star, but of someone who leaves intensive dance study somewhere along the way. The answers to why they leave, and what they take with them, remain unknown.

The authors are indebted to Martha Myers, dean of the American Dance Festival, for her invaluable help in preparation of this manuscript.

References

1. Kirkland G. Dancing on my grave. New York: Doubleday, 1986.
2. Anderson J. Dance. New York: Newsweek Books, 1974.
3. Humphrey D. The art of making dances. New York: Grove Press, 1959; 15–22.
4. Humphrey D. America's modern dance. Theatre Arts 1950; 39(9):48–50.
5. Gurley V, Neuringer A, Massee J. Dance and sports compared: effects on psychological well-being. J Sports Med 1984; 24:58–68.
6. Leste A, Rust J. Effects on dance on anxiety. Percep Motor Skills 1984; 58:767–72.
7. Puretz SL. A comparison of the effects of dance and physical education on the self-concept of selected disadvantaged girls. In: Priddle RE, Ed. Psychological perspectives on dance. New York: Congress on Research in Dance, 1978.
8. Calabrese LH, Kirkendall DT, Floyd M et al. Menstrual abnormalities, nutritional patterns and body composition in female classical ballet dancers. Phys Sportsmed 1983; 11:86–98.
9. Schnitt JM, Schnitt D. Eating disorders in dancers. Med Probs Perf Art 1986; 1(2):39–44.
10. Druss RG, Silverman JA. Body image and perfectionism of ballerinas: comparison and contrast with anorexia nervosa. Gen Hosp Psychiat 1979; 1:115–21.
11. Garner DM, Garfinkel PE. Sociocultural factors in the development of anorexia nervosa. Psychol Med 1980; 10:647–56.
12. Lowenkaupf EL, Vincent LM. The student ballet dancer and anorexia. Hillside J. Clin Psychiat 1982; 4:53–64.
13. Forsyth S, Kolenda PM. Competition, cooperation, and group cohesion in the ballet company. Psychiatry 1966; 29:123–45.

14. Arieti S. Creativity: the magic synthesis. New York: Basic Books, 1976.

15. Babikian HM. The psychoanalytic treatment of the performing artist: superego aspects. J Am Acad Psychoan 1985; 13(1):139–48.

16. Maloney MJ. Anorexia nervosa and bulimia in dancers: accurate diagnosis and treatment planning. Clin Sports Med 1983; 2:549–55.

17. Garfinkel PE, Moldofsky H, Garner DM, Stancer HC, Coscina DC. Body awareness in anorexia nervosa: disturbances in ''body image'' and "satiety." Psychosom Med. 1978; 40:487–98.

18. Garner DM, Garfinkel PE, Stancer HC et al. Body image disturbances in anorexia nervosa and obesity. Psychosom Med 1976; 38:327–336.

19. Braisted JR, Mellin L, Gong EJ, Irwin CE. The adolescent ballet dancer: nutritional practices and characteristics associated with anorexia nervosa. J Adol Health Care 1985; 6:365–71.

20. Azmukler GI, Eisler I, Gillies C, Hayward ME. (1985) The implications of anorexia nervosa in a ballet school. J Psychiat Res 1985; 19:177–81.

21. Schnitt JM, Schnitt D, Del A'une W. Anorexia nervosa vs "thinness" in modern dance students: comparison with ballerinas. Ann Sports Med 1986; 3(1):9–13.

22. Weeda-Mannak WL, Drop MJ. The discriminative value of psychological characteristics in anorexia nervosa. clinical and psychometric comparison between anorexia nervosa patients, ballet dancers and controls. J Psychiat Res 1985; 19:285–90.

23. Grinker J. Behavioral and metabolic consequences of weight reduction. J Am Diet Assoc. 1973; 62:30–34.

24. Jette N. The effect of modern dance and music on body image in college women. Am Correc Ther J 1981; 35:104–06.

25. Van der Velde CD. Body images of one's self and others: developmental and clinical significance. Am J Psychiat 1985; 142:527–37.

26. Slusher HS. Perceptual differences of selected football players, dancers and nonperformers to a given stimulus. Res Q Am Assoc Health Phys Ed 1966; 37:424–28.

27. Huff J. Auditory and visual perception of rhythm by performers skilled in selected motor activities. Res Quart 1972; 43:197–207.

28. Rotter JB. Generalized expectancies for internal versus external control of reinforcement. Psychol Monogr 80, no 1 (Whole No. 609), 1966.

29. Levenson H. Activism and powerful others: distinctions within the concept of internal-external locus of control. J Person Assess 1974; 38:377–83.

30. Reid WJ, Ware EE. Multidimensionality of interest vs external control: addition of a third dimension and nondistinction of self vs. other. Can J. Behav Sci 1974; 6:131–42.

31. Dasch CS. Relation of dance skills to body cathexis and locus of control orientation. Percept Mot Skills 1978; 46:465–66.

32. Schnitt JM, Schnitt D. Del A'une W. Health locus of control in modern dancers 1986 (submitted for publication).

33. Wallston KA, Wallston BS. Development of the multidimensional health locus of control (MHLC) scales. Health Educ Monog 1978; 6:160–170.

34. Schnitt JM, Schnitt D. Psychological aspects of dance. In: Clarkson P, Skrinar M, eds. The science of dance training. Champaign IL: Human Kinetics Press, 1987.

35. Brennan MA. Comparison of female dancers, gymnasts, athletes, and untrained subjects on selected characteristics. Percept Mot Skills 1980; 51:252.

GLOSSARY

ADAGE (Fr.), ADAGIO (Ital.). 1. A series or combination of dance exercises, usually performed in the center of the classroom to a slow musical tempo, comprising *pliés, tendus, dégagés, coupés, rond de jambes, développés, battements* and controlled pirouettes in all of the basic ballet positions and directions. The purpose is to display the grace, balance, line and skill of the dancer during slow, sustained movements. 2. In performance, that portion of the *pas de deux* in which the ballerina, supported, lifted or carried by her partner, performs delicately balanced *développés,* pirouettes and poses in attitude and *arabesque* along with a wide variety of lifts.

À LA SECONDE À LA HAUTEUR. See HAUTEUR.

ALLEGRO. A quick, lively musical tempo to which all springing and jumping movements, such as *jetés, sautés, entrechats,* and turns in the air are performed.

ARABESQUE. The dancer arches the body, balancing it over the supporting foot with the other leg extended posteriorly and the arms and hands extended forward to make the longest possible line from the tips of the fingers to the toes of the working leg. There are 2 to 5 basic variations, depending upon the particular style, involving different positions of the arms, the body, and the relative extension of the supporting knee.

ASSEMBLÉ. A step of elevation in which the dancer brushes one foot into the air, pushes off the floor with the other, brings both legs together in the air, and lands in fifth position.

ATTITUDE. The basic pose in which the dancer stands on one leg and brings the other leg up behind or forward at an angle of 90° from the midline, with the knee bent and the extremity externally rotated. The arms are raised, and one may parallel the position of the raised leg in the same or the opposite direction.

BALLERINA. A principal female dancer in a ballet company. The first principal of a company may be called a prima ballerina.

BALLET. 1. A classic form of theatrical dance characterized by specialized movements, technique, traditions, and vocabulary (See also CLASSICAL BALLET). 2. A theatrical spectacle that combines ballet dancing with specially composed music, costumes, scenery, and lighting.

BALLET CLASS. The typical 90-min. classical ballet class is divided into an established sequence of exercises performed at the barre and in the center. Various combinations of *pliés, battements, tendus, battements dégagés, frappés, ronds de jambe, fondues, petits* and *grand battements,* and *adagio* are incorporated into both phases of the class. Center work also involves an assortment of jumps, *batterie, pirouettes* and *tours* in *adagio, petit allegro* and *grand allegro* combinations.

BALLET MASTER OR MISTRESS. The person responsible for teaching classes, conducting rehearsals, and reconstructing or creating the choreography of ballets in the repertoire.

BALLON. A desirable characteristic of elevation in which the dancer appears to ascend lightly, to sustain this position in the air, especially over some distance, and to land very softly.

BARRE. The round horizontal bar, usually wooden, that is fixed to the wall of the classroom, studio, or rehearsal wall at a height of about 3½ ft. to provide hand support for the preliminary exercises of the class. These exercises have the general purpose of developing strength in the body, thighs, legs, and feet and of freeing the limbs for a full range of rapid, easy motion. They may include *pliés, battements, développés, dégagés, fondues,* and *frappés,* each of which has a special function. The bar is usually placed directly in front of a mirrored wall so that the dancer and ballet instructor may observe the movements clearly.

BATTEMENT. A beating movement of the working leg usually closing against the supporting leg. In a *grand battement,* the entire leg is raised from the hip into a position in the air (*en l'air*). A *petite battement* is a small beating by the foot against the ankle of the supporting leg. *Petites* and *grands battements* are performed at the barre and in the center. Many varieties may be performed at the bar: *arrondi* (circular), *dégagé* (outward up and down), *développé* (unfolding), *fondue* (sinking down), *frappé* (striking floor), *retiré* (foot withdrawn upward), and *tendu* (stretched working leg).

BATTERIE. A scissor-like movement of the legs during a jump. *Petite batterie* are small, sharply beaten movements of the legs as in *entrechats, brisés* and *je-*

tés battus. Grande batterie involve more exaggerated beats and greater elevation.

BRAS, PORT DE. *Bras* is the French word for arms. The 4 basic positions of the arms in the Vaganova (Russian) school, the 6 in the French school, and the 9 in the Cecchetti method combine with the basic positions of the feet and placement of the head and shoulders *(épaulement)* to make up the stereotypical poses that are characteristic of ballet.

BRISÉ. Basically, a traveling *assemblé* with a beat. The dancer jumps from one or two feet, briskly beats the legs together while moving forward, backward, or sideways, and lands on one or two feet. Although there are a number of variations on the basic step, the most spectacular is the *brisé volé,* a combination of forward (*en avant*) and backward (*en arrière*) brisés that have a light "flying," or fluttering, appearance.

CABRIOLE. A beating movement of the fully extended legs in the air that starts and ends on the same foot. The dancer brushes the working leg either forward, backward, or sideways into the air, jumps off of the supporting foot, and strikes it against the top leg, propelling it higher, then lands on the original supporting foot.

CHAÎNÉS. A series of small half turns or *tours* on each foot performed in a straight line or while making a circle. May be done on *pointe* or *demi-pointe.*

CHANGEMENT DE PIEDS. The dancer springs up from the fifth position, changes the position of the feet in the air, and lands with the opposite foot in front.

CHASSÉ. A gliding or sliding step in which one foot appears to chase the other out of position. May be performed in any direction.

CHOREOGRAPHER. The person who designs and composes ballets or dances. Quite often the choreographer is also responsible for teaching ("setting") the sequence, style, and intent of the movements or choreography to the dancers.

CLASSICAL BALLET. Historically, the classical ballet is characterized by such 19th century ballets as *The Nutcracker, Sleeping Beauty, Coppelia, Giselle* and *Swan Lake.* However, the term also refers to a 350-year-old tradition of a highly formalized and stylized ballet technique.

CORPS DE BALLET. The dancers who make up the bulk of the company or who appear only in groups in support of the principals on stage. Although their function was originally chiefly decorative and reactive, in recent times they have frequently been given individual and expressive roles. They now represent a school of performance from which some develop into featured dancers.

COUPÉ. A step in which one foot "cuts" the other away and takes its place.

CROISÉ. A standing position of the body in which the dancer forms an oblique angle or three-quarter view relative to the audience, and the extended leg appears crossed. *Croisé* is the opposite of *éffacé,* an open position of the legs seen from a three-quarter view.

DANSEUR, PREMIER. A principal male dancer in a ballet company.

DANSEUSE, PREMIÈRE. A principal female dancer in a ballet company.

DÉGAGÉ. The fully arched foot is pointed toward an open position in any direction.

DEMI-PLIÉ. The knees are bent as far as possible while keeping the heels on the floor.

DEMI-POINTE. The dancer rises onto the balls of the feet. Also referred to as three-quarter pointe.

DÉTIRÉ. The dancer holds the heel of the working leg in the air, extends the leg to the front (*en avant*), and carries it to the side (*à la seconde*).

DÉVELOPPÉ. A gradual unfolding of the leg as it is raised from the floor into full extension in the air.

ÉCARTÉ. The dancer presents a three-quarter or oblique view of the body to the audience with the working leg extended to the side.

ÉFFACÉ. The dancer faces one of the two front corners of the stage or studio and either extends the leg nearest the audience to the back or the farthest leg to the front.

ELEVATION. The ability of the dancer to raise the body from the floor and appear to sustain this movement.

ENCHAÎNEMENT. A combination of dance steps performed to a particular musical phrase.

EN DEDANS. A movement that originates in the back and circles to the front. In a pirouette, the turn is made toward the supporting foot.

EN DEHORS. A movement that originates in the front and circles toward the back. In a pirouette, the turn is made toward the working foot.

EN L'AIR. Any movement made in the air, as in *tour en l'air* or *rond de jambe en l'air.* Also, a raised position of the leg with the working foot elevated to the level of the hip (*à la hauteur*).

ENTRECHAT. A weaving or scissoring movement of the legs in the air. The dancer jumps into the air and rapidly crosses the legs in front and back. Each opening and closing of the legs is counted a beat. Performing 6 (*entrechat six*) and 8 (*entrechat huit*) beats in a single jump is fairly common; 10 (*entrechat dix*) is quite unusual.

ÉPAULÉ. The dancer presents a three-quarter view of the body with the arm and shoulder nearest the audience extended forward and the leg on the same side extended in *arabesque.*

FONDUE. The finish of a step or jump in which the dancer lowers the body by rolling down through the instep and bending the knee, ending in a *demi-plié* on one leg.

FOUETTÉ. A whipping motion in which the working leg moves the dancer around the supporting leg. These movements are usually performed *en l'air.*

FRAPPÉ. In the *battement frappé,* the dancer stands with the working foot wrapped around the ankle and forcefully extends that leg, allowing it to strike the floor during extension. It is the basic preparation exercise for developing a strong *jeté.*

GLISSADE. A gliding movement of the legs that often precedes a jump from a *demi-plié.* It may proceed forward or backward.

GRAND BATTEMENT. See BATTEMENT.

GRAND BATTERIE. See BATTERIE.

GRAND PLIÉ. See PLIÉ.

HAUTEUR. The working leg raised at a 90° angle to the hip (*à la hauteur*). An angle of 135° to the front, side (*à la seconde*), or back is considered a good extension.

JETÉ. A jump from one foot to the other in which the dancer brushes the working leg into the air before landing upon it. It may be done in any direction and in a number of variations.

LINE. The aesthetic conformation or projected image created by the shape and proportion of the dancer's body as well as the positioning of the head, shoulders, arms, body, and legs.

NOTATION. A system for recording dances in a series of symbols that can be interpreted to reproduce them without the presence of the choreographer who designed them. The system of Rudolf von Laban is most widely used.

PAS. The measured step of the dancer that may involve a simple or compound movement. A solo dance is a *pas seul* and a dance by two persons is a *pas de deux.*

PASSÉ (RETIRÉ). One leg is drawn up until the toes touch the back of the other knee. When the position is held as a pose, it is known as a *retiré.*

PETITE BATTEMENT. See BATTEMENT.

PETITE BATTERIE. See BATTERIE.

PIROUETTE. A complete turn of the body performed on one foot, either on *pointe* or *demi-plié.* Usually, the working leg is bent so that the foot touches the side of the knee of the supporting leg, but it may also be in *seconde* position, attitude, or *arabesque.* Pirouettes may rotate either clockwise (outward, or *en dehors)* or counterclockwise (inward, or *en dedans)* relative to the supporting leg.

PLIÉ. The *plié* is a simple bending movement of the knees while bearing weight and maintaining external rotation of the lower extremity, as in a squat, and is the most fundamental movement in ballet. It is performed in all of the basic ballet positions and exercises. In the *grand plié,* the thighs are parallel to the floor at the lowest point of the *plié.* The heels remain on the floor only in the *seconde* position.

POINTE. The female dancer on *pointe* is dancing on the tips of her toes, principally the first and second digits. The aesthetic purpose is to create a straight line from the ends of the toes to the hip; an elongated, delicate image of the lower extremity.

PORT DE BRAS. See BRAS, PORT DE.

POSITIONS, BASIC BALLET. In the first position, the legs and thighs are turned outward at the hips so that the feet make an angle of 180° and the heels are touching. The second position is similar, but the heels are a shoulder width apart. In the third, the thighs and legs are the same but one foot is crossed in front of the other to make a right angle to it at the instep. The open fourth position is the same as the first, but with one foot forward of the other by a foot. The closed fourth position is taken from the third or fifth position, with one foot a foot in front of the other. In the fifth position, with the same turn-out the feet are parallel and close together, with the heel of the front foot at the joint of the great toe of the back foot.

RELEVÉ. Raising the body to a *pointe* or *demi-pointe* position. It may also be used to describe lowering of the heel of the working foot from *pointe* to the floor and raising it again to that position.

ROND DE JAMBE. A circling motion of the foot in which the dancer, moving the leg from the knee, inscribes a circle on the floor (*rond de jambe à terre*) or in the air (*rond de jambe en l'air*) with the pointed toe of the working foot. The movements are performed *en dedans* (counterclockwise) or *en dehors* (clockwise). A *grand rond de jambe en l'air* is a sweeping movement of the entire leg from the hip in a semicircle from front to back, or vice versa.

SAUTÉ. Basically, a hop using both legs or only one leg for propulsion. There is no jumping from one foot to the other as in the *jeté.*

TEMPS LEVÉ. Raising the body into the air by a spring from the feet.

TENDU (BATTEMENT TENDU). A pointing of the foot on the ground either to the front or to the side or to the back.

TOUR EN L'AIR. A movement in which the dancer jumps vertically in the air and turns one, two, or three revolutions. Usually, the *tour en l'air* starts and finishes in fifth position; however, it may also end in other poses such as *arabesque* or by dropping onto one knee.

TURN-OUT. External rotation of the lower extremities in dance. Perfect turn-out entails a total of 90° of external rotation in the hips, knees, leg, ankle, and foot of each extremity so that when the heels are brought together they make a 180° angle. Although perfect turn-out is aesthetically desirable, it is not an anatomical or biomechanical commonplace.

For further reference to terms used in ballet, consult Technical Manual and Directory of Classical Ballet, *by Gail Grant (Dover:New York), 1982.*

INDEX